68

WITHDRAWN

LONG-TERM CARE:
PRINCIPLES, PROGRAMS, AND POLICIES

Rosalie A. Kane, D.S.W., is a professor of social work and public health at the University of Minnesota. Previously she was a social scientist at The Rand Corporation in Santa Monica, California and a faculty member at the University of California at Los Angeles and, before that, at the University of Utah, from which she also received a doctoral degree in social work. Her research emphases center around health and social services for the elderly and other dependent groups, quality of care issues, and, more recently, the study of values and ethics. She is past editor of the professional journal *Health and Social Work,* and she served on the Institute of Medicine's Committee on Nursing Home Regulation.

Robert L. Kane, M.D., is a graduate of Harvard Medical School and board-certified in preventive medicine. Currently he is Dean of the School of Public Health at the University of Minnesota. Prior to assuming that post, he was a senior researcher at The Rand Corporation and a Professor at the UCLA Schools of Medicine and Public Health. An early recipient of a Geriatric Academic Award from the National Institute of Aging, he has been associated with the developing field of geriatric medicine in the United States, and is senior author of *Essentials of Clinical Geriatrics,* a text designed for practicing physicians.

Rosalie and Robert Kane both are active on editorial boards, as consultants to a wide variety of national and international agencies, and as members of advisory groups. They have written extensively, both individually and collaboratively. Previous books coauthored by the Kanes include *Long-Term Care in Six Countries: Implications for the United States* (1976); *Assessing the Elderly: A Practical Guide to Measurement* (1981); *Values and Long-Term Care* (1982); and *A Will and a Way: What the United States Can Learn from Canada about Caring for the Elderly* (1985).

Long-Term Care: Principles, Programs, and Policies

Rosalie A. Kane, D.S.W.
Robert L. Kane, M.D.

With the assistance of
James Reinardy and Sharon Arnold

SPRINGER PUBLISHING COMPANY
New York

Springer Publishing Company, Inc.
536 Broadway
New York, New York 10012

87 88 89 90 91 / 5 4 3 2 1

Library of Congress Cataloging-in-Publication Data

Kane, Rosalie A.
   Long-term care.

   Bibliography: p.
   Includes index.
   1. Aged—Long term care—United States. I. Kane, Robert L., 1940-   . II. Title. [DNLM: 1. Long Term Care. WX 162 K161L]
RA564.8.K36   1987   362.1'6   87-16353
ISBN 0-8261-6010-7

Printed in the United States of America

To our children, now adults,
Miranda, Ingrid, and Kathryn

Contents

Preface   ix

PART I: Introduction

Chapter 1   What Is Long-Term Care?   3
Chapter 2   Evidence about the Need for Care   12
Chapter 3   The Current State of Long-Term Care   53
Chapter 4   Long-Term Care Issues: Quality, Access,
             and Cost   83

PART II: Evidence About Effective Long-Term Care

Chapter 5   Effective Long-Term Care   103
Chapter 6   Home Care and Day Care   111
Chapter 7   Other Community Long-Term Care Services   163
Chapter 8   Nursing Homes   223
Chapter 9   The Relationship Between Long-Term Care
             and Acute Care   279
Chapter 10   Systems of Long-Term Care   306

PART III: Conclusions

Chapter 11   Synthesizing the Evidence   353
Chapter 12   Improving Long-Term Care: Next Steps   366

References   384
Index   414

Preface

In the past few decades, long-term care has been a growth field. An impressive amount of research has been done, funded by agencies of the federal government, as well as by state governments, foundations, and private organizations. Unfortunately, the results are often inaccessible, hidden in elusive final reports. At the same time, published material about long-term care has proliferated; much of it is descriptive or exhortatory, but empirical work has also come into print. All this material seemed to cry out for synthesis and interpretation.

A grant from the Administration on Aging to The Rand Corporation, where we were employed from 1977 to 1985, and later to the University of Minnesota enabled us to assemble, review, analyze, and synthesize evidence from several decades of research about the effects of various long-term programs (both institutional and community-based) on specific target groups.

Members of a national advisory committee assisted us in the early formulation of this project: Nancy Gerlach, Philadelphia, PA; Edward Sage, Salem, OR; Daniel Laver, San Diego, CA; Charles Reed, Olympia, WA; Jon Looney, Batesville, AR; Donna Falcomer, Baltimore, MD; and Shirley Wester, John Mather, Diane Justice, and Nancy Gorshe, all of Washington, DC. Thanks also to Carl Serrato of The Rand Corporation in Santa Monica, CA, who assisted with the initial review. We appreciate the early encouragement of Gene Handelsman, then of the Office of Human Development Services, and Byron Gold of the Administration on Aging. Finally, our gratitude to our two project officers, Barbara Fallon, and before her, Irma Tetzloff, both of whom went out of their way to facilitate the project.

We are also indebted to the many people who shared their manuscripts and unearthed their unpublished reports to supply the raw material in this synthesis. Necessarily, however, the review has been filtered through our own particular consciousness about long-term care issues, and we take responsibility for all the opinions expressed.

Ann Mulally and, in later stages, Marilyn Eells, Shelley Cooksey, and Sarah Hazen patiently and carefully typed and retyped the manuscript, including its elaborate tables. We are especially grateful for their attention and support.

When Robert Kane first dedicated a book to them in 1974, Miranda, Ingrid, and Kathryn were barely old enough to read it. Now they are grown and have introduced us to many books and ideas. They continue to bring us delighted pride, and to them, our future long-term care system, we dedicate this book.

ROSALIE A. KANE, D.S.W.
ROBERT L. KANE, M.D.
University of Minnesota

PART I
Introduction

1
What Is Long-Term Care?

Long-term care concerns the details of the life and death of people in this country. It is, therefore, vitally important to all citizens. In the final analysis, decisions about the proper goals of a long-term care system and what constitutes an acceptable standard of provision are political and social decisions rather than empirical ones. It is urgent that such decisions be considered and discussed at all political and administrative levels. At each level, information is needed to guide policy, and so too is a common understanding of the issues. We have sought to review the field to glean information and to look at that information critically. Our aim was also to synthesize the information in a way that demystifies it, strips it of jargon, and keeps in the forefront the reality that long-term care is not about placements, cases, and target groups, but about people, their families, their communities, and their lives.

Directed at providing continuing care for the functionally impaired in the least restrictive environment, long-term care sits uncomfortably on the boundary between health and social services and includes elements of both. Although long-term care is an expensive problem and program for public health and welfare officials, the term is likely to be unfamiliar to the general public. For policy-makers, long-term care is caught between the unassailable good of health and the stigma of "welfare," while for most of the public the term conjures up no image at all.

We believe this situation needs to be changed. The concept of long-term care is too important to remain in the hands of technocrats. It ultimately concerns how and where people with disabilities will live and die.

DEFINING LONG-TERM CARE

In dry, professional terminology, long-term care is a set of health, personal care, and social services delivered over a sustained period of time to persons who have lost or never acquired some degree of functional capacity. (Capacity in such cases is usually determined by an index of functional ability.) In layman's terms, long-term care is the assistance that is needed to manage as independently and as decently as possible when disabilities undermine capacities.

Most often the need for long-term care arises among the elderly—particularly the very old—as the result of their diminishing abilities, but some people need long-term care because of physical or mental limitations that they experienced in their youth—or even at birth. Consider persons under 65 with spinal cord injuries, advanced multiple sclerosis, or other chronic debilitating conditions; young men and women who survive traumatic brain injuries to return disabled to their parental homes; developmentally disabled adults; and the chronically mentally ill. Even persons with AIDS present a particular challenge for long-term care.

The key to long-term care is functioning. Therefore, long-term care authorities have given considerable attention to defining minimal components of independent functioning. At the very least, people must manage their most basic survival needs. These include eating, toileting, dressing, bathing, and locomotion, activities that long-term care personnel often group together as Activities of Daily Living (ADLs). But many other functions are important to independence, and indeed these functions seem to multiply and become more complex in modern urban societies. At the minimum, independent persons may require the abilities to cook, clean, do laundry, handle household maintenance, transport themselves, read, write, manage money, use equipment such as the telephone, and comprehend and follow instructions. (Such activities have become known as Instrumental Activities of Daily Living or IADLs.)

Not everyone needs to perform all the activities just listed, whereas some need to perform others not listed. For example, apartment dwellers do not need to handle yards and snow. Married men of a certain age may not need to cook meals. With enough income, anyone can purchase many of these services. Indeed many people without functional impairment purchase housekeeping services for their own convenience, and such purchased services cannot be called long-term care. But if a person is too physically or mentally incapacitated to do whatever of these tasks are necessary in his or her environment, that person becomes a candidate for long-term care. And if the person's own resources—including income to purchase long-term care services, physical and mental abilities to identify the needs and arrange the services, and/or family and friends to assist—are insufficient to solve the problem, society becomes involved. With organized societal efforts, publicly sponsored long-term care programs are born.

In the shorthand of human service programs, long-term care is often equated with the places where it is given or the programs that provide it. Because programs develop in response to funding, service definitions become quickly linked to eligibility and coverage. Thus, for many, long-term care has come to mean nursing homes (the place where most public money for long-term care is spent). To those familiar with a wider range of possibilities, long-term care may also mean home health care, homemaker services, adult day care, and various other services. Analysts have, in fact, come to accept the packages of care defined by payors and refined by providers. But imaginative reform of long-term care programs will never occur without recognition that the concept refers to the range of services needed to compensate for functional problems, not the places where they are offered. Such services should also afford protection when necessary and enable the functionally impaired person to live as full a life as the disability permits.

Long-term care is thus a hybrid—part health and part social service. How health and social services in a community are managed will influence the effectiveness and the costs of the narrower range of long-term care programs targeted to assist the functionally impaired. Some of the services needed to prevent and minimize the need for long-term care in the first place and to manage chronic functional disability are health services. They require doctors, nurses, pharmacists, and others readily identifiable as health professionals. But many of the necessary components are social services concerned with aspects of living. Moreover, the way health care is provided—in hospitals and physicians' offices and mental health programs—and the way social services are conceived and organized—through housing programs, transportation programs, information services, income programs, aging services, and counseling—will vitally influence the shape and effectiveness of long-term care.

Income maintenance policies (including both Social Security and Supplemental Security Income [SSI]) loom large for any population largely retired from the workplace. Housing policies and programs will influence long-term care needs and costs. Adult social services (which include in-home supportive services for people of low incomes; adult protective services for vulnerable adults who are abused, neglected, or exploited; and a variety of counseling programs) are surely relevant. These are administered under block grants to the states and vary widely from place to place.

Every community in the country offers services to and on behalf of the elderly under the mandates of the Older Americans Act. Although not exclusively directed at the functionally impaired, these programs include senior centers (where those needing long-term care might be identified), information and referral programs (which could be a vehicle for effective allocation of long-term care), congregate and home-delivered meals, transportation and escort service, homemaking and chore service, and nursing home ombudsman service (much of which might be directly considered long-term care).

NATURE OF LONG-TERM CARE

Inherent in its definition are some complications for anyone who would design a long-term care program.

- Functional impairment should be the trigger for service. This means that functional impairment needs to be measured precisely enough that service may be initiated, increased, decreased, or stopped on the basis of agreed upon definitions of functional disability.
- Long-term care services are inherently desirable. The services needed to compensate for functional impairment are also useful and desirable for unimpaired persons and indeed are often purchased by those who can afford them regardless of disability. Policy-makers are naturally leery of introducing benefits so desirable that they may be hard to control.
- Long-term care services are provided mostly by and within families. Throughout most of life, people take care of their own everyday needs, and these tasks are often allocated within families. When a family member needs long-term care, the first recourse is usually another family member. Sometimes the long-term care involves little more than a slight intensification of the housekeeping, cooking, and laundry that a spouse has always done or that an individual has always purchased. Sometimes it involves enormous additional labor or expense from family members within or outside the household. In any event, most long-term care for people living outside institutions is done by family members, and public policy requires that much of this unpaid labor continue. The challenge is to develop policies that are fair to all concerned (the person needing care and the caregiving family members, the functionally impaired persons with family and those without family).
- Long-term care services are labor-intensive and relatively unspecialized. Service for people with functional impairment can entail a wide variety of activities—for example, cooking, cleaning, shopping, driving, bathing, assistance with locomotion. When provided by family members such service may involve much time and little division of labor. Some of these tasks are physically taxing; others are unpleasant. They are best done humanely, with warmth and kindness. They must be performed reliably. When family cannot perform any or all of the long-term care services needed, the challenge is to produce an efficient and high-quality

long-term care program that mirrors what a conscientious and effective family might do.

- Long-term care services should be flexible. The need for long-term care follows the rhythms of everyday life. People who lack the capacity to transfer out of bed need help in the early mornings when they first awake and in the evenings when they prepare for bed. The need for meals follows a predictable pattern, toileting less so. Help will almost certainly be needed on weekends and holidays, and some persons will need help during the night. The widespread use of nursing homes for long-term care is eloquent testimony to the difficulty of organizing flexible and responsive community services that meet the actual human need. Unfortunately, however, the problem is not usually conceptualized in this manner and, therefore, the effort has not been squarely undertaken.
- People of all ages and circumstance may need long-term care. As already indicated, the elderly are the most frequent long-term care users, but adults with a wide variety of physical and mental conditions may need some long-term care. (Some children also need long-term care, but the issues differ enough that we exclude minor children from consideration.) Should a community or state develop a single set of programs to serve all adults with long-term care needs? Should it develop a single set of guidelines for functional impairment? For that matter, can elderly long-term care users, an extraordinarily diverse group in income, education, interests, and physical and cognitive abilities, be well served by the same programs? If not by the same programs, might they all be served by the same entitlements?

VARIATIONS IN LONG-TERM CARE

Long-term care today in the United States is extraordinarily diverse. Moreover, its amorphous boundaries make even more variation theoretically possible. For example, long-term care varies or could vary in at least the following ways:

- *The goal for functioning.* Some long-term care programs have as a goal defining and correcting functional impairment; some aim to compensate for functional impairment through services; some strive to prevent functional impairment; and some claim all three goals. Moreover, a program may or may not incorporate meaningfully a goal of permitting dignity and autonomy despite dependency.
- *Focus of service.* The focus of long-term care may be the person with functional impairment, the entire family, the environment, or some mixture of all three.

- *Locus of service.* Long-term care may occur in the functionally impaired person's own home or apartment, some specially designed congregate living environment, or an institution such as a nursing home or a mental hospital.
- *Mix of services and service providers.* Long-term care can be organized with a wide variety of services provided by a wide variety of agencies and personnel. For example, a problem with meal preparation and laundry could be solved by separate meal-delivery and laundry take-out services or by an assistant who comes to the home to accomplish both tasks, or the person needing care might live in a complex where laundry and meals are provided as part of the rent.
- *Duration and intensity.* Once begun, long-term care can be construed as a permanent service with the assumption that clients, at the very least, need lifetime monitoring (though the amounts and types of services needed may vary), or it can be construed as a service that is started to meet an immediate definable need and stopped once that need no longer exists. Long-term care also varies in how generous or parsimonious the services will be.
- *Nature of public sector involvement.* Long-term care may be construed as a private matter, where governments are involved only when the problems cannot be solved within the constraints of private income. Definitions may also differ on when the threshold of private risk has been crossed. Part of this question involves the extent to which family income and labor should be considered available to fulfill an individual's long-term care needs.

Is it best to conceptualize long-term care as a distinctive system of policies and programs for the functionally impaired, or should long-term care span conventional programmatic boundaries? When a physician or nurse visits a long-term care recipient at home to diagnose or treat an illness, is this an instance of primary health care or of long-term care? When special long-term care benefits and programs are designed, which health and social services should be incorporated into long-term care and which should the long-term care recipient still receive through customary channels? Should long-term care be defined by exclusion, as is sometimes now the case? For example, post-acute hospital care, which may extend over a limited period, is lumped with long-term care for many benefit packages.

These questions are more than a lapse into semantics. The person who is functionally impaired has need for income, housing, health care, recreational and other social goods in common with all citizens. Some approaches to long-term care include one or another of these components. For example, the nursing home, which is America's major long-term care program, provides housing and some health care as well as the housekeeping and personal care services directly addressing the functional impairment (and much of nursing home care is paid for through health programs). Sometimes people identified as receiving long-term care are cut off from timely and appropriate access to other health and social services. (A nursing home resident will find it equally difficult to summon a physician or a transportation service subsidized by the Older Americans Act to the nursing home doors.)

On the other hand, sometimes people known to health programs and/or social service programs fail to receive available long-term care. The focus of many service providers is too narrow to consider functional results or environmental needs. Many service providers cannot or will not take responsibility to arrange long-term care. For example, senile dementia is a progressive disorder that is associated with the need for long-term care, but it is highly possible that persons with dementia may be known to a hospital, a physician, a mental health center, and/or an adult protective service program without any of these agencies organizing and monitoring a program of care.

However the boundaries of long-term care itself are drawn, other health and social welfare policies must affect the long-term care recipient. Generous income policies allow the functionally impaired more money to purchase their own services. Effective hospital-based rehabilitation may minimize the need for long-term care. Policies that foster rapid discharge from the hospital may precipitate undesirable long-term care arrangements. By definition, residents of nursing homes may be declared eligible or ineligible for a host of social services. These few examples could be multiplied. They highlight the importance of looking at related systems and programs when looking at long-term care.

FOCUS OF THIS BOOK

This book is the direct result of a fact-finding mission about long-term care. Over the last two years, we collected voluminous documentary evidence about long-term care in the United States, particularly studies of the effects of programs and services. Our purpose was to examine what is known about long-term care under differing circumstances and for different target populations. We sought to assemble, review, evaluate, and synthesize evidence about long-term care.

The overall questions guiding us were these: What have several decades of research and demonstration taught us that could help us decide how to spend the next dollar for long-term care? How might each community's particular history and characteristics affect such decisions? As much as possible we limited our attention to data—data about those needing long-term care, data about those providing it, and, most important, data about the effects of care. But the data do not speak for themselves; they require a context. Thus, we were interested in framing issues as well as scrutinizing evidence. Perceiving a dynamic relationship between issues and evidence, we approached the data with the hope of illuminating some of the key issues we considered to be important, but we also sought a better articulation of issues from reviewing the data.

The bulk of this book presents evidence about the effects of various long-term care programs, evidence gleaned from several decades of research, demonstration, and thought. But first we introduce long-term care—its importance, its characteristics, and current problems. That discussion occupies the first four chapters and comprises the introductory section of the book. In the remainder of this chapter, we explore some logical ramifications of long-term care and elaborate on our method of study. Chapter 2 describes the population needing long-term care; using the most current available data, we discuss the size and characteristics of the group likely to need service, their personal and family resources, and the effects of caregiving on family members.

Chapter 3 describes the existing long-term care programs, entitlements, financing mechanisms, and quality controls. The information is based on the most current descriptive data we could locate. We describe the financial and social costs of long-term care at present and the difficulties in encouraging a more desirable kind of care while simultaneously curbing costs. Chapter 4, the final part of the introductory section, delineates issues that underlie any review of evaluative data. Throughout we recognize that the way questions are posed profoundly affects likely answers.

Part II, divided into six chapters, presents our synthesis of information on the effects of long-term care programs. This is the heart of the book—the place where we discuss what has been learned about nursing home care, home care, and a host of other community services, and what has been learned about systems of long-term care. In Part III, we draw some conclusions about optimal long-term care—conclusions drawn from our joint exploration of issues and evidence.

EVIDENCE REVIEWED

We make no claims to being exhaustive in assembling information about long-term care. There is simply too much material to be successful in that effort. However, we did attempt to be thorough in assembling studies about programs and their effects, particularly large-scale studies done in the past decade or so. Many such studies were funded by one or another government agency and are available only in elusive final reports. We were able to assemble lists of research funded by the Administration on Aging, the National Institute on Aging, the National Center for Health Services Research, the Health Care Financing Administration, and other governmental agencies. Similarly we identified major work sponsored by state governments or by foundations. For the most part, we limited ourselves to studies, excluding purely descriptive or polemical material. We did, however, collect major opinion pieces that addressed long-term care policies from the vantage-point of their author's own review of research. We did an extensive computer-assisted bibliographical search to identify material in the published literature, and we sought the advice of members of our study's advisory committee and other colleagues about work in progress. Although we may have missed some items, we are satisfied that we have garnered sufficient data to depict the field as a whole.

2

Evidence About the Need for Care

In determining the need for care, we confront a series of difficult and confusing issues. As with all planning, long-term care planners must extrapolate from the present patterns of need and service use yet recognize that the future will be different. They must be sensitive to the potential for change among both the clients and the providers of care and indeed may wish to stimulate change through deliberate policies.

In this chapter, we examine the principles and pitfalls of projecting the need for long-term care. We discuss the prevalence of functional impairment. We also review efforts to predict nursing home use. This entails a look at patterns of informal care, because the availability of unpaid assistance from relatives and friends has been consistently considered a major factor in an individual's ability to remain in the community.

HOW LONG-TERM CARE NEED HAS BEEN DEFINED

"Needs assessments" are based on the assumption that the condition of an individual can be translated into a set of services corresponding to the deficiencies identified. In practice, however, the conclusions are drawn from some combination of induction and imputed judgment. Very few well-grounded formulas based on solid research are available for translating needs into services. Economists reject the term "need" in favor of the term "demand," arguing that need is simply a professional judgment, inherently no better than the consumer's judgment and in many ways less useful. At least the consumer usually pays some kind of price to express his preferences.

Planning services for a community is easier than planning for an individual. For example, age is an excellent predictor of the needs for a variety of services for a population but a poor predictor of what a particular person might need. Gerontological research has consistently found that variation within a group increases with the age of the members. Whether one looks at physiologic, psychological, or social characteristics, the older the population under study, the greater the variation found. Although the risks of most negative events increase among groups of older persons, it is difficult to predict which individual in the group is at personal risk. This observation is especially pertinent to the difficult task of translating research into practices designed to prevent untoward events, such as entering a nursing home. Because the predictive equations are much more potent for groups than for individuals, expensive effort may be lavished on persons who were not at high risk for the event.

Demonstrated Need

Functional ability is the key to defining the need for long-term care. An emphasis on functioning taps into the behavioral consequences of chronic disease or ill health, rather than focusing upon the disease itself. The same disease can have different consequences for how persons carry out the routine tasks of day-to-day living. Multi-dimensional measurement of functional limitations recognizes that limitations can be physical, social, and/or psychological (Hedrick, Papsidero, and Maynard, 1984). For planning purposes, the concept of need as functional limitation is best specified as dependence on the assistance of others (Weissert, 1982; Eustis, Greenberg, and Patten, 1984). For example, the Katz Index of ADL, one of the best known and most frequently used measures of ability to perform activities of daily living, distinguishes between independence or the need for assistance in carrying out basic tasks like eating, toileting, bathing, and getting in and out of bed (Katz et al., 1963). Much more elaborate functional assessment instruments, such as the OARS Multi-dimensional Functional Assessment Questionnaire (Duke University, 1978), have also been widely used to determine the incidence and prevalence of functional limitations in populations.

However, a review of functional assessment and survey instruments used in a number of studies (Hedrick, Papsidero, and Maynard, 1984) suggests that despite a common language, several sources of incompatibility must be resolved before policy can be addressed from existing data bases. These include items seeking subjective judgments regarding "trouble" or "difficulty"; differences in response alternatives concerning use of equipment and use of personal assistance; questions appearing to assess functional ability ("can you"), in contrast to functional performance ("do you"); differences in the time periods to which instruments refer.

Table 2-1 presents 1982 National Long-Term Care Survey (NLTCS) data on functional dependencies by age and sex for those living in the community (Soldo and Manton, 1985). The data demonstrate the high functional dependency rates of the "old" old. Three times as many people aged 85+ report needs for ADL help as people in the 65 to 74 group. Table 2-2 presents a variety of studies that used ADL measures to look at need for care. Many of these confirm the relationship between increasing age and increasing need found in the NLTCS. Cornoni-Huntley et al. (1985), for example, found that age- and sex-specific rates of need for assistance in at least one ADL tended to double with each successive 10-year age group.

Translating Needs into Services

One of the most difficult challenges in long-term care is translating a set of functional disabilities and assistance needs into a prescription for a package of services. Several factors impede this translation. We lack a good taxonomy of services. A group at Duke University, working with the OARS data

TABLE 2-1 Percentage of Persons 65 Years of Age and Over Living in the Community with Functional Dependencies, by Age and Sex: 1982

Age/Sex	ADL (activity of daily living limitation) Score[b]				
	Only IADL Limited[a]	1 to 2 (mildly disabled)	3 to 4 (disabled)	5 to 6 (severely disabled)	Total
65 to 74					
Male	4.2	3.4	1.7	2.4	11.7
Female	4.8	4.7	1.9	1.9	13.3
75 to 84					
Male	7.1	6.5	2.5	4.6	20.9
Female	8.5	10.3	4.3	4.4	27.6
85+					
Male	9.9	15.7	7.7	7.5	40.8
Female	10.3	18.2	7.9	11.8	48.2

[a]Needs assistance with the instrumental activities of daily living (IADL): managing money, shopping, light housework, meal preparation, making a phone call, taking medication.
[b]The score is the sum of the number of activities of daily living (ADL) with which respondent requires assistance: eating, bathing, dressing, toileting, etc.
Source: Tabulations from the 1982 Long-Term Care Survey prepared by the Center for Demographic Studies, Duke University. Reported by Soldo and Manton, 1985.

from a population-based study done in Cleveland, has developed a system for classifying services (Laurie, 1978). Table 2-3, based on that study, illustrates the effort to create hierarchies and clusters, as well as the difficulties inherent in such a step. Definitions are difficult to formulate. One area tends to blend into the next. The needs in one context may mandate different service packages from those in another setting. Informal services remain hard to quantify. When is a visit a visit? If a caregiver helps someone physically and talks to her at the same time, is that a social contact as well? The network of sponsorship and coverage results in a tangled web of services characterized by the overlapping jurisdictions, complex eligibility requirements, and benefits packages unique to each program. Definitions of what must and cannot constitute a service vary from program to program.

At present, there is no technology to translate needs into services. Should we rely on the opinions of persons served today? If so, persons served by which programs? Or rather should we insist that the correct translation can be best demonstrated by showing that the level of unmet need is substantially reduced after the service is rendered? To use a familiar analogy, the test of a drug lies in its ability to produce a cure (or at least an improvement) in a specified condition. A drug shown to do this consistently is then approved for use in treating that condition. Just as with drugs, we can look at the effects of a single ingredient or a combination. Should we not apply the same methods to testing long-term care services? But if policy were to dictate the evaluation of long-term care services by change in unmet needs, the current research data base is insufficient.

Need from Current Patterns of Use

One of the most popular approaches to forecasting future need relies on extrapolating from present use. The technique assembles data about use of service organized by as many demographic parameters as possible (e.g., age, sex, race, socio-economic status). The specific rates for each of these characteristics for each subgroup are calculated, weighted, and used to estimate their prevalence in some future population. This approach has two obvious weaknesses: (1) It relies on an ability to project demographic change accurately (the consistent underestimates of the Census Bureau's projections of the elderly population suggest that this is harder than it seems). (2) It assumes that the relationship between demographic and utilization variables will be constant (we have already noted the important role of supply as a critical intervening variable, to say nothing about sociological changes or changes in technology). Nonetheless this approach is used quite often, in part because it is rather easy to accomplish and can be done under a number of alternative demographic scenarios.

Special caution about extrapolations is in order. Gerontologists have observed a discernible trend of increasing life expectancy after age 65. As

TABLE 2-2 Dependency Measures: Selected Studies and Findings

Source and Population/sample	Design	Measures	Selected Findings
GAO (1977) Random sample of 1,609 non-institutionalized Cleveland residents (65+); interviewed in 1977 and one year later.	Scores in 5 areas of human functioning were combined in an 8-level *total* score of well-being (e.g., level 5, "generally impaired," represents those "mildly or moderately impaired in four areas."	The OARS Multi-dimensional Functional Assessment Questionnaire rated persons in 5 areas of functioning—social, economic, mental, physical, activities of daily living.	ADL/IADL disabilities were indirectly reflected, along with other dimensions, in a total score. 21% were "unimpaired"; 23% were "generally impaired" or worse.
Branch (1977, 1982) Statewide area probability sample, initially comprised of 1,625 non-institutionalized elderly, 65+ (1974–75).	A longitudinal study with 15-month (Time 2) and 5-year (Time 3) intervals between measurements. 825 interviews were completed at Time 3 (1980–82). Focus was upon the prevalence of needs and extent to which they were unmet in such areas as transportation, personal care assistance, housekeeping, social activities, emerging assistance, food shopping and preparation.	Operational definitions differentiated needs into four major categories (e.g., 1 = Need currently met and no apparent problems; 4 = Need currently unmet with unmet problems). Subcategories of behavioral and evaluative items provided specific response profiles. Measures of functional disability included adaptations of the Rosow-Breslau scale and Kietel range-of-motion test.	Emphasized the short-term (15-month) stability and similarity of response patterns over time. Individuals measured at Time 2 have changed but overall percentages remained the same. Third wave data showed only 5% to 10% of the sample in need of intensive support, e.g., 91% were independent in bathing, 97% in walking inside, 3% of the sample had unmet needs for assistance in two or more areas of instrumental activities.

Community Council of Greater New York (1978) Random sample of about 450 non-institutionalized NY City residents aged 65+ (preliminary data from U.S./U.K. Cross National Geriatric Community Study).	Data obtained from in-home examinations were related to Personal Time Dependency (PTD) variable, including disabilities in ADLs, IADLs, emotional autonomy, social initiatives, awareness.	Comprehensive Assessment and Referral Evaluation (CARE).	Only in the 90+ group were the majority of persons dependent, with a need for SNF-equivalent care; below age 75, half of the PDTs require limited home care (e.g., shopping, cooking).
Branch and Jette (1981) 2,654 community individuals aged 55–84 from the original cohort of the Framingham Heart Disease Longitudinal Study; noninstitutionalized sample.	Interviews (1976–78) in person/ by phone regarding social disabilities (house-keeping, transportation, social interaction, food preparation, grocery shopping) and physical disabilities.	Social disabilities measured through four grades of need (need met, no problem [1] to need unmet, current problem [4]) similar to Mass. Health Care Panel; unmet needs and high risk indices also constructed. Physical disabilities were measured using modified Katz ADL scale, items from the Rosow-Breslau functional health scale and from Nagi.	Social disabilities: A 3-fold increase in the proportion with *unmet* social needs with advancing age; 2% for men 55–64 and 6% for men 75–84; in contrast, 6% of women 55–64 and 15% of those 75–84 have unmet social needs. House-keeping and transportation were areas with the most unmet need. Physical disabilities: For all ADL items but eating, the 75–84 group was more likely to use help but over 90% of these were independent. Overall, women appeared to be more disabled than men with each age cohort.

TABLE 2-2 Continued

Source and Population/sample	Design	Measures	Selected Findings
Weissert (1982) Nationwide sample of 11,730 household elderly (1979 Health Interview Survey).	Secondary analysis of the survey data on items of functional dependency; subjects hierarchically classified according to most severe dependence.	Katz ADL scale; items on mobility and need for help in meal preparation, money management, household chores, shopping, need for health services at home (e.g., shots).	Total of 12.7% dependent in personal care, mobility, household activities, or health services.
Scanlon and Hamke (1983) Self-weighting representative sample of aged 65+ from four local surveys in Cleveland; eastern Kansas; Lane County, Oregon; Virginia.	Data combined/analytically compared to describe prevalence of dependency, social services available to the population, service use.	Each survey used the OARS Multi-dimensional Functional Assessment Questionnaire (Duke).	Total dependency prevalence estimate of 35.2% (personal care, 12.9%; mobility, 12.9%; IADL, 9.9%).
Weissert and Scanlon (1984b) Nationwide sample of households (1977 Health Interview Survey) with 1,168 aged 65+; stratified 2-stage nationwide probability sample of nursing homes (1977 National Nursing Home Survey) with a sample size of 1,698 facilities.	Both data sets were merged directly to produce prevalence rates and characteristics of functional dependency for the dependent population. Focus of the analysis in defining LTC needs was upon ADL and mobility items.	NNHS and HIS contain ADL items on bathing, dressing, toileting, eating; HIS has items on mobility assistance in and outside the house and NNHS has an item on walking assistance.	24.1% of dependent prisons were in nursing homes; 30 times as many of these were dependent in personal care has in mobility. Those dependent in mobility only had little likelihood of institutionalization.

Cornoni-Huntley et al. (1985)	Descriptive baseline data on cognitive disabilities were given for 3 coordinated 5-year longitudinal studies designed to study risk factors and predictors of mortality, hospitalization, nursing home placement.	Physical disability measured by limitations in mobility and ADLs, using items from Katz, Rosow & Breslau, Nagi, Jette & Branch; Mental Status Questionnaire measured cognitive disability.	Proportion of people needing assistance in at least one ADL tended to double at each age level for each sex, e.g., East Boston males, prevalence was 9% (65–74), 17% (75–84), 36% (85+).
3 noninstitutionalized, aged 65+ populations in East Boston (3,812); Iowa and Washington counties, Iowa (3,673); and New Haven (3,420).			
Manton and Soldo (1985)	Secondary analysis of data through multivariate grade of membership (GOM) analysis isolated 4 homogeneous groups of the LTC population on socio-demographic and disability variables; disability levels were projected (1980 to 2040) assuming both constant and reduced disability rates.	33 socio-demographic and functional-limitation measures (variables) used for GOM analysis; Katz's ADLs used; other functional measures included shopping, managing money, climbing stairs, making phone calls, washing hair, getting around outside.	The most disabled GOM group was not distinguished by age, and had a greater than average chance of being married. Two other disability groups were characterized by cognitive vs. physical independence, suggesting different service delivery options.
Household survey of a sample of 5,580 noninstitutionalized aged 65+ with confirmed ADL or IADL limitations (1982 National Long Term Care Survey).			

TABLE 2-3 Generic Service Components

Home Help	*Medical Help*
Personal care	Medical care
Checking	Psychotropic drugs
Homemaker	Supportive devices
Administrative and legal	Nursing care
Meal preparation	Physical therapy
Continuous supervision	Mental health
Financial Help	*Assessment and Referral*
Financial	Coordination, information, and referrals
Housing	Overall evaluation
Groceries and food stamps	Outreach
Social/Recreational	*Transportation*
Social/recreational	Transportation

shown in Figure 2-1, life expectancy for older persons has steadily inched forward regardless of sex or race. In fact, the difference in life expectancy at age 65 due to race has essentially disappeared. Recent data suggest that this trend toward increasing survival is continuing.

The implications of this increased life expectancy for functioning are less clear, and indeed controversial. One group argues that the causes of improved survival will equally contribute to reduced morbidity and that the gained years will be vital ones. The so-called "compression of morbidity" into the period close to death offers an attractive scenario (Fries and Crapo, 1981; Fries, 1980; Fries, 1984). But this optimism is rejected by several informed sources, who argue that the gain in mortality means that more of the disabled survive. In this view, the older population is likely to be *more* disabled, not less so (Schneider and Brody, 1983; Manton, 1982). The correct answer most likely incorporates both points of view. Some disabled who would have died survive, and many who survive are healthier than their forebears.

Data from the National Health Interview Survey suggest that the prevalence of reported disability among noninstitutionalized elderly has increased (Colvez and Blanchet, 1981). However, when these data are examined in finer subgroups (those 65 to 74 and those 75 or older), the patterns of change over time are not so clear. Figure 2-2 depicts the rates for several measures of chronic disability. For some there appears to be a trend upward as described by Colvez and Blanchet, but the pattern is inconsistent. When the use of medical resources is examined in Figure 2-3 the problem is compounded; there is no obvious corresponding increase in use over time, at least at this level of aggregation.

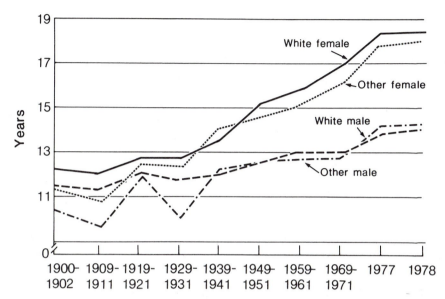

FIGURE 2–1. Life Expectancy at age 65, 1900–1978. (Source: Allan and Brotman, 1981.)

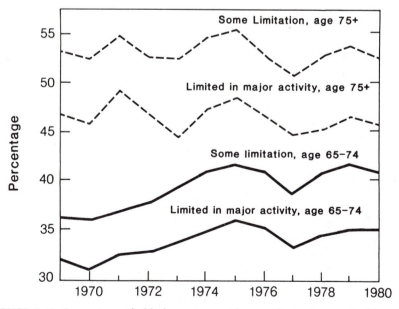

FIGURE 2–2. Percentage of elderly persons with some limitations and with major activity limitations, 1970–1980. (Based on data from the National Center for Health Statistics.)

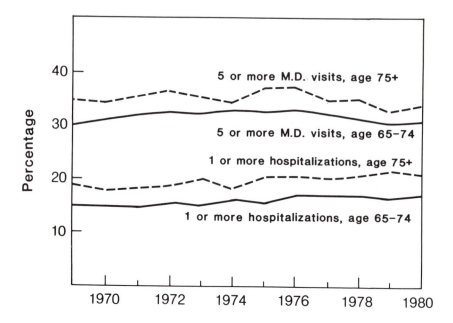

FIGURE 2–3. Percentage of elderly persons with one or more hospitalizations and five or more M.D. visits, 1970–1980. (Based on data from the National Center for Health Statistics.)

THE EXTENT OF LONG-TERM CARE NEED

Data for estimating the extent of need for long-term care come from a number of surveys and secondary analyses of surveys. Most of these are cross-sectional rather than longitudinal efforts and, therefore, provide no information on the progression of needs as they change within populations.

Two important surveys of the noninstitutionalized elderly are the 1982 National Long-Term Care Survey (NLTCS) and the 1979 National Health Interview Survey (NHIS). More recent data on this population will soon be available from the 1984 Supplement on Aging of the National Health Interview Survey. Although the most complete data on the institutionalized elderly are found in the 1977 National Nursing Home Survey (National Center for Health Statistics, 1979), preliminary data are now available from the 1985 NNHS, the third in this series of periodic surveys of nursing home residents (Hing, 1987; Strahan, 1987). In addition to these cross-sectional studies of functional disability, a few community or statewide longitudinal studies have been done, such as the Massachusetts Health Care Panel Study (Branch, 1977, 1982) and the cohort studies launched under National

Institute on Aging contracts in three areas of the country (Cornoni-Huntley et al., 1985).

One of the richest longitudinal data bases on general need for long-term care in the elderly comes from Canada. The province of Manitoba has established an ongoing data resource, which surveys a random sample of the older population and tracks it via the automated files of the centralized health insurance system. This link permits longitudinal studies of morbidity, mortality, and utilization (Mossey et al., 1981; Roos and Shapiro, 1981). For example, in a study of the cohort comparing the use of physician and hospital services over successive years, the high average rates of use with age are the result of a markedly disproportionate distribution, with a small group accounting for most of the use. Moreover, the non-users in one year are likely to be non-users in the subsequent year (Roos and Shapiro, 1981; Mossey and Shapiro, 1985). Smaller studies in the United States also show that a small group of users accounts for a disproportionate share of medical service and that such utilization patterns tend to persist over time (McCall and Wai, 1983). Thus, the best predictor of future use may be an individual's past use record. The Manitoba researchers also found that one of the best predictors of subsequent mortality among the elderly respondents was the individual's perception of his or her own health status (Mossey and Shapiro, 1982).

Cross-sectional data on almost any parameter of impairment demonstrate a pattern of increasing frequency with age after 65. The usual inflection point in the curve is around age 75. Table 2-4 summarizes data from a national survey of community-living elderly. For each of the dependency

TABLE 2-4 Dependency Rates for Community-Living Elderly, 1983

Type of Need	Rate per 1,000 Persons		
	Age: 65 to 74	75 to 84	85+
Needs help in one or more basic physical activities	52.6	114.0	384.4
Needs help in one or more home management activities	57.3	141.8	399.0
Usually stays in bed	11.3	25.6	51.2
Has device to control bowel movements or urination	5.3	10.8	28.5
Needs help of another person in one or more of the above	69.9	160.3	436.5

Source: Feller, 1983.

TABLE 2-5 Utilization of Acute and Long-Term Care Services by Age Group

	45 to 64	65 to 74	75 to 84	85+
MD visits per year[a]	6.1	7.4	8.4	
Acute hospital discharges per 1,000 persons[b]	192	334	504	615
Days of hospital care per 1,000 persons per year[b]	1461	3069	4980	6798
Number of persons in nursing home per 1,000 persons[c]	—	12.5	57.7	219.4

[a]National Center for Health Statistics, Health Interview Survey, unpublished tabulation, 1983.
[b]1983 Hospital Directory Survey, National Center for Health Statistics.
[c]Preliminary data from the 1985 National Nursing Home Survey, National Center for Health Statistics.
Sources: [a,b]Adapted from tables in United States Special Committee on Aging (1986a). [c]Taken from Hing (1987).

measures shown, the general pattern of at least a doubled rate with each decade of age can be observed.

Cross-sectional data on the 5% of the elderly population aged 65 or older living in nursing homes present a somewhat different picture. Since dependency triggers institutionalization, increased dependency with age is less pronounced for this group. The 1985 NNHS shows only a gradual increase in dependency with age, varying from 10% to 15% depending on the item. Nursing home residents as a whole were highly dependent; 63% needed help in transferring in and out of bed or chair, 54% were incontinent, and 40% needed assistance in eating. A full 63% were said to be disoriented or have memory impairments.

The pattern of increasing use of services with age holds for health care utilization. Although utilization of acute care services (shown in Table 2-5) does not quite double with each decade after age 65, the progression is steady. Because all patients over age 65 are essentially covered by the same health insurance benefits, the increase in use can be attributed safely to increasing need. Days of hospital care go up by about 50% per decade. The rate of nursing home use belies the oft-quoted rate of 5% of the elderly; it more closely approximates the pattern of functional disability, with a marked increase in the decade after age 65 and an enormous increase after age 85. On the other hand, some increases with age are less than one might expect. Visits to physicians rise only by about one visit per year per decade.

RISKS OF INSTITUTIONALIZATION

In the last 20 years, much of the discussion about need for care has been stimulated by the search for alternatives to nursing home care. For mixed humane and frugal motivations, government has hoped to identify those needing so much care that they are likely candidates for nursing homes. To prevent unnecessary nursing home admissions without inordinate expenditures, one needs to focus efforts upon that specific group of elderly persons who are most likely both to enter nursing homes and to stay there.

How can we determine the risks of nursing home admission? One convenient approach might be to use a multi-dimensional instrument, such as the Older American Resources and Services (OARS) instrument, to identify those at risk, but such instruments have thus far not proven to be effective in targeting those at institutional risk (Stassen and Holahan, 1981). The research literature offers some guidance in identifying this subgroup of the elderly population.

Table 2-6 summarizes the major information available on "risk factors." These risk factors are internal and environmental characteristics of community and nursing home residents that have been associated with greater probability of admission. The table identifies a variety of them, including advanced age, ADL impairment, living alone, poverty, use of ambulatory aids, senior citizen retirement housing, mental deterioration, and use of IADL assistance. A glance at the table suggests two questions: (1) What are the characteristics or factors that research consistently finds to be associated with entering institutions? (2) How powerful are they in helping us predict institutionalization?

The bar graph in Figure 2-4 presents a rough gauge of the commonality among factors. Characteristics that appear to have the greatest commonality are age, diagnostic condition, limitation in ability to perform daily activities, living alone, marital status, mental status, race, and lack of social supports. Three of the risk factors, living alone, marriage, and social supports, are to some extent measuring the same reality.

Searching for commonalities in risk factors among the studies presents a number of problems. Not all of the studies were targeted to samples representing the same populations: The variety of populations included community residents only, combined nursing home and community residents, welfare recipients, discharged hospital patients, homemaker and day care recipients. The Shapiro and Tate (1985) study surveyed a population in Manitoba, Canada, where long-term care is covered as part of a universal health insurance program.

The table excludes information about nursing home use among the control group members in various demonstration projects. Such demonstrations (addressed in Chapter 10) deliberately selected their clientele and

TABLE 2-6 Risk Factors for Nursing Home Admission

Source	Sample	Risk Factors	Explanatory Power
National Center for Health Statistics (1979)	Survey of nursing home residents in 1977 (compared to those age 65+ living in the community).	Age, female, white, unmarried.	Not applicable.
Brody, Poulshock, and Masciocchi (1978)	Survey of disabled home-health elderly agency clients and nursing home residents (urban/rural county).	Living arrangement, living with spouse/child, social support.	Not applicable.
Vincente, Wiley, and Carrington (1979)	Nine-year follow-up of residents age 55+ in Alameda County, California.	Age, poverty, white, lack of social supports.	Not applicable.
Palmore (1976)	Twenty-year follow-up of residents age 60+ in Piedmont, North Carolina, area.	Unmarried, white.	Marital status explained 9% of the variance in whether or not a person was institutionalized; race explained 4%.
Weissert et al. (1980a)	One-year study of daycare recipients and controls in six sites.	Primary diagnostic conditions, impairment prognosis, hospital outpatient or other ambulatory use.	Hospital outpatient use explained 5% of the variance in whether or not a person was institutionalized, other ambulatory care use explained 1%, and impairment prognosis explained 1%.

Weissert et al. (1980b)	One-year study of home-maker recipients and controls in four sites; patients were hospitalized for at least three days during the two weeks prior to the study.	Primary diagnostic conditions, ADL prognosis, hospital outpatient or other ambulatory use.	Bed disability prognosis explained 8% of the variance in institutionalization; outpatient hospital use explained 2%; other ambulatory use, 2%; ADL prognosis, .8%.
McCoy and Edwards (1981)	National sample of welfare recipients age 65+.	Age, functional impairment, white, living alone or with non-relatives, lack of social supports.	Those who are 85+ were about four times as likely to be institutionalized in comparison with other elderly persons; whites were about twice as likely; those living with non-relatives were four times as likely to be institutionalized as those living with spouse only; those in everyday contact with friends and/or relatives were almost half as likely to be institutionalized as those without such contact.

TABLE 2-6 Continued

Source	Sample	Risk Factors	Explanatory Power
Branch and Jette (1982)	Six-year panel study of 1,625 Massachusetts elders living in the community.	Age, use of ambulation aids, mental disorientation, living alone, using assistance in ADL.	The six risk factors explained about 10 percent of the total variance in institutionalization. Compared to those without any of the risk factors, those using ambulatory aids had 4.1 times the likelihood of institutionalization; those mentally disabled, 3.6 times; those 80+, 2.8 times; those using ADL assistance, 1.9; those living alone, 1.7; those using IADL assistance, 1.3.
Kane and Mathias (1984)	Random samples of hospital patients (PRSO data) from four areas (West Los Angeles, CA; Riverside, CA; Utah; South Carolina) who had entered the hospital from home.	Age, sex, mental diagnosis, and orthopedic surgery.	Age was the only consistently strong predictor for all four areas. Other factors selected to predict institutionalization varied, suggesting that their relative importance differs among geographical areas.

Weissert and Scanlon (1984c)	Combined samples of community and nursing home elderly from 1977 National Nursing Home Survey and 1977 Health Interview Survey.	Personal care dependency, diagnostic conditions, poverty, advanced age, heating-degree days.	The probability of institutionalization for those 65+ who are toileting-eating dependent was .91; for those with mental disorders, .81; for cancer, blood metabolic, or genitourinary disorders, .31; for poverty, .19; for advanced age, .12; for those living in a colder climate (heating-degree days), .05.
Wachtel et al. (1984)	50 hospitalized elderly (65+) with 50 controls, all discharged to home or nursing home.	Men: no spouse at home, mental, respiratory or nervous system disorder; multiple meds. Women: mental disorder, musculoskeletal disease; prior hospital admission reduced probability of placement.	Not applicable.

29

TABLE 2-6 Continued

Source	Sample	Risk Factors	Explanatory Power
Shapiro and Tate (1985)	3,902 community elderly, 65+, in the province of Manitoba studied over a short (2½ years) and long (7 years) period.	For those institutionalized within a 2½-year period: age, senior citizen apartment residency, living without a spouse, admitted to hospital in year of interview, ADL problems; for those admitted in a 7-year period: above factors plus being female, low self-rated health, and frequent contact with relatives.	Of those 65+ institutionalized within 2½ years, those 85+ were 7 times as likely to be institutionalized; those 75–84, 3 times as likely; those residing in senior citizen housing and living without a spouse, 2½ times; those hospitalized in the year of the interview and those with 1 or more ADL disabilities were more than 2 times as likely to be institutionalized; those with mental impairment, 1.7 times as likely. These were also the major risk factors for the seven year period.
Soldo and Manton (1985)	6,393 community based elderly (65+) with limitations in ADLs or IADLs.	Of four analytically defined subgroups, the homogeneous group most likely to be institutionalized consisted of unmarried women of advanced age, with IADL limitation and deficiencies in their informal support networks.	The probability of a person in this group being on a nursing home waiting list was .021; the probability of having been a nursing home patient at any time was .084.

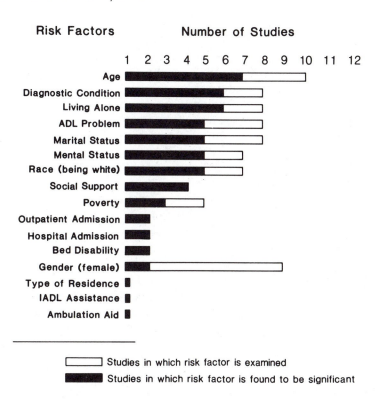

FIGURE 2–4. Commonality of risk factors for entering a nursing home among 12 studies. (Source: All studies that are referenced in Table 2–6, excluding Soldo and Manton, 1985.)

comparison groups to be groups at high risk of entering nursing homes. Although "community" is variously defined in the studies included in Table 2-6, all represented efforts to predict nursing home use in a general population of community-dwelling elderly. Data from the experimental study of homemaking and day care (Weissert et al., 1980a, 1980b) are included because the sample was drawn from the general Medicare rolls rather than a population assumed to be at risk.

Nor did all of the studies investigate the same risk factors. The use of ambulatory aids, for example, has only been studied by Branch and Jette (1982). There are a number of other differences that make cross-comparisons difficult. Only some of the study designs were longitudinal, allowing for the prospective study of characteristics as they occur prior to admission. Not all of the studies used statistical methods that isolate the impact of each factor, controlling for other characteristics. Finally, the studies differed in the way factors such as "poverty" are defined and in the sensitivity with which they are measured.

The predictive powers of these risk factors—and prediction is the key if we want to identify most of those at risk—have thus far proven to be quite limited. The combination of the risk factors identified by the Branch and Jette study (Branch and Jette, 1982; Branch, 1984), for example, explains only about 10 percent of the variance in admission to nursing homes. Furthermore, one needs to distinguish risk factors related to the client (e.g., functional ability, age) from those related to the environment (e.g., social support). The latter may become important only when the former are a problem.

Of the studies listed in Table 2-6, the Shapiro and Tate (1985) study is particularly interesting because it is one of the few that followed a relatively large sample (3,383) of community elders over a long period (seven years). Looking at 28 different variables, the authors found that advanced age, living arrangements, mental deterioration, problems with ADLs, and senior citizen apartment housing were the major factors that increase the odds of institutionalization.

In another longitudinal study, Branch and Jette (1982) followed a cohort of Massachusetts elderly community residents over a six-year period. They suggested that the very old (e.g., aged 80 to 99), those living alone, those using ambulation aids, the mentally disoriented, and those using assistance to perform IADLs are potential target groups for programs seeking to replace institutional with non-institutional services.

Among cross-sectional studies, the Soldo and Manton study (1985) is noteworthy because of its large sample and sophisticated analysis. The researchers used the "grade of membership" statistical technique (GOM) to determine groups that are homogeneous with respect to socio-demographic, disability, and service utilization patterns. Of four analytically derived groups thus identified, the group most likely to enter a nursing home tend to manifest IADL dependencies rather than more extreme functional disabilities. Persons in the group were uniformly unmarried women of advanced age and those disproportionately dependent upon children and relatives for daily assistance. The group's risk appeared to be primarily a function of deficiencies in their informal support system, in contrast to another group with risks more directly related to their ADL or care needs.

INFORMAL CARE AND SOCIAL SUPPORT

Long-term care is highly personal, stemming directly from a particular person's functional limitations. The majority of long-term care services in the United States continue to be provided by the family. Services are often purchased when family help must be supplemented or when no family members are available or willing to help. As the previous section showed, the nature of the family and household combines with functional disabilities to predict nursing home use. We cannot predict the amount of purchased care necessary or the amount of care that will need to be provided at public expense without understanding what can be expected of family.

In part, of course, the future behavior of family members will be influenced by the generosity of public provision. For example, if a public benefit for personal care of the chronically impaired were universally offered to persons in their own homes, adult daughters, spouses, and other family caregivers might withdraw from physically and emotionally taxing tasks such as bathing elderly family members. Whether such expanded benefits are viewed as a foolhardy waste of the taxpayers' money, a wise investment in human resources, or something in between, depends partly on ideology and partly on our understanding of the *effects* of caregiving on family members. Providing long-term care may eventually have negative consequences for the caregiver and ultimately increase societal costs.

With typical professional parochialism, care rendered by relatives or other volunteers has come to be known as "informal support" or "informal care," in contrast to the "formal care" offered by agencies and paid providers. Similarly, this large topic is often called "social support," as if the natural course of family and social arrangements came into being in an adjunctive or supportive capacity to help meet professionally identified needs. Table 2-7 summarizes studies on informal care in three groups: those describing the extent of informal care, those describing the role relationships between caregivers and care recipients, and those describing the effect of giving care on the caregiving family members.

The Extent of Informal Support

Soldo (1984) estimated that 73% of the care provided to elderly dependent persons in the community came from relatives, friends, or neighbors; that 16% of these dependent persons received care from both formal and informal caretakers; and that only 9% received assistance exclusively from formal providers. There was virtually no difference in the rate of informal care received among those with and without formal services. Although one might speculate that there would be some substitution of informal service for formal help, most of the additional care seemed to come in the form of technical and medical services outside the expertise of informal caregivers. Formal assistance was less available in nonmetropolitan areas. Nearly twice as many informal caretakers in farm areas contrasted with urban areas received no formal assistance when caring for persons with multiple care needs. This substantiates the belief that the supply of service dictates demand.

Social research has by now dispelled the myth that the elderly have little contact with family and friends, highlighting the importance of family and friends in providing long-term care (Shanas, 1962, 1979; Brody, 1978; Callahan et al., 1980; Sauer and Coward, 1985). Elaine Brody (1985) recently summarized dozens of studies of her own and others to illustrate

TABLE 2-7 The Role of Social Supports: Selected Studies and Findings

Source	Population/Sample	Design	Selected Findings
THE EXTENT OF INFORMAL CARE: GAO (1977)	Random sample of 1,609 noninstitutionalized Cleveland residents (65+); interviewed in 1977 and one year later.	The OARS questionnaire has a Social Resources dimension and a Utilization of Services Section to determine type of help and supports as well as major source of help.	Children were the primary available source of help for 42%; friends, 8%; medical and recreational services were provided mostly by agencies; home help and transportation by informal services; financial and assessment/referral services were split evenly between formal and informal.
Wan and Weissert (1981)	Community sample of 1,871 Medicare recipients randomly assigned to experimental (day care and housekeeping services) and control groups.	The 1,871 subjects were measured five times during the one-year demonstration period; 3-year follow-up data on 1,119 were also included. Regression was used to determine the impact of such variables as demographics, physical status (ADLs), mental functioning (MSQs), social networks on institutionalization. A 6-item scale measured the presence of social supports, including children, siblings, grandchildren, other relatives, and friends.	The availability of social support had a positive association with both physical and mental functioning. Availability of children/grandchildren had positive impact on reducing SNF institutionalization but not short-term hospitalization.

Author	Sample	Method	Results
Weissert (1982)	Nationwide sample of 11,730 household elderly (1979 Health Interview Survey).	Secondary analysis of the survey data on items of functional dependency; subjects were hierarchically classified according to most severe dependence.	Personal care dependents who were unmarried living alone, and poor were underrepresented in the community. Proportion of those whose needs were at least mostly met: needs help eating (97%), transferring (86%), toileting (77%), dressing (65%), bathing (48%), mobility (31%).
Branch and Jette (1983)	Third follow-up of Massachusetts random panel of elders enrolled in 1974. This third wave in 1980 included 825 survivors, aged 71–91.	Multiple regression was used to determine the extent to which use of informal help in ADL and IADL was influenced by nature and composition of support networks, level of physical disability, age, living situation, and total household income.	22% had no living children and 41% had no nearby children; 35% had no other nearby relatives living; 80% received no ADL help but 82% received some help with IADL; at 85+, 42% received ADL help; divided between formal (38%), informal (50%), or mixed (12%); 86% of IADL help came from informal sources. Physical disability, age, and living with someone associated most with women getting informal ADL help. For men physical disability and living with another were associated with informal ADL help. Similar results were found for informal IADL help.

TABLE 2-7 Continued

Source	Population/Sample	Design	Selected Findings
Soldo (1984)	National probability sample of 5,756 household elderly; 457 LTC elderly (bed-fast or mobile with self-care limitations).	Secondary analysis of data from the 1975 National Survey of the Aged, LTC elderly sample; cross-tabulations of elderly with functional family supports; indices of service-use patterns and IADL support were developed to show distribution of service by living arrangement, sex of children, number of children, elderly's incapacities for self-care.	40% of elderly with daughters did not have a "functioning" helper in terms of frequency of contact; one-third in terms of proximity. Among the disabled ambulatory, the presence of adult children associated with residence in the community supported by informal services; presence of daughters may be proxy indicator of depth of commitment.
ROLE RELATIONSHIPS: Gurland et al. (1978)	Random sample of about 450 non-institutional NY City residents aged 65+ (preliminary data from U.S./ U.K. Cross National Geriatric Community Study).	Analysis of informal system included a 4-level hierarchy of the magnitude of support system, time commitment and skill level of supports, 1977 dollar equivalents of services by primary providers.	Daughters provided 34% of primary support services; spouses, 29%; other family, 14%; formal providers (nurses, aides, home helpers) constituted about 1 in 6 of primary providers. Major demand for primary provider services was short sessions (8 hr per week), but daily care (40 hr per week) was also prominent. Greatest demand was for housekeeping, with personal care second.

Cantor (1979, 1981)	Randomly stratified matched samples; 1,552 inner-city New York residents, aged 60 or over.	2,180 households identified and 71% interviewed (1970) regarding socioeconomic and health variables, extent of kinship support system. Analyses included forced multiple regression on the predictive effect of ethnicity, controlling for social class, income, etc.; descriptive data on contact and help with "functional" children, neighbors, friends; elderly's preferences of support agents were grouped according to 10 hypothetical incidents of need.	Blacks, Hispanics, other working poor were more likely to have highly developed patterns of child-parent interaction arising out of economic and social necessity than the more well-to-do elderly. Data suggested that, regardless of task, kin were generally seen as the most preferred support giver; when the preferred group was absent, other groups acted in compensation.
Stoller and Earl (1983)	753 non-institutionalized elderly, stratified to represent rural focus.	Comprehensive Assessment, Referral, and Evaluation Instrument (CARE) used to measure demographic as well as psychiatric, medical, nutritional, economic, and social problems; data collected on up to three helpers on relationship and type of assistance. Descriptive statistics and multivariate techniques used to describe prevalence of helpers by task capacity, distribution of assistance, source of assistance.	Spouses were primary sources of help for married elders, and adult daughters were the major source when spouse was not present; helping networks increased in size and scope as functional capacity declined.

TABLE 2-7 Continued

Source	Population/Sample	Design	Selected Findings
Townsend and Poulshock (1986)	101 community elderly (60+) in need of ADL/IADL assistance together with the adult children caregivers.	Data collected on size, composition, structure of social networks through separate interviews with caregivers and care receivers. Analysis of variance and t-tests for matched samples were used to determine differences between group responses.	Data suggested unique generational perspectives between children and elders on caregiving and decision-making networks. Children reported larger networks with a greater variety of sources, and greater centrality of themselves and kin within the networks. Both agreed on general hierarchy of help.
Morris and Sherwood (1983/84)	Purposive sample of six subgroups (institutional applicants, urban blacks, urban Puerto Ricans, rural samples, urban ethnics, congregant housing residents) of 700 vulnerable elderly and 500 informal helpers.	Interviews with both elders and helpers focusing on help given by four most important persons in the network; personal ADLs measured by Katz ADL scale; measures of help concerned how helping relationships are functioning, types of help provided regarding crucial daily activities.	Most helpers interviewed were not sole providers: a minimal shell of informal support existed; formal members were seen as ancillary to informal; in the absence of children, other relatives, friends, neighbors assumed increased roles; most informal networks included helpers who were fully aware of elders' problems (85%). Only 12% of elders were not confident that current levels of help could be counted on, but 29% were not confident that help in new areas could be provided if needed.

| Mitchell and Register (1984) | 334 blacks and 1,813 whites 65+ who had living children; community sample. | Secondary analysis of data from 1975 Lou Harris national survey; three composite measures constructed to represent receiving help, giving help, socio-economic status. Chi-square and analysis of variance used to test if blacks saw children more often, received more help (e.g., money, errands, help when ill), gave more help than whites. | Evidence for extended family hypothesis supported by findings that blacks more likely take children/grandchildren into their homes and are more likely to receive help from their children. Only slight, though statistically significant, differences found between whites and blacks. |
| Chappell and Havens (1985) Chappell (1985) | 400 homecare users and 400 non-users, aged 65+; random sample from community (Winnipeg). | Analysis of samples (weighted to represent community) regarding functional limitations, size of total and available networks, assistance received and given; t-tests showed differences between users and non-users. Chappell (1985) also showed difference between groups in availability of supports, interaction with support system, satisfaction with relationships, receipt of assistance. | Non-users had more individuals available to them than users (48.2 versus 33.2); almost half of the sample was either both giving and receiving help or neither giving nor receiving assistance; home care users received more help from informal sources than non-users, suggesting that they complement rather than substitute for each other. |

TABLE 2-7 Continued

Source	Population/Sample	Design	Selected Findings
Travelers Employee Caregiver Survey (1985)	A 20% sample of employees aged 30+ of Travelers Insurance Company Home Office in Connecticut; 52% returned questionnaire (N=739).	Cross-sectional study using written questionnaire to determine extent of care responsibilities for friends and relatives age 55 and over.	Study concluded that at least 20% of employees aged 30+ had caregiving responsibilities for one or more persons aged 55+. Women gave more care than men; most frequent caregiving activities were companionship/checking (76% of caregivers), transportation (62%), and household chores
EFFECTS OF CAREGIVING ON CAREGIVERS: Horowitz and Shindelman (1983)	203 persons identified as primary caregivers of older persons getting home care or day care in New York City, included spouses (average age 71), children (average age 51), and others; 21% of sample black and 18% Hispanic.	Four scales used (caregiving involvement, caregiving consequences, affection, and reciprocity) to determine the relationship between present caregiving and past relationships.	15% not close to dependent person. Most frequent reasons for giving care were family obligations (58%) and affection (51%). Reciprocity for past help mentioned by 17%. Reciprocity was related to amount of help given but not impact of caregiving. Affection was positively related to commitment and negatively to perceived stress.

| Birkel (1984) | 40 pairs of impaired elders (60+) and their primary caregivers; noninstitutional volunteer sample. | Comparative analysis between a group of elders with physical impairments and those with cognitive impairments; levels of physical, cognitive, behavioral functioning determined through use of nine measures including Lawton's IADL scale. Mental Status Questionnaire, PGC Morale Scale; groups compared on time-dependency, caregiver strain, predictors of caregiver strain determined. | No significant differences between groups in measures of caregiving time (28 hours for physical group and 30 hours for mentally disabled group). Caregivers of dementia group suffered more strain on personal stress and negative feelings towards the elder. A larger group of household members appeared to help alleviate strain for the dementia group, perhaps because the tasks demanded were basically custodial; larger households appeared to create more stress for the caregivers of the physically disabled. |

TABLE 2-7 Continued

Source	Population/Sample	Design	Selected Findings
Benjamin Rose Institute Survey (Poulshock and Deimling, 1984; Deimling and Bass, 1984; Noelker, 1983; Wallace and Noelker, 1983)	Purposive sample (stratified re geographic area, race, generational configuration) of 614 caregiving families from 2,000 referrals.	Four separate studies involved inter-item analysis to determine conceptual dimensions of burden (Poulshock and Deimling); regression of physical, mental disabilities upon measures of stress (Deimling and Bass); correlations between physical and mental impairments and marital tension (Wallace and Noelker); and multivariate analysis to explore relationship between types of incontinence and characteristics of elders, stress effects upon caregivers (Noelker).	Studies suggested a multi-dimensional relationship between disability and caregiver burden. Wandering behavior was particularly associated with caregiver depression, health, activity restriction, relationship between caregiver and elder; mental, not physical, disability was associated with marriage tension; caregivers with incontinent elders had significantly greater stress effect on six measures than those with continent elders (time restriction, social activity restriction, group activity restriction, health deterioration, negative affect in caregiver-elder relationship, negative affect among family members).

Snyder and Keefe (1985)	117 primary caregivers, 81 females and 36 males; non-random sample; 70% in San Francisco Bay area counties.	21 item self-report questionnaire regarding caregivers' health problems, sources of support, use of formal services by caregivers, need for additional services. Functional level of adult dependents measured on a three-point Likert scale. Descriptive statistics provided.	Weak correlation between caregiver health and disability of disabled adult ($r=.13$) and between length of caregiving and receipt of help from family and friends ($r=.14$); those caregiving for the longest time were least likely to report receipt of formal services ($r=-.26$). Male caregivers most frequently used housework services; women most frequently used support groups. The service most requested by men and women was regular respite.
Brody and Schoonover (1986)	Elderly widows, their daughters, and sons-in-laws from 150 families living in the community (Philadelphia area). Respondents were volunteers selected on the basis of working ($N=78$) or nonworking ($N=72$) status.	Personal interviews used to examine the affects of women's work-force participation on the care of elderly widows; patterns of care to the aged were explored as they vary when daughters are employed and not employed outside the home.	Employed and non-employed daughters provided equal amounts of help with shopping and/or transportation, household tasks, money management/service arrangement, and emotional support. Working daughters provided fewer hours of care with personal care and meal preparation, but this was offset by the combined help of the informal network and helpers paid by the family.

TABLE 2-7 Continued

Source	Population/Sample	Design	Selected Findings
Fitting et al. (1986)	A nonrandom sample of 26 female caregivers (mean age of 65) and 28 male caregivers (mean age of 70) living in the Baltimore area. The subjects are well-educated, middle-class caucasians.	Structural interviews and scales were used to compare the wife and husband caregivers of dementia patients on the key variables of burden, family environment, psychological functioning, functional impairment, and social networks.	Men and women had similar perceptions of their social environments. Increasing severity of the spouse's illness was associated with higher burden in younger wives and older husbands only. Wives experienced significantly more depression, and more women than men (16 vs. 7) reported that their spousal relationship had deteriorated since the onset of illness.
George and Gwyther (1986)	A sample of 510 family caregivers of memory-impaired adults (obtained from the Duke University Family Support Program mailing list; average age 57; socioeconomic level was higher than that of the general population.	A mailed survey was used to examine the impact of caregiving upon the caregiver's mental health, physical health, social participation, and financial resources. Correlates of caregiver well-being were also explored.	Compared to the general population, caregivers were more likely to experience mental health problems. Caregivers reported substantially lower levels of social participation and higher uses of psychotropic drugs (28% vs. 19%). Living with the patient was related to use of psychotropic drugs, stress symptoms, low levels of affect and life satisfaction. Patient illness was not related to caregiver well-being.

| Zarit, Todd, and Zarit (1986) | A sample of 33 caregiver wives and 31 caregiver husbands taken from patients at a clinic offering support for caregivers or from the membership of an Alzheimer's disease advocacy group. All the demented spouses met DSM-III criteria for dementia. | In a longitudinal study, caregivers were measured at baseline and two years later regarding burden, spouses' severity of impairment, social support quality of relationship with spouse, and, at Time 2, reasons for institutionalizing spouse, when applicable. | Subsequent nursing home placement for 11 spouses was more strongly associated with caregiver's perceived burden than with the severity of the dementia. Wives had initially reported more burden than husbands but there was no significant difference at follow-up. |

that care to the "grandparent" and "parent" generations is given extensively and is accompanied by sacrifice and emotional stress. Recent studies, usually based on data from local surveys or upon secondary analysis of national data, have presented specific information on the role of informal care: the supply of care provided by such networks, the extent to which it meets the needs of the elderly, and the impact of long-term care needs and informal caregiving upon the family and social network. A number of those studies are summarized in Table 2.7.

Determining the supply of informal long-term care services requires operational definitions and assumptions about who in the social network is available for caregiving. Presence of kin is a crude indicator of the supply of long-term care help. According to Shanas (1979), 80% of the elderly have at least one adult child; 75% have children who live less than one-half hour away. However, Soldo (1984) argued that the presence of kin overestimates the supply of true long-term care providers. Availability of kin for caregiving varies by the relationship to the person needing care, the proximity, intensity, and duration of needs, and the competing demands on the potential family caregiver. Given that adult daughters appear to provide more "instrumental hands-on services" than adult sons, she tried to identify those with daughters available to help. Of the elderly sampled, 20% had no daughters and of those with daughters, 40% did not have a "functional daughter" who had sufficiently frequent contact and one-third did not have a functional daughter who lived reasonably nearby. Kulys and Tobin (1980) have shown that the potential sources of informal support cited by older persons may be overly optimistic reports of actual availability.

In his analysis using data from the 1979 National Health Interview Survey, Weissert (1982) found that for the elderly community population—most of whom receive only informal assistance—those whose needs are most severe are most likely to get help. Thus, of those who needed help eating, 97% received help most or all of the time, while of those who needed help with mobility, only 31% received the same level of help. Interpreting such data is difficult because many of those with major needs and unavailable or ineffective assistance may have already entered nursing homes. A cross-sectional sample under-represents the poor and those living alone. However, in a controlled study of community elderly receiving day care and homemaker services at three sites, Wan and Weissert (1981) concluded that social support networks have a positive impact upon physical and mental functioning status, as well as a preventive impact upon nursing home admissions.

Branch and Jette (1983) provide data about a population aged 71 to 91 from the third wave of the Massachusetts population study. More than a fifth had no living children, and a substantial number had either no children or no other relatives in the geographic vicinity (41% and 35%, respectively). Although most performed basic ADL activities with no help (over 80%), all but 18% used help with IADL activities. Those using help with ADL received it from informal sources (50%), formal sources (38%), and a mixture of both (12%), whereas overwhelmingly help with IADL activities came from informal sources (86%).

In the Cleveland study (General Accounting Office, 1977), probably the most well known and most often quoted survey, most older persons (87%) stated that they had a primary source of help if they should become sick or disabled. The types of services most often mentioned as being provided by families and friends were transportation (60%), personal care (56%), checking (44%), and administrative and legal support (15%). Services most frequently provided by agencies were medical care (75%), housing (12%), and social/recreational services (30%).

In their study of personal time dependency in New York City, Gurland and his colleagues (1978) found that 77% of primary support services (services most critical to maintaining the elderly person at home) were provided by daughters, spouses, and other family members. Morris and Sherwood (1983/84) studied a purposefully selected sample of 700 vulnerable adults and 500 of their informal helpers; they found that only 8% relied solely or primarily on formal resources, with 64% of those in need using informal helpers primarily or solely.

Role Relationships of Informal Caregivers

Family—especially spouses, daughters, and daughters-in-law—provide the majority of informal care services for the elderly. In the Cleveland study (GAO, 1977), the most frequently mentioned source of primary care was the older person's children (42%), followed by spouse (27%), sibling (10%), and other relatives and friends (17%). An Alameda County study of the caregivers of disabled persons over 65 found that daughters helped more than sons, that helpers were more likely to be unmarried and unemployed than other siblings, and, most notably, as the number of adult children in a family rose, the proportion of children helping decreased (Wiley, 1983).

Friends and neighbors appear to play a backup role at best (Gurland et al., 1978), helping with emergencies and time-limited tasks. In Cantor's study (1979) of 1,552 elderly inner-city New York residents, respondents were asked to whom, other than a spouse, they would most likely turn for assistance: child, other relative, friend, neighbor, formal organization. For almost all options, particularly health and personal care, kin were either clearly preferred or the only option possible.

A note of caution is appropriate, however, about the danger of extrapolating too far from respondents' reports of potential sources of support. Kulys and Tobin (1980) described considerable loss of potential support when they attempted to verify the postulated sources of assistance reported by a sample of community living elderly. Morris and Sherwood

(1983/84) suggested that although children were a more certain resource, other relatives and friends had about an equal probability of participating in the support systems of the vulnerable elderly with whom they have contact. When relatives or friends and neighbors assisted, they were more likely to be the only type of persons present in the network, suggesting that they acted only when children are unavailable.

Data on size and composition of social networks may vary, depending upon whether the source of the data is the adult child or the elderly dependent person. Townsend and Poulshock (1986) found that size and composition differed, depending upon whether reported by the impaired elderly or their adult children. Children consistently mentioned more helpers than the elders did. Also, although married elderly generally mentioned their spouse as the one primary caregiver, widows and their children were likely to not name any primary caregiver.

Although it is often assumed that the supportive networks of the long-term elderly population are small, usually with one primary caregiver, the evidence is not definitive. Morris and Sherwood (1983/84) found that elderly persons reported two or more individuals within their informal caregiving network in 86 percent of the cases sampled. Interviews with those named as part of the caregiving network identified additional helpers in 48% of the cases. In contrast, Stoller and Earl (1983) found that the majority of 753 northeastern New York elders had networks that were either empty or had only one helper. The sample studied, however, was relatively unimpaired, almost all respondents reporting that they accomplished personal care activities alone or with minimal assistance. The authors also discovered that the number of caregivers increased as functional disability increased.

Using a sample of 800 elderly home care users or non-users in Winnipeg, Manitoba, Chappell and Havens (1985) studied the size of the total social network (all persons generally available in their lives) and found that most (55%) reported that anywhere from 11 to 40 people were available in their lives. In an additional analysis, Chappell (1985) reported that users and non-users of home care differed in the size of the available network, but that users had fewer social supports available only among the young elderly and non-widowed.

Findings on the size of social networks and amount of informal care as related to ethnicity are limited, but suggest that socio-economic status rather than race is the basic determinant of aid from children to parents. Cantor (1981) used ethnicity and socio-economic status as key variables in a study of white, black, and Hispanic New York residents. Social class and income were the major determinants of aid, although Hispanic elderly persons did appear to be more likely to have children from whom they received a greater amount of help. Analysis of Harris survey data based on a sample of 334 blacks and 1,913 whites found that black elders received more from their children than white elders; however, the difference, although statistically significant, was slight (Mitchell and Register, 1984).

Thus far, at least one large-scale employer has conducted a survey to determine how its employees are affected by the need to care for older relatives and friends (*Travelers Employee Caregiver Survey*, 1985). A 20% sample was drawn from the company's home office staff over age 30 ($N=1,412$), and a 52% response rate was received (739). Almost 30% of the respondents indicated that they were currently caring for somebody 55 or over, and assuming at least some of the nonrespondents also gave care, the researchers concluded that about one in five of their employees had caregiving responsibilities. Mothers were the recipients of care in 46% of the cases, and in 62% of the cases the care recipient lived alone. Interestingly, in 15% of the instances, the employees perceived that they gave care to someone in a nursing home. Female employees were more often primary caregivers than male employees. The latter were more likely to report that their wives or paid employees gave care. On the whole, the sample felt they received very little information useful to them as caregivers. They particularly wanted information on community resources and how to select them and on public and private insurance coverage. Much less interest was expressed in information about caregiver support groups.

Effects of Caregiving on Caregivers

Unlike the large surveys on the prevalence of functional impairments, surveys and studies on what has come to be called caregiver "burden" or "strain" are local studies, with relatively small sample sizes. Although this limits generalizability, it also allows for more specific and diverse exploration of the area.

One of the largest such studies is the Benjamin Rose Institute survey of 614 families who were residing with and caring for impaired elders. Based on those data, Poulshock and Deimling (1984) suggested that both the elderly persons' impairments, and their consequences upon caregivers, need to be studied and measured from a multi-dimensional perspective. Different impairments may lead to different experiences of burden, having different consequences upon family life. Preliminary findings suggested that measures of elder mental impairment and corresponding burden measures were substantially correlated with the negative impact on elder caregiver/caregiver family relationships, whereas ADL impairments were more highly correlated with restrictions in caregivers' activities. Another analysis of the same data (Deimling and Bass, 1984) assessed the impact of elders' physical and mental impairments on caregiver stress, finding that elders' disruptive behavior—in contrast to physical disabilities and cognitive incapacity—had a significant impact upon all four stress measures used: caregiver changes in level of depression, physical health, restrictions in activities, and elder-family relationships. Yet another examination of the Benjamin Rose data (Wallace and Noelker, 1983) found an association between mental impairment of the elder and caregiver-spouse marital tension, but no such relationship for physical impairment of the elder.

In the Benjamin Rose sample of dependent elderly, 57% had urinary/fecal incontinence. Incontinent elders had more numerous and severe functional limitations than continent elders, and those with both isolated urinary and combined incontinence evidenced more mental impairment and disruptive behaviors than the continent elderly. Incontinence was credited with burdening caregivers' personal time, imposing activity restrictions, reducing health status, and creating negative family relationships. Caregivers whose elders had combined incontinence more often considered alternative placements for the elders, such as nursing homes (Noelker, 1983).

Two other studies are of interest. A survey of 117 San Francisco caregivers found that those who had been caregiving the longest length of time were least likely to report receiving social services; the service most frequently requested by both male and female caregivers was respite care (Snyder and Keefe, 1985). The second study found no significant difference in the time required to care for elders with dementia as opposed to those with physical disabilities, but that, nevertheless, the caregivers of the dementia group experienced more personal stress and negative feelings toward the elderly and were more likely to consider placing them in a nursing home (Birkel, 1984). For the physically disabled group, caregiver strain was positively associated with increased numbers of household members, whereas for the dementia group, strain and household size were negatively related. The author speculated that large numbers of helpers create opportunities for tension in working with the physically disabled.

The findings of three additional studies emphasize the close association between stress and caring for the demented elderly (George and Gwyther, 1986; Zarit, Todd, and Zarit, 1986; Fitting et al., 1986). George and Gwyther, for example, found that caregivers of memory-impaired adults were more likely than the general population to report mental health problems, lower levels of social participation, and higher levels of drug use. The relationship between stress and caregiving, however, is more complicated than one might at first think. From clinical research with caregivers, Zarit and his colleagues concluded that burden is somewhat subjective, based more on the caregiver's perceived burden than on the severity of the dementia itself. Also, Fitting's comparative study on male and female caregivers found the increasing severity of the demented person's illness to be associated with higher burden in only younger wives and older husbands.

Some authors have addressed the motivations for providing care and the associated stresses. In a review of voluminous related literature, Hanson and Sauer (1985) concluded that both affection and a sense of obligation operate in the bonds that cause adult children to help their parents. Cicirelli's study of 164 adult children and their elderly parents in Lafayette, Indiana (1981), suggested that the amount of care and attention given increased with parental dependency, but feelings of attachment remained the same regardless of a parent's health. Giving care was perceived as more stressful by sons than daughters, and care to fathers in the absence of attachment was more stressful than care to mothers. However, this study involved largely healthy parents with few personal care or homemaking requirements. Another study with a large population of primary caregivers found that reciprocity, in the sense of having previously received help from the now dependent relative, was associated with the amount of help given, but not the accompanying stress. In contrast, affection for the care recipient was associated with reduced caregiver stress (Horowitz and Shindelman, 1983).

Brody's phrase "women-in-the-middle" has been seized upon to depict the multiple stresses in parent care, which is still largely women's work. From her study of the females in three generations, she pointed out that the elderly still expect more care from daughters than sons and that women also expect this duty of themselves. Nonetheless, women of all three generations believed it was better for a working woman to pay someone to care for her parent than to leave her job to do so (Brody, 1981). Another study of married female caregivers of elderly widowed mothers dramatized the meaning of care for many women. Almost half the sample had helped an elderly father before his death, and one-third had helped other elderly relatives. Almost two-thirds had children living at home, and the authors speculated that many would undoubtedly care for spouses in the future. Thus, care of their mother at this time was an episode in an extended phase of caregiving that spanned decades. More than a quarter of the nonworking women had quit their jobs for parent care, several others were contemplating doing so, and others had cut back on the amount of work. Despite their commitment to caregiving and their considerable sacrifices, three-fifths of the women felt guilt that they were not doing enough for their mothers (Brody, Kleban, and Johnsen, 1984). In a further analysis of data from the same study, however, the authors found that elderly mothers were suffering neglect due to increased work-force participation of daughters. Working daughters were found to contribute equal amounts of help to their mothers in areas such as transportation/shopping, money management, and emotional support. Although working daughters did provide less personal care, this was offset by increased support from the informal network and helpers paid by the family (Brody and Schoonover, 1986).

Brody's study suggests that there is a long time horizon for caregiving, and indeed little research is available that follows caregivers longitudinally. It would be of interest to know what circumstances are associated with the continuation of care and what causes people to relinquish responsibility. An early study of long-term care recipients in Massachusetts is suggestive; it reported a sharp drop-off in the percentage of relatives willing to provide care in the community after a second hospitalization compared to after a first. Perhaps a hospitalization provides a convenient and face-saving time to reassess the feasibility of giving care (Eggert et al., 1976).

SUMMARY

Determining the need for long-term care is an inexact process, as this long chapter suggests. But fortunately, we are not in complete ignorance. Quite safe predictions can be made for community groups based on functional impairment levels, which in turn rise markedly with age. Long-term care at rock-bottom is a necessary response to functional dependency.

Interpreting the need for formal service provision, and in turn the need for public provision of those services, is more complicated; it reflects public policy. At the very least, the proportion of elders with no living or nearby relatives are candidates for outside help. Those who depend on caregivers who are themselves frail, those who are in need of heavy or highly technical care, or those falling into both categories probably need some help from outside the family. As we noted, it is typical that those receiving substantial family help also receive some additional purchased care at either their own or public expense. The extent to which families are hurt by their care of spouse or parent is unclear, but the help comes at monetary and opportunity costs and is often accompanied by emotional stress and social disruption. How the need for non-family care to reduce family stress is defined is a political and ethical decision.

We have emphasized that the current use of formal service is a most imprecise indicator of need. Furthermore, we urge that discussions about the risks of entering a nursing home be disentangled from discussions of the need for long-term care. The former is a vital subject in its own right. Research to date has identified only relatively weak and insensitive predictors of the likelihood a person will enter a nursing home. In any event, long-term care can often be given interchangeably by nursing homes or a range of community programs; therefore, the likelihood of entering a nursing home cannot be equated with the likelihood of needing care.

3

The Current State
of Long-Term Care

The present is a major determinant of the future. Supply of services strongly influences service utilization. Present providers, moreover, are active advocates in any discussions about the shape of change. This chapter describes long-term care programs, policies, and financing mechanisms as they presently exist. We include information about the supply of services and the policies that give rise to that supply. When possible, we describe the ownership and structure of long-term care industries in the United States and the variation in programs and policies.

A few caveats are necessary. First, in a field as fluid as long-term care, information about the supply of services is inevitably somewhat outdated by the time the data are published. Second, information based on reimbursement records is easier to gather than general information about the availability of services for purchase. This is particularly true if the vendors are not required to be licensed. Therefore, we can generate information more confidently about nursing homes and certified home health agencies than about board-and-care homes or providers of homemaking, for example. Similarly, we can more easily generate information about the public costs of long-term care than the private costs. Third, long-term care policies are in considerable flux; it is not yet clear what patterns will emerge as a result of new opportunities for flexibility in state Medicaid plans. Fourth, and most important, the availability of community long-term care will respond to payment sources. Many such programs require little capital start-up costs. For example, when Canadian provinces began funding home health care and homemaking services for the functionally impaired, the services rapidly became available even in rural areas (Kane and Kane,

1985). Thus, we must not regard the current configuration of long-term care provision and policy as immutable.

COMPONENTS OF LONG-TERM CARE

Facilities

Nursing homes are the bulwark of current long-term care provision. Attempts to describe the nursing home industry have often been frustrated by rapid change and unwillingness to disclose. Information about the supply of nursing home beds certified by Medicare and Medicaid is public information. The most remarkable feature is the wide variation among states in bed-to-population ratios, and in many other characteristics of the nursing home industry.

Preliminary data from the 1985 National Nursing Home Survey, summarized in Table 3-1, provide the most recent estimates on facility characteristics such as ownership, certification, bed size, and affiliation. The number of nursing homes was estimated at 19,100, a 22% increase since the first survey was done in 1973–74. Most of the growth occurred before the 1977 survey; since then only about 200 homes have been added. This dramatic decline in the growth rate may be attributed to certificate-of-need requirements, moratoria on construction in some states, more stringent standards, and tightened reimbursement policies (the latter perhaps deterring investors). Although state officials are generally alert to the dangers of "overbedding," neither they nor federal authorities have developed guidelines for a desirable supply of nursing home beds in a region. According to a 1983 study (Isaacs and Goldman 1984), state officials widely perceived they needed improved methods for deciding how many nursing home beds to authorize.

Although the rate of increase of homes has declined, the percentage of elderly persons using them at any one time has remained relatively constant at about 5% of the population over 65. The declining growth rate for nursing home beds coupled with the increase in the elderly population has led to an increase in occupancy rates. In 1984, homes operated at 92% of capacity, compared to 85.6% in 1972 (Strahan, 1987).

Table 3-1 indicates that almost 76% of nursing homes were certified as either skilled nursing facilities (SNFs), Intermediate Care Facilities (ICFs), or dually certified. Care in SNFs and ICFs is covered by Medicaid, whereas Medicare coverage is allowed only in SNFs. Although SNFs have stricter regulatory requirements, the differences in the care needs of residents at the two levels of care are notoriously obscure.

According to 1981 Medicare–Medicaid data (Institute of Medicine, 1986), the distribution of SNF and ICF beds shows wide regional variation. In some states this category comprises only 6% or less (Idaho, Massachu-

TABLE 3-1 Selected Nursing Home Characteristics, 1985

Facility Characteristics	Nursing Homes		Nursing Home Beds	
	Number	Percent Distribution	Percent Distribution	Beds per Nursing Home
Total	19,100	100.0	100.0	85.0
Ownership				
Proprietary	14,300	74.9	69.0	78.4
Voluntary Nonprofit	3,800	19.9	22.8	97.6
Government	1,000	5.2	8.1	131.9
Certification				
Certified Facilities	14,400	75.8	88.8	99.4
SNF Only	3,500	18.3	19.0	88.0
SNF/ICF	5,700	29.8	44.6	127.0
ICF Only	5,300	27.7	25.2	77.2
Not Certified	4,700	24.6	11.3	38.9
Bed Size				
Less than 50 Beds	6,300	33.0	9.3	23.9
50–99 Beds	6,200	32.5	27.4	71.7
100–199 Beds	5,400	28.3	43.2	130.0
200 Beds or More	1,200	6.3	20.1	272.3
Census Region				
Northeast	4,400	23.0	22.8	84.4
North Central	5,600	29.3	32.7	94.9
South	6,100	31.9	30.1	80.0
West	3,000	15.7	14.4	78.6
Affiliation				
Chain	7,900	41.4	49.3	101.5
Independent	10,000	52.4	41.9	68.1
Goverment	1,000	5.2	8.1	131.9
Unknown	100	0.5	0.7	116.0

Source: 1985 National Nursing Home Survey. Adapted from National Center for Health Statistics data (Strahan, 1987).

setts, Oregon) whereas in others it is over 90% (Alabama, Arizona, California, Florida, New Mexico, Ohio, Rhode Island). The proportion of ICF only facilities correspondingly varies from zero (Arizona) to 98% (Oregon). These differences less likely reflect real differences in residents' needs for services than they reflect factors such as the state's criteria for appropriate staffing in nursing homes and its approaches to Medicaid funding. If a state's reimbursement rate differs significantly between ICFs and SNFs, for example, there is an incentive to control costs by licensing more ICF beds. In the last analysis, the designation of the levels and the rate at which each is funded are political decisions.

Nursing homes are businesses—often big businesses. In 1985, almost 75% of the homes, containing 69% of the nation's bed supply, were proprietary. The average bed capacity was 85; voluntary nonprofit facilities and government facilities, though fewer, tended to be larger than proprietary homes.

The increase in chain ownership and the consolidation of homes in enormous chains is striking. In 1985, 41% of all facilities were affiliated with chains, an increase from 28% in 1977, and chain-owned homes accounted for about half the nation's bed capacity (Strahan, 1987). The three largest nursing home corporations—Beverly Enterprises, ARA, and Hillhaven—together accounted for 2.2% of the country's beds in 1973, 6.4% in 1980, and by 1983 they owned, leased, or managed close to 10% of the beds. In 1983, Beverly Enterprises alone controlled 90,000 beds. In some regions of the country, concern has arisen because a very large proportion of beds is controlled by just a few firms (Food & Beverage Trades Department, 1983; Hawes and Phillips, 1986). In 1983, 32 corporations controlled 17% of the beds, most of their new ownership having been achieved through the acquisition of existing homes (LaViolette, 1983). Such consolidation produces powerful leverage and can confound client choice and regulatory control.

The wide variations in licensed nurses per nursing home bed and in RN/LPN staffing ratios among states point not only to differences in state regulations and the willingness of nursing homes to invest in staff, but also to the need for more evidence and data before prescribing sophisticated staffing standards (Institute of Medicine, 1986). If standards are to be more than arbitrary, better data are needed to link these rates to patient outcomes.

Home Care

Home health care is the provision of preventive, supportive, rehabilitative, or therapeutic health care in a home setting. Considered more broadly, it also includes supportive social services such as homemaker and choreworker services, homedelivered meals, friendly visits, and telephone reassurance (Levit et al., 1985). A few recent legislative initiatives, such as the Medicaid waivers authorized under Section 2176 in the 1981 Omnibus Budget Reconciliation Act, encourage the broader concept of home care for those who would otherwise be institutionalized. For the most part, however, home care is targeted to the acutely ill on a short-term basis and provided by Medicare-certified home health agencies (HHAs). These agencies must offer skilled nursing and at least two more services from a list of six specified services.

As shown in Table 3-2, there were 4,258 certified HHAs in 1983. However, there are probably more home health agencies. According to the National Home Caring Council, there are somewhere between 6,000 to 8,000

TABLE 3-2 Medicare Certified Home Health Agencies by Ownership Type 1972, 1982, and 1983

Type of Ownership	1972		1982		1983		Percent Change	
	#	%	#	%	#	%	1972 to 1982	1982 to 1983
VNA	531	24.0	517	14.2	520	12.2	−2.6	+0.6
Combination	55	2.5	59	1.6	58	1.4	+7.3	−1.7
Official Health Agency	1,255	56.7	1,211	33.3	1,230	28.9	−3.5	+1.6
Rehab Facility-Based	11	0.5	16	0.4	19	0.4	+45.5	+18.8
Hospital-Based	231	10.4	507	13.9	579	13.6	+119.5	+14.2
SNF-Based	7	0.3	32	0.9	136	3.2	+357.1	+325.0
Proprietary	43	1.9	628	17.3	997	23.4	+1360.5	+58.8
Private Nonprofit	No Listing		632	17.4	674	15.8	—	+6.6
Other	79	3.6	37	1.0	32	0.8	−53.2**	−13.5
TOTALS	2,212	100.0	3,639	100.0	4,258*	100.0	+64.5	+17.0

*Includes 13 unclassified HHAs.
**This decline is due, in part, to the reclassification of private nonprofits into a separate category.
Sources: *Home Health Line*, Vol. IX, February 6, 1984; Callender and LaVor, 1975, both cited in Williams, Gaumer, and Cella (1984), p4.

HHAs in the United States (Williams, Gaumer, and Cella, 1984)—almost a doubling since 1972. Most of the growth, especially within the last few years, has taken place in the proprietary and SNF-based home care, which now represent over 25% of the agencies. On the other hand, Visiting Nurse Associations (VNAs) and official government health agencies have remained relatively stable in number throughout the period. The number and percentage of types of agencies, however, do not necessarily give an accurate picture of market share. Government agencies, for example, constitute almost half of all HHAs but only accounted for 16% of total Medicare visits in 1980. VNAs, on the other hand, tend to be larger than other agencies and provide a proportionately larger number of home visits and services.

The growth has been geographically uneven. Between 1977 and 1981, for example, the number of HHAs decreased in the New England area by 10.5% while the Pacific and South Atlantic regions both experienced an increase of over 35% (Christensen, Mistarz, and Riffer, 1984). The growth patterns are somewhat related to the type of ownership. Hospital-based HHAs appear to have grown primarily in the Mountain and Pacific areas while non-hospital investor-owned growth has occurred primarily in the Mountain, South Atlantic, and West South Central regions. Much of this growth has been due to chain and corporate investment.

Much of this growth appears to be the result of Medicare's recently enacted prospective reimbursement policy, where set rates per hospitalization are tied to diagnostic related groups (DRGs). The policy provides an incentive for hospitals to discharge patients as soon as possible, creating a demand for home care services. Thus, the survey found an increase in services for the acutely ill, such as intravenous therapy and hyperalimentary feeding, rather than in services directed towards the chronically ill.

Williams and her colleagues (1984) provide some information on the service and staffing patterns of HHAs. Table 3-3 shows that, in addition to skilled nursing, the services most likely to be provided by an HHA are home health aides/homemakers, physical therapy, speech therapy, and medical social services. Most of the agencies provide these services themselves, although some services, particularly speech and physical therapy, may be subcontracted. On average, HHAs employ 19.2 full-time-equivalent staff members (1982 data). Eight of these are RNs or LPNs; 4.8 are homemaker/ health aides. Nonprofit agencies such as church-related HHAs or VNAs have the highest staffing levels for all types of employees, whereas government agencies have a lower-than-average number of nurses (7 full-time-equivalents) and the fewest aides (2.6 full-time equivalents).

Adult Day Care

The concept of adult day care originated in Britain, where day hospitals were used to provide medical care to persons with chronic disabilities. As developed in the United States, adult day care centers offer a wide range of

TABLE 3-3 Proportion of Home Health Agencies Providing Various Types of In-Home Services January 1984

Type of Service Offered	% Providing the Service	% Providing Services By:	
		Staff	Arrangement
	(N=4271*)		
Skilled Nursing	100.0	98.6	1.4
Physical Therapy	83.0	52.0	31.0
Occupational Therapy	49.3	28.9	20.4
Speech Therapy	65.4	35.7	29.7
Medical Social Services	52.8	40.4	12.4
Home Health Aide/Homemaker	94.5	84.4	10.1
Interns and Residents	0.8	0.5	0.3
Nutritional Guidance	23.8	17.8	6.0
Pharmaceutical Service	6.4	3.5	2.9
Appliances and Equipment	23.0	11.6	11.4

*Data on services provided were missing for 13 of the 4,284 HHAs operating January 1984.

Source: Health Care Financing Administration, Providers of Service File, unpublished; as cited in Williams, Gaumer, and Cella (1984).

services, varying in emphasis upon programs following medical and/or social models (Huttman, 1985). A generic definition of adult day care is a protective setting offering services on a less than 24 hour per day basis. The services may include physical therapy and other types of rehabilitation, health maintenance programs, assistance with activities of daily living, and social and recreational activities. An adult day center may be in a hospital, a nursing home, a social service agency, or it may be freestanding. The programs have had a slow and uncertain development in the United States and data about their ownership and sponsorship are limited (Padula, 1985).

Mace and Rabins (1984) compiled a list of 980 centers from the mailing list of the National Institute on Adult Day Care (a professional unit of the National Council on the Aging). Their 1983 survey of 353 of these centers as well as a recent nationwide survey of 222 centers (Wallace, n.d.) provide limited information on the clients, services, and staffing characteristics of four adult day care centers.

Adult day care centers are most commonly sponsored by nonprofit human services organizations such as government or non-sectarian programs. Thirty-six percent of the larger list of centers surveyed by Mace and Rabins were under the auspices of human services programs, 20% under nursing homes, and 7.5% under medical centers. Other organizations sponsoring day centers included state psychiatric hospitals, churches, senior centers, and life care communities. About 10% percent of the centers were independent freestanding entities. Proprietary day centers seem rare as yet, perhaps reflecting lack of reimbursement combined with an unenthusiastic buying public.

The Mace and Rabins study found that the 353 centers that they surveyed in detail served an average of 21.7 clients per day; 70% to 80% of the centers operated under capacity. This phenomenon was attributed to the long start-up time required before centers become fully operational, insufficient third-party funding, and the public's failure to recognize adult day care as a resource. The average client/staff ratio was 5 to 1, although centers in which more than half of the clients were demented averaged about 20% more staff. Nurses and social workers were the most commonly reported paid professional staff members and were most often the program directors. Forty-five percent of the centers had both a nurse and social worker on staff; 10% had neither.

In the Wallace survey, the typical day care client was found to be 75.5 years old and attending a center 3 to 3.2 times per week. The three most dominant medical problems of participants were heart disease, diabetes, and Alzheimer's disease. Many clients had accompanying psychological problems, such as depression and loneliness/isolation.

According to the Mace and Rabins study (1984), the services and activities most frequently offered included crafts (97% of centers), current events discussions (94%), family counseling (87%), reminiscence (84%), nursing assessment (81%), physical exercise (78%), nursing care (77%), and ADL rehabilitation (74%). Thirty-six percent of the centers offered psychiatric assessment and medical care, 28% percent offered psychiatric treatment, and 10% offered neurological treatment. Average daily fees charged by the centers were just over $20.

Respite Care

Most services are designed to benefit specific recipients. Respite services have as their primary objective giving temporary relief to those family members who provide care. Incidentally, of course, they may benefit the person receiving the service too. Almost any service can be offered as respite. For example, home care and day care can be provided on a respite basis, and short-term stays in nursing homes may also be arranged.

Respite programs are still in an early phase of development and differ across communities as well as states. No national data on the number and characteristics of such services are available. Two studies, a 1984 survey of 32 selected states (Isaacs and Goldman, 1984) and a 1983 nationwide survey of respite care with only a 36% response rate (Bursac, 1983), give some indication of the state of service in this area.

Bursac found that a third of the 32 responding states had begun to implement respite care services as part of their community-based long-term care programs. The remaining states were in the process of planning or initiating demonstration projects. Although adult day care/day hospital programs were most frequently cited as eligible providers of respite care, a majority indicated that most respite services were being provided in the home. Of the 18 responding states with programs, 15 provided respite care services in the home, 10 provided them in institutional settings, 8 in adult day care centers, and 2 in hospitals. Connecticut, Maine, New York, Florida, Missouri, and Wisconsin appeared to have developed the most comprehensive approaches to establishing respite services on a statewide basis. For example, under its "Community Care for the Elderly Act," Florida allocates funds for respite care. In this program, respite care may be provided for up to 240 hours per client per project year, depending upon individual need. Service may be extended to 360 hours, if recommended by the client's case manager. In 1981 and 1982, 1,581 clients received respite care through this program.

In interviews with representatives of 32 states in early 1984, Isaacs and Goldman (1984) found 10 states where respite programs were underway or about to be initiated. Most of these programs were demonstrations with small budgets. New York, for example, was supporting eight respite care programs, using Medicaid and state funds. Delaware and Illinois were in the process of reserving beds for respite care in nursing homes or community residential facilities. New Jersey provided respite under a Medicaid waiver, but had also developed an additional $200,000 demonstration respite program for those not eligible under the waiver.

Housing

Although not long-term care per se, housing policy has a significant role in long-term care planning. At the least, convenient low-maintenance, specially designed, and/or low-cost housing will influence the kind of long-term care necessary for an individual and the cost of long-term care in a community. Certainly nursing homes provide shelter in addition to whatever services are clustered under their roofs. When housing for the elderly or the impaired includes hotel-like services such as meals in a common dining room or housekeeping, the housing program further encroaches on services provided by nursing homes. In Chapter 6, we discuss evidence about effects of particular housing programs on targeted long-term care populations. Here we simply summarize existing housing programs designed to make it easier for the functionally impaired to dwell in the community.

Housing for the elderly can be thought of as a continuum of resources or programs ranging from those geared toward enhancing the adequacy of independent living (equity conversion, home repair, shared housing) and extending through semi-independent and sheltered arrangements (congregate housing, board and care) to intermediate and skilled nursing facilities (Harmon, 1982). Table 3-4 summarizes the housing supply by the major housing programs.

TABLE 3-4 Housing Programs: Supply Side

Type of Program	Description	Estimated Supply
Low-Rent Public Housing Program	Federally financed public housing units for low-income households are operated by locally establshed, nonprofit public housing administrations. Originally, assistance was in the form of annual debt service contributions with tenant rents (now 30% of net income) used for maintenance. Recently, additional federal assistance has been required for maintenance.	Approximately 650,000 units are occupied by the elderly; more than 1.2 million have been produced (1985 data).
Section 8 of the 1974 Housing and Community Development Act	Created in 1974 to provide subsidized housing to low-income households. Payments made to owners and developers are used to make up the difference between what the renter can afford and HUD's fair market rent determination. In 1983 the Section 8 new construction program was repealed except for Section 8 funds used in conjunction with Section 202. The administration's current emphasis is upon the use of Section 8 vouchers for existing rental housing.	About 800,000 units under the program are occupied by the elderly (1985). 42,000 five-year vouchers were funded in 1985; 39,500 additional vouchers were appropriated in 1986.
Section 202 of the Housing Act of 1959	Originally authorized in 1959 and revised in 1974. Funds are allocated to private, nonprofit sponsors for use in developing Section 8 housing for the low-income elderly and handicapped. Funds are allocated on a geographical basis according to number of elderly households, households lacking plumbing facilities, poverty levels.	Less than 150,000 units are occupied by the elderly. 12,000 202 units were constructed in 1985 and an equal number appropriated in 1986.

Congregate Housing Services	The Congregate Housing Services Act of 1978 set up demonstration programs to provide public housing authorities and 202 sponsors with subsidies to provide nutritional meals and supportive services for clients. Program was set up as a 5-year demonstration program.	At the beginning of 1985, 64 projects were in operation serving over 2,700 elderly persons.
Low-Income Home Emergency Program (Community Services Administration and DHHS) and the Weatherization Assistance Program (Department of Energy)	LIHEAP provides financial assistance to SSI recipients and to states for the provision of supplemental energy allowances to low-income households. DOE provides states with funds to help nonprofit agencies purchase and install weatherization materials.	In 1985, states spent $1.48 billion to heat 6.8 million households (no age-specific data). DOE had weatherized 1.5 million homes by September 1985; about half had a person in the household 60 years or older.
Life Care Communities	Lifetime self-sufficient residential facilities, including medical and nursing services, as well as residential and social services. Admission is typically based on a one-time entrance endowment, plus monthly fees.	About 300 life care communities serve 100,000 residents with an average age of 80 (1981 data).
Home Equity Conversion Plans	There are two types. Reverse Mortgages or Reverse Annuity Mortgages (RAMs) are "debt plans" allowing homeowners to borrow against home equity with no payment until death, sale of the home, or a specified period; sale/leasebacks consist of selling a house and immediately leasing it back from the buyer.	About 100 home equity conversions financed by local organizations were made by the beginning of 1984. Three new programs with plans to provide financing beyond single community or state boundaries were established in 1984: Grannie Mae, American Homestead's Century Plan, the Older American's Consumer Cooperative.

TABLE 3-4 Continued

Type of Program	Description	Estimated Supply
Shared Housing	The housing of at least two unrelated persons in the same facility where common living spaces are shared. It may involve agency-sponsored facilities, or private home-shared situations where contracts are often facilitated by organizations.	Not available.
ECHO Housing (Granny Flats)	"Elder cottage housing opportunity units" that are small, freestanding, and removeable can be placed on the property of adult children or can be used to form cluster units.	Not available.
Home Maintenance Programs	Maintenance programs that generally concentrate on minor repairs and maintenance jobs for elderly/handicapped homeowner households. Most programs are under private nonprofit or city government auspices.	Not available.

Federal Housing. Approximately 1.5 million units assisted under federal housing subsidy programs are occupied by elderly households, although government sources estimate that there are an additional 2 million eligible families not being served (United States Senate Special Committee on Aging, 1986a). Of the subsidy programs, Public Housing and the Section 8 New Construction/Substantial Rehabilitation Program (repealed in 1983) have been the principal new construction programs to benefit the elderly. Over half of the 2.5 million units constructed through these programs are occupied by older Americans. The elderly occupy about 650,000 of the nation's housing units in the Public Housing Program, paying no more than 30% of their net income for rent. Under the Section 8 program (Title II, Section 8 of the Housing Assistance Payment Program, the 1974 Housing and Community Development Act), about 800,000 housing units are occupied by the elderly (United States Senate Special Committee on Aging, 1986b).

The Section 202 program of the Housing Act of 1959 is considered the nation's flagship housing production program, although it represents less than 10% of federally assisted units for the elderly. Section 202 is used by churches, service clubs, and limited-profit groups to obtain below-market interest loans to build housing for the elderly. The 99th Congress appropriated funding for construction of 12,000 units in 1986, about the same number as those built in 1985. The Congregate Housing Services Program (CHSP), authorized in 1978, represents one model for combining Section 202 housing with supportive services (Urban Systems Research, 1976). Through it, HUD awards grants to provide nutritional meals and supportive services for tenants in their housing projects. At the end of 1984, 64 CHSP projects serving about 2,700 elderly persons were in operation (United States Senate Special Committee on Aging, 1986b).

More recently, the Housing Act of 1983 put the emphasis upon existing housing stock rather than new construction. Some officials have advocated the use of vouchers to allow low-income families to choose where they live. Critics are concerned that this approach will not address the country's shortage of decent, low-cost housing and may result in higher rents for low-income people. In 1984, Congress approved less than 20% of the 87,000 vouchers requested by the Administration.

Board and Care. The country abounds in boarding houses and retirement homes, some spartan and some deluxe. Such homes are not certifiable for Medicaid; residents pay for the service themselves. Social service departments may supplement the income of the poor to help finance such accommodations. Often the rates are set at the level of SSI payments. This general board and care category varies from state to state and is known under a number of names, including domiciliary care homes, adult foster care homes, sheltered care facilities, and halfway houses. In general, it refers to the provision, by non-relatives, of food, shelter, and oversight/personal care that is nonmedical in nature. The personal care and oversight responsibilities are determined by state regulations. The service may extend to obtaining medicine and supervising medication, linking residents to community services, and helping with ADL and IADL tasks (Harmon, 1982). Anecdotally it is said that some board and care homes house persons more frail than some nursing homes.

The numbers and types of board and care homes and the characteristics of their residents are difficult to determine. The number of unlicensed homes, for example, is unknown. The development of reliable descriptive data is also hindered by the variety of programs, administrative auspices, and funding sources. A national survey of state regulatory board and care programs (Stone, Newcomer, and Saunders, 1982) identified 142 distinct board and care programs administered by 92 state government agencies.

Reichstein and Bergofsky (1983) identified 30,000 board and care homes in the United States, 5,000 of which were unlicensed. They found these facilities to range in size from 1 to 500 beds, with a median of 14 beds per home. Most of the homes were family owned and operated. An estimated 370,000 persons resided in these facilities; about half of them 65 years or older.

A telephone survey with representatives of state agencies (Stone and Newcomer, 1985) attempted to identify the number and type of licensed board and care beds in 1983. Although data were incomplete from at least five states, the survey identified 382,207 residential care beds, 28,638 foster care beds (beds falling under specially licensed programs), 6,396 apartment beds (freestanding facilities that include units to provide board and care), and 41,272 unclassified beds. Data on the populations served by these beds were also sparse, but 92,343 beds were targeted to a distinct mentally ill population and 289,864 were set aside for a distinct aged population (65+) or a mixed population of aged and nonaged disabled.

Based upon a 1979/1980 nationwide survey of 118 state programs, Mor, Sherwood, and Gutkin (1986) presented a descriptive analysis of residential care homes (RCHs) providing elderly persons with room, board, *and* personal care. They found that medical access and medication supervision were almost universally required by the programs (82%); assistance with ADLs was required by about 60% and help in developing and maintaining relations with community agencies only by 44% From a sample of homes located in five states, the authors found that RCHs regulated by departments of health were structurally different from those under integrated health and welfare auspices regulated by social service departments. The former were more likely to have over 21 beds, be corporately owned, have six or more residents per bath, have heat-sensitive sprinkler systems, have paid staff, and not be occupied by the owner. The integrated homes, operating under the aegis of welfare departments were more akin to small family foster homes and yet tended to house more medically and mentally impaired persons.

Other Housing Programs. In addition to traditional housing programs, there are a number of newer approaches toward housing the elderly aimed at maintaining the elderly in independent living situations. These include life care communities, shared housing, elder cottage housing opportunity (ECHO) units, home maintenance programs, and home equity conversion plans (Day-Lower, Bryant, and Mullaney, 1982; Myers, 1982; Federal Council on the Aging, 1983; Hodges and Goldman, 1983; Reiger and Engel, 1983). National statistics on the majority of these programs are non-existent. Either programs are at an initial stage of development or, as in the case of federally funded programs such as weatherization assistance, reporting requirements have recently been relaxed and many states no longer maintain age-specific data.

Life Care Communities. Life care communities generally involve a lifetime contract between an elderly person and a self-sufficient residential community. In exchange for a usually substantial entrance fee and a monthly fee, the person is guaranteed medical and nursing services, as well as residential and social services. Estimated numbers vary according to the definition of life care facility that is used. In 1981 there were about 300 life care communities in the United States, serving 100,000 residents with an average age of 80 per life care community (United States Senate Special Committee on Aging, 1986b). A later study (Pies, 1984) estimated that there were between 300 and 600 community care retirement communities in the nation. Those oriented principally toward "life care" rather than "nursing care" were mainly located in the southeastern or western United States and typically had more than 200 apartments each. The median entrance fee for a one bedroom unit was $44,475.

Home Equity Conversion Programs. Home equity conversion programs allow elderly home owners to convert part of their home equity into cash without having to leave their homes. Strictly speaking, they are long-term care financing programs rather than housing programs per se, but theoretically the plans offer lifetime use of the home to people who might otherwise need to sell to afford care (Scholen and Chen, 1980). Reverse annuity mortgages (RAMs) are "debt plans" allowing homeowners to borrow against home equity with no payment until death, the sale of the home, or a specified number of years. Sale/leaseback programs involve selling the home to an investor who immediately leases it back to the seller. By early 1984, only about 100 home equity conversion transactions had taken place (Weinrobe, 1984). The San Francisco Development Fund's Reverse Annuity Mortgage Program and Buffalo's Home Equity Living Plan, both started in 1981, have been pioneers in the field. Three new equity conversion programs, which planned to service multi-city and multi-state areas, began in 1984: Grannie Mae (Oakland, CA), the American Homestead Century Plan (New Jersey), and the Older Americans Consumer Cooperative (United States Senate Special Committee on Aging, 1985).

Shared Housing. Shared housing involves at least two unrelated persons in a home where common living spaces are shared. Such housing can be agency-sponsored or may simply involve a private, home-shared situation. Benefits include economic savings, companionship and care for the elderly, and the possible postponement and/or avoidance of institutionalization. Shared housing programs have developed in many major United States cities. Most match elderly householders with other elderly persons, but some, such as Homeshare in Madison, Wisconsin, match younger persons, especially college students, with the elderly. The programs appear to be small. One study, reviewing data from six home-sharing programs, found that the number of individuals "matched" in a given year varied from 87 to 300 persons. The paid staff per program varied between one and three persons (Howe, Robins, and Jaffee, 1984).

ECHO Housing. Often referred to as "granny flats," the name under which they were introduced into the United States from Australia, ECHO is an acronym for "elder cottage housing opportunity" units. Echo housing units are small, freestanding, and removable units that can be located on the property of adult children or used to form community cluster units. Thus far, the development of these units, as well as additions to home structures such as accessory apartments, have been hindered by strict zoning laws and concerns over loss in property values.

Home Maintenance. Home maintenance programs have developed using a number of public and private funds, including Community Development Block Grant Funds, Older Americans Act (Title III) funds, Social Security Act (Title XX) funds, and Department of Energy Weatherization funding. Like home equity conversion programs, they are geared toward helping the poor elderly maintain their independent living with the community. It is estimated that about 65 percent of all elderly poor are homeowners and that three-fourths of all elderly-headed households are owner-occupied (Jacobs and Weissert, 1984). We could not locate age-specific national data on the types and amounts of services that these programs provide to the elderly. One 1982 national study of 190 home maintenance agencies found that 58% of the agencies were private, nonprofit agencies such as Community Action Agencies, and that 27% were administered by county or city government agencies. Most of the programs had fewer than 10 full-time employees, and about 10% had no paid staff at the time of the survey (Ferguson, Holin, and Moss, 1983). Seventy percent of the programs relied on only one source of income, and a majority obtained funding on a tenuous year-to-year basis (Ferguson and Holin, 1983). A two-year study of seven home maintenance programs for the elderly located in six states determined that an average of 600 repairs to homes were made per program per year for 1980 and 1981. Repairs to the interior of the homes (e.g., installation of smoke alarms and grab bars, ceiling and wall repairs) and plumbing repairs were most frequent, followed by door, window, and weatherization repairs.

Senior Centers and Congregate Dining

"Senior center" is a loosely defined concept and therefore presents difficulties when attempts are made to describe the number and characteristics of centers. In the Older Americans Act they are described as multipurpose facilities for the provision of a broad spectrum of health, social, and educational services to the elderly (Estes, 1979). The National Institute of Senior Centers describes them as focal points where older persons can come together for services and activities. Such definitions make it difficult for studies to operationally differentiate between "centers," "clubs," or "groups" (Krout, 1983). The one national study of centers, conducted by the National Council on Aging in 1975, surveyed a broad pool of potential centers and had the respondents classify themselves as "senior centers" or "clubs." Of the 4,870 organizations studied, 51% classified themselves as senior centers (29% of these as multipurpose), and 46% as clubs (Krout, 1983). Estimates done in 1981 place the number of senior centers at over 5,000, with an additional 4,000 senior clubs that meet less than once a week (Huttman, 1985).

A 1975 National Council on Aging study found that senior centers were evenly divided between public agencies and voluntary/nonprofit organizations, and that about one-half of the centers—excluding the 29% that were multipurpose—had no full-time staff. Forty-two percent of the centers provided less than three services; the most common services provided are education, recreation, I&R or counseling services, and, in many cases, additional volunteer opportunities and health services.

The most recent broad-scale survey of senior centers, conducted in late 1982, presents data on a stratified sample of 755 centers from 31 states (Krout, 1983). The data need to be interpreted with caution because the sample does not represent the total senior center population. Still, the survey presents comprehensive information on facilities, organization and budget, staffing, participants, and services. Included in the findings are the following:

- Of the 112 average daily participants at a senior center, half were between the ages of 65 and 74, and only 36% were 75 years or older. The large majority were female, not married, and reported incomes of less than $10,000 a year. Eighty-five percent were white, 20% black, and 9% Hispanic.
- Senior centers offered a mean number of 11 activities and 18 services to their participants. Activities included arts and crafts (87%), trips (82.1%), lectures (75.2%), newsletter (56%), and discussion groups

(59%). Most frequently services offered included: access (I&R, outreach, transportation), health and nutrition (screening, education, group and home-delivered meals), and information and assistance (e.g., consumer information, crime prevention). Eighty-eight percent of the centers offered information and referral; 85% offered group meals; 84% offered transportation; 78% nutritional education; and 76% home-delivered meals. Services and activities least offered included adult day care, programs for the handicapped, income supplement programs, home health, and leadership opportunity training.

- Community size was positively associated with the number of activities and services. Metropolitan and central city centers offered an average of 18.5 services, while non-metropolitan and rural centers averaged 10.8 services.
- One-half of the service centers had no paid or volunteer staff except an administrative head; 60% to 70% had no paid staff for services and activities other than nutrition. Centers had an average of 6.3 full- or part-time paid staff persons, and 27 full- or part-time volunteer staff.

Additional information on senior centers and other supportive services offered through Title III of the Older Americans Act is provided by the yearly Program Performance Reports submitted yearly by State Units on Aging to the Administration on Aging. Reports for 1984 show that there were a total of 7,915 "community focus points" in the United States, including 3,860 multipurpose centers, 3,162 congregate meal sites, and 937 "other" focal points (breakdown exceeds the total due to duplicate counting). Although again reflecting duplicate counting, the reports provide data on the estimated number of persons served by various programs. Estimates for the proportion of minorities served by the various programs range from 17% to 19% (United States Senate Special Committee on Aging, 1986a).

Senior centers and congregate meal programs cannot be construed as long-term care. They serve a clientele that begins at age 60; only about a third of the users are over 75, and few are likely to be functionally impaired. The importance of senior centers to long-term care provision rests in their potential as a focal point for information and referral and support to family caregivers of the frail elderly. If users of senior centers maintain their associations, the average age of members will probably increase and more of the clientele will be at risk for long-term care.

FINANCING LONG-TERM CARE

Public Sector Financing

Table 3-5 lists 1985 costs and 1986 cost estimates of federal outlays benefiting the elderly. Together these are estimated to be a little more than a quarter of all federal expenditures. Social Security for income maintenance

TABLE 3-5 Federal Outlays Benefiting the Elderly[a] (dollars in millions)

Program	1985 actual	1986 estimate
Medicare	60,907	64,417
Medicaid	8,057	8,878
Other federal health	4,573	4,662
Health subtotal	73,537	77,957
Social Security	137,852	146,235
Supplemental Security Income (SSI)	3,649	3,719
Veterans compensation/pensions	5,745	6,113
Other retired, disabled, & survivors benefits	24,634	25,863
Retirement/disability subtotal	171,880	181,930
National Institute on Aging	126	132
Older American volunteer programs	102	106
Senior community service employment	320	323
Administration on Aging	825	836
Subsidized housing	9,166	4,870
Section 202 elderly housing loans	501	490
Farmers Home Administration Housing	55	84
Food stamps	615	612
Social services (Title XX)	369	369
Low-income home energy assistance	642	606
Other miscellaneous	1,185	1,193
Other subtotal	13,906	9,622
Total elderly outlays	259,322	269,505
Percentage of total federal outlays	27	26

[a]Much of the data used to compile this table are based on unsubstantiated estimates and preliminary program and demographic information. Most estimates are for recipients aged 65 and over, include the effects of proposed legislation such as COLA, and include rough estimates of the effect of Gramm-Rudman-Hollings on fiscal year 1986 outlays. Some federal programs (e.g., consumer activities, USDA extension services, national park services) have been excluded due to lack of data. *Source:* United States Senate Special Committee on Aging, 1986b (Volume 3).

is, of course, by far the largest federal expenditure on the old. Medicare (Title XVIII), Medicaid (Title XIV), and social services (Title XX) of the Social Security Act along with Title III of the Older Americans Act comprise the major programs that finance health and long-term care services for the elderly, and together they account for 28% of all federal outlays. Table 3-6 briefly outlines these four programs, including eligibility criteria, benefits, and copayments/deductibles where applicable.

Medicare. Medicare is one of the federal government's most costly domestic programs, second only to Social Security. As shown in Figure 3-1, it is directed toward acute rather than long-term care and specifically

TABLE 3-6 Summary of Major Federal Programs for the Elderly

Program	Services Covered	Eligible Population	Copayments/User Charges
Medicare (Title XVIII of the Social Security Act) Part A - Hospital Insurance	In each benefit period (beginning with admission and ending 60 days after hospital or SNF discharge), 90 days of inpatient hospital care plus 60-day lifetime reserve; 100 days post-hospital SNF care; intermittent skilled home health care; limited hospice services. Hospitals are paid prospectively per admission according to patient's classification into one of 471 diagnosis related groups (DRGs). SNFs and home health agencies are paid per day and visit respectively.	All persons eligible for Social Security, younger persons with permanent disabilities or end-stage renal disease; also voluntary enrollees, 65 and over; most persons over 65 are covered.	The 1986 hospital deductible is $492 plus a daily copayment of $123 for days 61–90; lifetime reserve days 61–90 have a copayment of $246. SNF care has a daily copayment of $61.50 for days 21–100.
Part B - Supplemental Medical Insurance	80% "reasonable and customary charges" for physician services, diagnostic tests, medical devices, outpatient hospital services, and laboratory services.	Those covered under Part A who elect coverage and pay monthly premium of $15.50 (1986). Medicaid pays premium for its recipients.	$15.50 monthly premium, $75 annual deductible and 20% copayment of reasonable or customary charges. In 1985, only 29.8% of physicians were "participating" physicians who accepted Medicare rates as payments in full. Extra charges beyond Medicare rates can be high.

| Medicaid (Title XIX of the Social Security Act) | Mandatory services for categorically needy: Inpatient hospital, outpatient, SNF, limited home health, lab and x-ray, family planning, early and periodic screening, diagnosis and treatment for children through age 20; Optional services (vary from state to state): Dental care, therapies, drugs, intermediate care facilities, extended home care, private duty nurse, eye-glasses, prostheses, personal care services, medical transportation, home health services and homemaking. State can establish limits on the amount, duration, and scope of services. Under section 2176, as of 1982, DHHS can also waive certain Medicaid requirements to broaden coverage for a range of community services to those who could otherwise require nursing home care. | Those who are known as "categorically needy" are automatically eligible: those who qualify for Supplemental Security Income (SSI), state supplementary Payments (SSP), or Aid to Families with Dependent Children (AFDC). States have the option of covering certain needy families with unemployed parents, pregnant women with no eligible children, children under 18 and in school by including them in AFDC or covering them though they may not be eligible for AFDC. They also have the option of including the medically needy: those who do not qualify for public assistance by income but whose medical expenses effectively reduce their available income to categorical levels. | None, once recipient spends down to eligibility. |

TABLE 3-6 Continued

Program	Services Covered	Eligible Population	Copayments/User Charges
Title XX of the Social Security Act	The title authorizes reimbursement to states for social services distributed via the Social Services Block Grant (SSBG). States have freedom to spend funds on state-identified needs, which for the elderly might include day care, substitute care, protective services, counseling, home-based services, employment, education and training, health-related services, information and referral, transportation, respite, legal services, home-delivered and congregate meals. States can choose to pay vendors on fee for services, through contracts, and/or voucher system.	Largely for low-income population. Criteria vary from state to state. SSBG allows states to design their own mix of services and to establish their own eligibility requirements. Previous Title XX requirements regarding allotment of services to categorically poor as well as income eligibility criteria have been eliminated.	Determined by state programs.

Title III of the Older American Act	Three separate federal allocations are made to states for supportive services and senior centers (Title III-B), congregate meals (Title III-C-1), and home-delivered meals (III-C2). Supportive services include transportation, outreach, information and referral, housekeeping, personal care, chore, visiting and telephone reassurance, legal services, residential repair, escort services, health services, physical fitness programs, pre-retirement and second career counseling. State units have authority to transfer amounts of funds among the three allocations.	All persons 60 years and over regardless of income; special emphasis upon targeting low-income, minority, and isolated older persons.	By statute services are free. Voluntary contributions are requested.

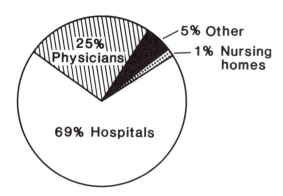

FIGURE 3–1. Where the Medicare dollar for the elderly went: 1984. (Source: United States Senate Special Committee on Aging, 1986a.)

excludes custodial care. In 1985 it expended only $600,000 on nursing home care, in contrast to $48.5 billion and $17.1 billion on hospital care and physicians' care, respectively (Waldo, Levit, and Lazenby, 1986). Currently, home health care is the fastest-growing component of Medicare, with expenditures of about $2.3 billion in 1985. This growth will probably continue, particularly in relationship to the increasing number of shortened hospital stays caused by the new prospective payment system for hospitals. Again, the emphasis of Medicare home health here is on post-hospitalization as a less expensive mode of care than longer hospital stays. To be eligible the patient must require at least one of the following: skilled nursing, physical therapy, or speech therapy; occupational therapy, medical social work, and home health aide services are also available. Eligible patients must be homebound and in need of intermittent (not continuous) care. These rules guarantee that Medicare's home health expenditures will be for acute episodes. Custodial care is explicitly excluded from Medicare coverage.

Medicare beneficiaries seem poorly informed about what the program covers. A widely quoted study commissioned by the American Association of Retired Persons indicated that 80% of respondents thought that Medicare covered nursing homes costs on a much less restricted basis than it actually does. Similarly, Medicare recipients understand very little about Medicare benefits or the benefits under their privately purchased supplementary "medigap" insurance policies (McCall, Rice, and Sangl, 1986). Private planning for long-term care is hampered if those likely to need care assume a false sense of protection. Moreover, concerted political action to change the nature of public policy is also unlikely to arise if citizens are misinformed about existing conditions.

Medicaid. In contrast to Medicare, Medicaid is designed for the poor; therefore, the elderly must deplete their savings and become poor before being eligible for benefits. The shape of Medicaid expenditures for the elderly is largely the product of the gaps left by the restrictiveness of Medicare. Thus, Medicaid for the elderly has been largely a long-term care support program. The Medicaid program spent $14.7 billion on nursing home care for the elderly in 1985 (Waldo, Levit, and Lazenby, 1986). (See Figure 3-2.) Expenditures on home health care—although potentially expandable to broader coverage in areas such as personal care—are less than a third of Medicare costs, $597 million in 1983. In 1982, the most recent year for which data are available, home health benefits accounted for more than 1% of total Medicaid expenditures in only nine states. New York spent 78% of all Medicaid home health dollars (Williams, Gaumer, and Cella, 1984). Established in 1966 by Title XIX of the Social Security Act, the program is administered by the states, with matching funds from 50% to 78% provided by the federal government. Although all participating states must offer certain mandatory services, they have flexibility in determining eligibility, choosing optional services, and establishing limits on the amount, duration, and scope of services.

Title XX Funds. Title XX of the Social Security Act authorizes funds for support services to the elderly through the Social Service Block Grant (SSBG). Changes in the original Title XX legislation of 1975, enacted as part of the Omnibus Budget Reconciliation Act in 1981, have eliminated most restrictions, allowing states to determine their own services, target groups, and eligibility criteria. Since federal reporting regulations have also been eliminated, it is difficult to determine what proportion of the Title XX budget, in 1985 frozen at $2.7 billion per year, is being spent on services for the elderly (General Accounting Office, 1984). The National Data Base on Aging reported that the SSBG in 1982 comprised about 6.3% of State Units on Aging budgets and 4% of Area Agency on Aging budgets (United States Senate Special Committee on Aging, 1985).

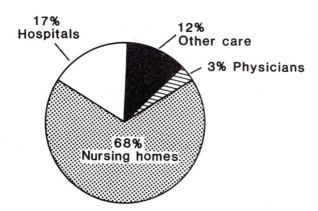

FIGURE 3-2. Where the Medicaid dollar for the elderly went: 1984. (Source: United States Senate Special Committee on Aging, 1986a.)

Title III Funds. Title III of the Older Americans Act also provides allocations for community services to the elderly. Title III's contributions are relatively modest: a total of $669 million in 1985. Fifty percent of the funds were for congregate nutrition services, and $68 million were for home-delivered meals. $265 million were for senior centers and for supportive services, including access, in-home, and community services. About 654,000 elderly persons, for example, received Title III homemaker services in 1985.

VA Funds. The Veterans Administration provides a number of important services for the elderly, in addition to the programs described above. Of the approximately three million veterans who used VA facilities in 1983, 14% were 65 years or older: They had an overall utilization rate three-to-four times that of younger veterans (Veterans Administration, 1984). The age distribution of veterans as the result of the wars means that the VA will be facing a more severe growth in the elderly than will the civilian population. In 1985 the VA spent $8.7 billion to finance health services for veterans (Waldo, Levit, and Lazenby, 1986), including the operation of 172 hospitals, 99 nursing homes, and 16 domicilaries (Mather, 1984); $.7 billion was spent on nursing home care, including care in VA facilities or purchased care in community homes. Recently the VA has begun to develop noninstitutional extended care programs. These include the financing of 30 hospital-based home care teams that served 7,423 patients in 1983, 12 respite care programs, and five Adult Day Health Care programs. The Veterans Administration has also established a network of inpatient and outpatient Geriatric Assessment Units.

Private Financing

Despite the large federal and state expenditures on health and long-term care for the elderly, the elderly and their families pay for a large proportion of the costs (Moon, 1983). Direct out-of-pocket costs for care averaged 15% of the elderly's income in 1984, the same proportion as before Medicaid and Medicare were enacted in 1965. According to the Health Care Financing Administration, direct out-of-pocket health care expenses for the elderly averaged $1,059 per person in 1984, excluding premium payments for Medicare Part B and private insurance (United States Senate Special Committee on Aging, 1986a). In that year, the elderly spent 42% of this sum on nursing homes, 21% on physicians, 6% on hospitals, and 31% on other care (Figure 3-3). Of the $32 billion expended on nursing home care, for example, $15.8 billion consisted of direct out-of-pocket payments (Levit et al., 1985).

Recorded out-of-pocket payments for home care appear small but are likely to be under-represented. The 1982 National Long-Term Care Survey

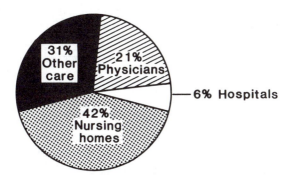

FIGURE 3–3. Where the out-of-pocket dollar for the elderly went: 1984. (Source: United States Senate Special Committee on Aging, 1986a.)

estimated that of the 4.7 million noninstitutionalized disabled Americans, 70% of these relied solely on unpaid sources of support—that is, the volunteered labor of families and friends. Those who were paying for home health care had costs ranging from only $360 to $1,680 per year (United States Senate Special Committee on Aging, 1986b). However, the private costs of home care are difficult to determine. Much of the expense in the form of cleaning services, yard work, convenience food, home improvements, and equipment probably does not get counted. One study of 2,500 frail elderly participants in a long-term care demonstration showed that 75% of all non-spouse primary caregivers provided some financial assistance. Purchase of clothing was most frequently mentioned, followed by help with medical bills, housing costs, and miscellaneous living expenses. The average expenditure rose from $84 a month when those giving no financial help were included to $190 per month among those providing some financial help. Almost half of the caregivers providing some financial help spent one-tenth or more of their income this way, and about 25% used one-fifth of their income in financial assistance to the person receiving care (Stephens and Christianson, 1984).

Private insurance covers only about 1% of the nation's long-term care costs. Although the majority of elderly Americans have supplemental medical insurance, these policies generally allow only for "medigap" coverage; i.e, they cover Medicare copayments and deductibles, but provide only the limited coverage for skilled care as defined by Medicare (United States Senate Special Committee on Aging, 1986b). Meiners (1984) found examples of 16 different insurance companies that cover long-term insurance in a more comprehensive manner than standard "medigap" policies.

According to Meiners, a major problem in the development of long-term care insurance benefits has been the lack of distinction between levels of care. Insurers have attempted to overcome this problem through policies such as limiting coverage to state-licensed SNF or ICF facilities or making benefits contingent upon prior hospitalization or SNF stay. Most policies were found to be indemnity policies that paid a specific sum for a specified number of service days. Few insurers were willing to guarantee policy renewal without escape clauses, and insurers reserved the right to raise premiums.

Waivers

Section 2176 of the 1981 Omnibus Budget Reconciliation Act permitted the Department of Health and Human Services to waive certain Medicaid requirements in order to allow states to finance a broad range of community-based long-term care services. The intent of the legislation is to allow states relative freedom in developing cost-effective systems as alternatives to nursing homes. Thus, the services are only for low income persons who would otherwise require ICF or SNF placement. The federal statute specifies seven services under the waiver: case management, homemaker, home health aide, personal care, adult day health, habilitation, and respite care. Other services can be approved by DHHS. In applying for a 2176 waiver, states must provide evidence that average per capita Medicaid expenditures under the waiver will not exceed average per capita expenditures if the waiver were not granted.

Greenberg, Schmitz, and Lakin (1983) studied all waivers that had been approved prior to February 15, 1983 (at that time 26 states had waivers approved). About three-quarters of the applicants had targeted their programs to serve the aged and the physically disabled; the others targeted the developmentally disabled or mentally ill. States generally took an experimental approach to their programs, all but two of the 26 states choosing not to offer them statewide. Some of the most common services offered were case management (24 states), homemaker services (16), respite care (17), and personal care (11). In their waiver proposals states projected aggregate annual savings of approximately $250 million. As of mid-June 1986, 47 states had filed requests for 188 waivers since the program began. Of the 40 states with waivers at that time, 35 programs covered the mentally retarded, 41 were for aged and disabled persons, and 3 were targeted to the mentally ill (Fackelmann, 1986).

CONCLUSIONS

As this chapter has shown, the number and type of long-term care programs in institutions and the community vary widely throughout the country. The institutional predominance in long-term care covered by public funds is dramatic, and, accordingly, community programs are dwarfed by institutional programs. Information about patterns of service is imprecise and inaccurate in both sectors, especially when programs are reimbursed by neither Medicare nor Medicaid. Even when public funding is present, however, information is less than perfect. We have been able to present only patchy information about key areas such as board and care homes, adult day care, and home health provision that is outside the orbit of Medicare. For-profit industry dominates both the nursing home and the board and care fields, and is rapidly growing in home care.

Financing of long-term care is about an even public-private partnership. The public portion is highly visible and political, and the private portion is largely invisible, hard to document, and taken directly out of the pockets of users. Medicaid—the health care program for the poor—finances most of the public share of nursing home costs and demands impoverishment of the persons it helps. Home care—which is widely considered the basic service in any long-term care system—gets much of its character from Medicare requirements designed for post-acute convalescence and rehabilitation. Socially oriented home care and homemaking are often provided by agencies whose staffing and procedures were developed to satisfy Medicare. Generally speaking, services have been shaped to meet the expectations of the dominant public funding mechanisms, with recently increased attention to what a private market is likely to find attractive. Despite the tilt of the current system toward institutions, community services have few capital costs and can be instituted relatively quickly once a payment source is available.

The suppliers of long-term care constitute an important and vocal constituency, which will be involved in any effort to change either the regulation of or financing of care. Moreover, without clearly established evidence about the effects of various programs on specific clientele, no clear basis exists to argue that one service is better than another. For example, it is difficult to say that nursing homes should be staffed a certain way, develop specific programs, or offer a particular kind of environment because there is little consensus about the efficacy of one program over another. Similarly, although home health agencies, as presently organized, seem overly medicalized and rigid, it is difficult to assert the outlines of a model program that would combine flexibility with competence. The wide variation from state to state reflects this inability to establish meaningful goals or standards, which in turn makes programs politically more vulnerable. This book was motivated by a desire to address that problem by sorting and arranging evidence about "good" programs, a task undertaken in Part II.

Interchangeability is also a hallmark of long-term care. A given client can feasibly be served at home, in a congregate housing complex with additional in-house services, or in a facility of some type. Moreover, community services can be combined in various ways—for example, home care, day care, and delivered meals can be mixed and matched. Theoretically, even facilities can mix the services they provide directly with those brought in from other service providers. Again, reconfiguration of services should be based on a sound rationale and evidence about the likely effects.

Given the high and soaring costs of long-term care, the arena has become a political mine field. Many proposals have been made to reduce public expenditures. One federal response has been to offer states more flexibility in exchange for fiscal responsibility. Another approach is to explore a similar tradeoff to provider consortia by creating capitated schemes that give the organization flexibility in exchange for financial risks. And a popular fall-back is the prevalent idea that citizens themselves could and should save more through their lifespan for long-term care, with the concomitant examination of insurance and other mechanisms that might infuse more private money and, one hopes, offer more private choice.

4

Long-Term Care Issues:
Quality, Access, and Cost

To conclude this introductory section, we now turn from statistics to issues. How can we create policies to promote humane and effective long-term care? What are the obstacles to such a desirable state? Is long-term care an intractable problem of uncontrollable public and private expenses and uneven quality, as it is sometimes presented in the media?

The problem is both less and more than it first appears. We may be exaggerating the difficulties of developing an affordable yet humane long-term care policy that will meet the needs of the increasing numbers of expected users in the next decade. Other, less wealthy countries have come closer to the mark; surely the United States can do as well. Adopting a desperate stance is counterproductive—it encourages satisfaction with holding operations, rather than a search for a desirable policy direction.

Yet, we should not minimize the qualitative problems and the high personal costs to United States citizens of the present system. The long-term care problem in the United States is not simply how our society can afford to care for all dependent people from available public and private dollars. The problem is how to develop an acceptable system with less physical, financial, emotional, and social toll on citizens when they or someone in their family needs care.

Long-term care presents problems of quality, access, and cost. Service should be of acceptable quality, however defined; those who need the services should have reasonable access without financial or other barriers; and the cost should be affordable by individuals and society. If quality is adequate and access is also adequate and equitable, it remains only to work toward greater efficiency without sacrificing the first two values. The practical issue is much more perplexing, however, if there is a simultaneous need to improve quality and access (perhaps by major reconfiguration of the services available) and to control accelerating costs. Working on both fronts at once is difficult, and the goals of proposed reform easily become murky. In some states, public policies have evolved to maintain the quality of long-term care, control the cost, or both. For example, suggestions for modifying financing or reimbursement policies in long-term care abound, but often it is unclear whether a given approach is designed to control overall costs, shift the burden of those costs, or change the quality of the service. The way we identify the problems significantly influences the kinds of solutions that are proposed and supported.

This chapter briefly discusses quality, access, and cost in long-term care, identifies mechanisms now in place to deal with the issues, and mentions strategies under consideration. (Demonstration projects designed to effect quality, access, or cost are reserved for discussion in Chapter 10.) We conclude by discussing unresolved issues in long-term care according to a conceptual framework that considers community and facility care as part of a coherent system. In our formulations, we give strong consideration to the preferences of the people long-term care programs serve and the consequences for their well-being.

QUALITY ISSUES

A service of acceptable quality must meet or exceed specified and agreed-upon minimum criteria. Acceptable quality also implies that the service is an appropriate approach to address the particular problem. For example, it would be pointless to applaud a surgical procedure for its technical characteristics if the wrong operation had been done. Therefore, in examining the quality of long-term care received by any individual, either in a nursing home or a community-based program, we need to consider whether the services are appropriate to the needs and preferences of the users and whether each service is of acceptable quality.

But minimum adequacy and appropriateness are difficult concepts. Who defines them? Do we rely on the judgments of professionals with vested interests? Whose values dictate the definition of success? What outcomes should long-term care providers be expected to emphasize? And do we have the data to know what does and does not work to enhance the desired outcomes?

In Chapter 2, we noted that older persons overwhelmingly prefer to receive care at home rather than in nursing homes as they know them or imagine them. If persons are inappropriately shunted to nursing homes because other care is difficult to arrange, a qualitative problem exists. As we also suggested in Chapter 3, some long-term care programs seem to be interchangeable. Where complete interchangeability of effectiveness and cost is possible, the choice should surely be up to the user. If various service packages can achieve the same results but at markedly different costs, public programs surely have some right to refuse to pay for the full cost of the more expensive option. Then the challenge becomes one of defining the acceptable minimum public benefit and developing fair ways by which persons can use private money to enhance their preferences.

Quality assurance has three sequential steps: defining quality, assessing programs to identify areas in which quality is deficient, and correcting any identified deficiencies. Without the correction step, the whole procedure is somewhat futile. Unfortunately, quality in long-term care has been inadequately defined (i.e., too much emphasis on structure, credentials, and written policies and too little on the quality of life of residents). Quality has also been inaccurately assessed. Surveys have been unreliable, and their validity is in question both because facilities are forewarned and because the residents themselves are not the usual source of data.

Despite these inadequacies of definition and assessment, clearcut problems have been identified. Few are satisfied that such problems can be expeditiously or permanently corrected under present policies. Poorly corrected problems include misuse of therapeutic drugs; inadequate diagnosis of acute illnesses and medical care for them; inadequate nursing care, resulting in the development of bedsores; misuse of physical restraints; insufficient rehabilitation programs such as activation, bowel and bladder training, and mental health services; insufficient social activities; poor food; and violations of civil rights (Kane et al., 1979a, 1979b).

Because nursing home care has been the dominant form of publicly financed long-term care, efforts to define and maintain quality have largely centered on care given to nursing home residents. Governments use a variety of mechanisms available to uphold quality:

- Licensing of facilities, which is the responsibility of each state. Licensing requirements vary from state to state. Most require minimum staffing levels, set educational requirements for the administrators, and require that the physical plant comply with safety and fire codes.
- Certification of the facility to receive payment from the Medicare and/or Medicaid program. State certification agencies (usually located in the department of health) perform annual inspections to ensure that facilities have met the federal standards for skilled nursing facilities and intermediate care facilities, as well as any additional standards the state may have developed. Federal inspectors have oversight responsibility to check the adequacy of this inspection process through "look-behind" inspections for a sample of facilities.
- Inspection of care. By federal law, the government must ensure that care reimbursed by Medicaid is both medically appropriate and of acceptable quality. The states fulfill this duty by annual review of each

Medicaid-funded resident's care. Fiscal intermediaries for Medicare undertake similar reviews for a sample of beneficiaries.
- Ombudsman program. Under the Older Americans Act, each State Unit on Aging funds a nursing home ombudsman program that has a responsibility to receive complaints, advocate for nursing home residents, and serve as mediator between residents and facilities.
- Regulation of personnel. States may require that nursing home personnel (such as administrators or nursing assistants) be licensed or certified and, thus, meet specified standards of preparation or performance.

Current certification standards are geared toward ensuring that facilities have the capacity to provide adequate care rather than ensuring that they in fact *do* provide good care. They require that the building itself meet safety specifications, that procedures be established for infection control, that facilities employ staff or consultants with certain formal credentials, that medical records meet certain requirements, and so on. Even standards applying specifically to professional personnel such as nurses, medical directors, rehabilitation specialists, dietitians, social workers, and activity directors largely establish the minimum expectations for training and duties rather than the expected outcome of their performance. Furthermore, standards are heavily weighted toward the residents' *physical* well-being. The survey process has tended to rely heavily on information gathered from records and staff, rarely on observing and interviewing residents. (In 1986, the Health Care Financing Administration (HCFA) modified the Medicare certification process, introducing a new Patient Care and Services (PaCS) instrument that gathers information directly from a sample of residents during surveys. This new system seems an important step in the right direction.)

Finally, and most disturbing, identified problems in care tend to be unresolved or recurrent. Presently, states have only draconian options to resolve problems. Closing facilities or withholding reimbursement are dramatic efforts that disrupt residents and, when bed supply is scarce, create a practical problem of relocation. More intermediate sanctions (such as fines or admission "holds") would help resolve deficiencies in care. In addition, personnel who violate standards willfully should be subject to revocation of license and even prosecution. As it now stands, such personnel may be fired from one facility only to show up in another.

Several descriptive studies of quality assurance underscore the problems with the current mechanisms. In a survey of 20 states, Polich (1983) found that only two had attempted to measure outcomes as an indication of quality. Studying the certification agencies in 47 states, the Institute of Medicine (1986) found that resources for inspection and follow-up activities were meager. The median sum allocated for regulatory activities was

$4,700 per nursing home, and the median number of nursing homes per field surveyor was 13 (with a range of less than one to 42). In half the states the survey department budget had increased between 1980 and 1984, and in half it had decreased. Most states combined the licensing and certification inspections and conducted them on an annual basis. Most states had intermediate sanctions available, but few used them with any regularity. Besides the universal authority to remove a facility's license, decertify the facility, and impose criminal penalties for patient abuse, 36 states had authority to remove residents, 32 to suspend admissions, and 26 to impose fines. Most of the actions in each category were concentrated in just a few states.

The ombudsman program has the potential to be a major force in quality assurance. Established under the Older Americans Act, it provides for a community presence in nursing homes to mediate between facility and residents on disputed matters and to advocate for residents (Buford, 1984). To date, however, its role has been ambiguous and variously interpreted from state to state. The skill and staffing levels around the country have been uneven. In 1985, all told, there were only about 1,000 paid staff and 5,000 volunteers in ombudsman programs. Typically, nursing home ombudsmen have had little authority, sometimes not even enjoying clear access to facilities and/or records, and some programs have interpreted the role as a cross between mediator and personal service volunteer rather than as advocate (Monk, Kaye, and Litwin, 1984).

While advocates complain about toothless regulation, the industry complains about excessive regulation that devours staff time and arbitrarily interferes with a homelike environment and creative programming. HCFA responded with demonstration projects to test the effects of more streamlined inspections and regulatory relief for facilities with a good history (Zimmerman et al., 1984).

The Institute of Medicine's thorough review of nursing home regulations (1986) also considered the influences of reimbursement and bed supply on quality. Although an adequate reimbursement rate seems a logical prerequisite to quality, the Committee noted that a wide range of state reimbursement rates now prevails and quality variation can be detected in nursing homes within states with the lowest and the highest rates for Medicaid reimbursement. Therefore the Committee concluded that adequate reimbursement alone was insufficient to assure an adequate quality of care. Apropos of the supply of nursing home beds, the Committee noted that most states have moved to constrict the growth of beds. This in turn gives consumers little possibility to reject facilities giving poor care. But many policy analysts believe that an ordinary competitive market cannot exist for nursing homes even if an oversupply of beds exist. Therefore, the marketplace is unlikely to assure the quality of care, even if the supply of beds were not restrained.

Thus, the Institute of Medicine's report endorsed a strong federal regulatory presence in nursing homes. It recommends consolidation of SNF and ICF criteria into a single set of standards, and revision of all standards to focus more on outcomes, quality of life, and civil rights. The Committee advocated a survey process that gathers information directly from residents, has an element of surprise, and uses streamlined annual inspections with an opportunity for in-depth follow-up when necessary. The report also contained many recommendations to strengthen the enforcement and correction aspect of quality assurance and to enhance the ombudsman program.

A number of quality issues remain:

- Regulations should be directed toward assuring that desirable and appropriate outcomes are achieved, leaving providers freer to be creative in their approach but still holding them accountable.
- To define quality adequately in facilities, tradeoffs must be made among desirable outcomes—for example, physical well-being, pain control, improvement of functioning, psychological well-being, safety, and social activities. It is unclear who should make those choices (the residents, the staff, the regulators, the payors). Perhaps it is possible to establish specific goals as desired by particular residents, or to develop facilities with differing emphases from which potential residents select.
- Facilities house an extremely heterogeneous group of residents. In particular, some residents are severely or moderately cognitively impaired. It is unlikely that quality of life can be assured for both the confused and the mentally intact in the same programs.
- Quality assurance has barely been explored for home care and other community long-term care programs. Given the difficulty in guaranteeing adequate care in facilities, the prospect for affording protections in the private settings of dispersed personal homes is daunting, especially when some of the clientele will be vulnerable and unable to report poor care or exploitation.
- Long-term care in facilities and at home depends on a cadre of personnel who tend to be ill trained and paid the minimum wage. Upgrading the quality of care without upgrading the skills and the salary of nursing assistants and homemaker/home health aides seems problematic, yet some argue the cost of any real change would be prohibitive.
- Once a true consensus on the expectations for a long-term care program of adequate quality is reached, the challenge remains to examine the incentives affecting the providers. Incentives should be present that drive the system to that goal, and, at the least, no perverse incentives that encourage negative results should be permitted. Because so much of long-term care is a proprietary industry, the payment system is a

candidate for positive incentives and should be examined for lurking disincentives to quality. Incentives are particularly desirable if they encourage providers to strive toward excellence rather than merely to meet minimum standards of acceptability.

ACCESS ISSUES

Long-term care is often branded as fragmented and uncoordinated. In the face of a confusing array of financial entitlements, many people remain without much financial coverage. At the time decisions are made about whether to enter a nursing home and which one, the potential resident and his or her family are usually in great stress. If in a hospital, they often have to make their decision in a matter of days or hours, and realistically they seldom have much choice of facility. Typically only a few beds are available.

Furthermore, facilities also make choices. Especially when paid a fixed daily rate for a class of patients (i.e., payment based on eligibility for skilled nursing care versus intermediate care or payment based on a more elaborate case-mix designation such as discussed in Chapter 8), facilities prefer to avoid residents needing heavy care, exhibiting a "behavior problem," having pre-existing bedsores, or financed by Medicaid. Because Medicaid regulations prohibit paying more than private rates, facilities typically charge private-paying patients more than Medicaid patients. (Only one state— Minnesota—has made it illegal for a facility to charge private patients more than Medicaid patients; those facilities charging higher rates than the state allows must opt out of the Medicaid program entirely.) A demonstration project that offered monetary incentives for accepting heavy care patients to participating facilities in San Diego, California, produced moderate changes in admission patterns. Nonetheless, a number of state Medicaid programs are moving to case-mix reimbursement as a means of encouraging heavier care admissions (Meiners et al., 1984). Blacks and other minority groups also tend to be under-represented in nursing homes, but it is uncertain whether this is due to discrimination, strong family attachments in minority communities, or both.

Consumers have great difficulty gathering information about community long-term care programs. Information and referral programs themselves tend to be poorly informed about long-term care. Even those who can afford to purchase care have poor access to information, partly because they may be too ill to make the search, partly because the subject is inherently confusing, and partly because the advertising that appears in the media is bewildering. Physicians tend to be able to provide little information, yet it is the physician who legally sets in motion requests for nursing home care or home care if it is to be financed by a public program.

Two strategies to improve access to long-term care for those who have genuine functional impairment, and to tailor the long-term care program to individual needs, are preadmission screening and case management. Both are popular strategies at present, and both are expected to contain costs as well as improve access.

Preadmission Screening

Preadmission screening services assess the appropriateness of nursing home placement prior to admission. Going beyond the determination of financial eligibility for a Medicaid-financed admission, they often entail a multi-dimensional assessment and an effort to help persons plan for their care. A nationwide study done in late 1985 found 31 preadmission screening programs operating in 29 states (Iverson, 1986); 68% operating on a statewide basis, and 32% affecting a region in a state. Ten of the programs screened only persons eligible for Medicaid, while six also screened persons who would become eligible quickly after paying for some months of nursing home care (typically, three months or six months); 15 states had programs in which all applicants to nursing homes may or must be screened regardless of their income or resources. In only three states was screening mandatory for persons entering nursing homes as private-paying residents. The cost of screening ranged from $28 to $148, perhaps reflecting the scope of services and the variety of financial arrangements. Two-thirds of the programs reported that they provided some form of case management or coordination of services in conjunction with the screening, including personal care, home health, homemaking, transportation, and nursing home placement. No information was available about the financial eligibility for the additional services.

In Chapter 10, we will discuss some of the preadmission screening programs that have been evaluated. One of the general issues to be raised here, however, is the extent of the real authority of any preadmission screening program to prevent persons from entering nursing homes with their own funds. Lacking the right to forbid those with less need to enter a nursing home and spend down to Medicaid levels, programs necessarily rely on their ability to assist people to piece together more desirable services in the community.

Case Management

Case management involves creating service packages to meet an individual person's need and allocating resources across a community or catchment area. The concept became well known in the 1970s in conjunction with 222 (Medicare) and 1115 (Medicaid) waiver demonstration projects. Such projects waived ordinary rules of eligibility or coverage to offer a package of community services at home in an effort to prevent unnecessary nursing home admissions. Projects with catchy titles such as ACCESS in Monroe County, New York, TRIAGE in Connecticut, Community Care Organization (CCO) in Wisconsin, and Alternative Health Services in Georgia all used forms of case management to coordinate the new benefits. Case management was also introduced in pioneering state programs where persons were eligible for homemaking and other socially oriented long-term care benefits financed from a pool of Title XX, Older Americans Act, and state funds. Massachusetts and Pennsylvania are notable for having instituted these programs, both under the direct administration of the Area Agencies on Aging in the state. Case management was at the heart of the largest social experiment in long-term care, the National Channeling Demonstration, begun in 1980. Funded jointly by HCFA and the Administration on Aging and administered from the office of HHS's Assistant Secretary for Planning and Evaluation, the channeling demonstration tested two variations of case management: a basic model consisting of case management with minimal ability to purchase extra services and a complex model that allowed case managers to purchase services for clients according to assessed needs and care plans but within budgetary restraints. Each model was implemented in five communities, involving ten cities and ten states. The lessons learned from long-term care demonstrations, including channeling, are discussed in considerable detail in Chapter 10.

As already indicated, the 1981 Omnibus Budget Reconciliation Act permitted states to apply for waivers to offer a range of community services for persons who would be eligible for nursing home care. Case management was one of the services listed under this provision and is a component of almost all the waivers that have been granted. In the law, case management was defined merely as "the coordination of a specified group of services for a specified group of individuals," and its component parts were further explained as casefinding or screening, comprehensive assessment, care planning, implementation, monitoring, and reassessment.

Case management is now being offered by many organizations (home health agencies, family service agencies, hospitals, Area Agencies on Aging, health maintenance organizations, and even privately practicing case managers). When case management is organized by the state (typically in conjunction with a preadmission screening program and a group of waivered community services), the state may designate a particular public or voluntary agency to do the case management or may farm it out to many agencies. In the confusion that has resulted, many questions beg a clearer answer:

- How can the advocacy function (making the best possible plan for the client) and the gatekeeping function (using the community's resources well) be combined? Are these roles inherently contradictory?

- Is case management useful without additional services or without additional money to pay for services? The answer to this question depends on whether the major problems of long-term care are getting information about services, finding enough services in the community, or paying for them.
- Can case management appropriately be done by organizations that also provide service? Does this introduce a conflict of interest?
- To what extent should case managers build expectations of family care into a plan?
- To what extent should case managers use the client's preferences as the basis for a plan?

COST ISSUES

The high cost of long-term care and the demographic projections forecasting even more future users are dominant themes for most policy-makers. In seeking a long-range solution for containing the cost of long-term care, two issues should be distinguished: financing, or the way money is raised, and reimbursement, or the way and amounts providers are paid. The solutions so far advanced often merge these two issues.

Because nursing home costs are the lion's share of expenditures, efforts have been concentrated on reducing this sector by various financing and reimbursement strategies, including limiting the supply of nursing home beds, changing the way nursing homes are paid, substituting less expensive community care for more expensive care in facilities, and/or putting providers at financial risk through capitated systems. Other popular cost-cutting strategies are deceptive because they concentrate on reducing public costs, without necessarily addressing overall costs. These include: stimulating long-term care insurance plans, encouraging private savings for long-term care, and developing inducements for even more family care to postpone nursing home use.

LIMITING SUPPLY

By 1980, all but three states had enacted certificate of need (CON) laws for nursing home expansion. These were aimed both at a rational distribution of resources and control of expenditures (Feder and Scanlon, 1980). As of July 1985, four states had extended or initiated moratoria on the building of new beds (United States Senate Special Committee on Aging, 1986b). A 1984 survey of long-term care initiatives in 32 states found that a number of CON agencies were tying the control of bed supply to payment mechanisms. For example, Florida and New Jersey had developed exemptions for private-paying life care communities (Isaacs and Goldman, 1984). Although limits on growth of nursing home beds will encourage the development of community programs, the resultant bed shortage reduces any genuine competition with homes of poor quality going out of business and discourages admitting heavy care patients. CON requirements for nursing homes are a financial mechanism designed to curb Medicaid costs, not a quality control mechanism. Unfortunately, no clear formulas exist for the correct bed-to-population ratio. Indeed the ideal figure may change as a result of policies in the acute care or mental health sectors.

CHANGING NURSING HOME REIMBURSEMENT

As Chapter 3 indicated, the SNF-to-ICF ratios and the Medicaid reimbursement rates for nursing homes vary widely. In the last decade, many states have moved from flat per diems for SNFs and ICFs to some form of prospective payment based on previous experience. In addition, as of 1985, seven states had begun paying nursing homes according to a case-mix formula. Usually only the component of the rate attributable to nursing service is adjusted by the characteristics of the resident, and such adjustments are usually based on studies of the number of nursing minutes required to care for types of residents (Schlenker, 1986). Case-mix systems are designed to address access issues and to make payments more equitable—theoretically, facilities should not lose money by accepting more difficult patients. Minnesota's case-mix system provides an additional incentive for economies in other areas that make up the rate; if a facility spends less than allowed for specified administrative and general services (excluding resident care and food), they keep a portion of the savings. On the whole, however, case-mix systems, including Minnesota's, contain perverse incentives regarding resident outcomes. If a resident becomes more mobile, needs fewer nursing procedures, and constitutes less of a behavior problem, the facility is paid less. Thus, it is in the financial interest of the facility to prevent the resident's functional improvement. Kane et al. (1983b) have advocated a contrasting payment system that links payment and quality by rewarding facilities for producing desirable resident outcomes over and above what might have been expected for the particular resident. Further discussion of these issues is found in Chapter 8.

The early 1980s saw the implementation of a prospective case-mix-adjusted reimbursement system for hospital care under Medicare. Instead of receiving their "reasonable" costs, hospitals are now paid a fixed rate according to which of 471 diagnosis related groups (DRGs) describes the patient. This system encourages hospitals to discharge quickly and to give less intensive or comprehensive services to its inpatients. The DRG approach is diametrically opposed to the principles of geriatric care of the frail elderly. Just when a multiproblem approach is needed, the system forces arbitrary focus. It has been suggested but not proven that DRGs have led to sicker persons entering nursing homes, sometimes for planned recuperation and rehabilitation. Thus, efforts to get nursing home costs under control may be hampered by events in the acute sector.

Home health agencies are paid by the visit or the hour (depending on the type of personnel making the visit), with retrospective audits of the appropriateness of care. According to a GAO study of randomly selected case records in 37 home health agencies, 27% of the visits were either for services that should not have been legitimately covered or were questionable. The report concluded that home health care under Medicare is a difficult program to control (General Accounting Office, 1981). However, it is feasible to pay Medicare-certified home health agencies according to a prospective flat rate rather than by the visit, as is now the case (Gaumer and Williams, 1984). Hay (1984) is now testing a system for Medicaid home health in Hartford, Connecticut, in which monetary incentives are given directly to the users in the form of rebates for each service rendered that is lower than the median cost, or (for a second experimental group) for overall service costs that fall below the median because of reduced length and intensity of service. Patients will keep half the savings accrued.

Presently discussions are underway about the merits of offering hospitals a prospective payment from which they would be responsible for whatever aftercare was needed in hospitals and home health settings. Bundling aftercare into hospital DRGs will be complex because social factors as well as health factors dictate the necessity and cost of such care. Moreover, it is uncertain what effects would be created by giving the hospital such prominence in long-term care.

ENCOURAGING ALTERNATIVES TO NURSING HOMES

Perhaps the most appealing cost-saving strategy is to prevent unnecessary nursing home admissions by providing less expensive home care. This solution can unite the interests of the most hardened cost-cutter and the most zealous advocate for human dignity. Most of the demonstrations already mentioned had that goal. Although we present findings from those studies in subsequent chapters, here we note the pitfalls inherent in the approach. Chapter 2 indicated that many persons need long-term care who never enter a nursing home or who delay admission as long as possible; most of these people receive care exclusively or largely from their families. Thus to save money through offering alternative services requires precise targeting of those likely to enter nursing homes in the near future to avoid substituting public home care benefits for free family care.

In addition to the issue of targeting the correct population and avoiding replacement of family care, several other factors influence the likelihood that increased home care will save money (General Accounting Office, 1982b). First, home care is more likely to save money if it is offered to people who require less than continuous services; people who need heavy and constant care can be served less expensively in nursing homes. Second, home care will be less expensive if one has flexibility in the amount of service authorized and the types of personnel reimbursed. Costs are rapidly inflated by minimum blocks of service or mandated professional participation. Third, home care will be less expensive for the public if the client needs no subsidization for rent or living expenses. And fourth, home care costs more if clients live in geographically dispersed homes, such as in rural areas, or in large, inconvenient homes that require extensive maintenance and adapt poorly to disability.

The rosy hope that home care would almost automatically reduce nursing home costs has now been thoroughly dispelled. The challenge becomes one of providing a range of services at home and in facilities, both of which are acceptable to clients and effective in maintaining their functioning while keeping a cost-conscious stance. It is still feasible that, with careful targeting and ceilings on how much can be spent at home, the overall costs of long-term care can be contained. However, yet another policy issue stands in the way. Thus far, the only people eligible for major services at public expense are poor or near poor. Yet the cost of privately purchased home care can be too high for middle-class families, and the problem of organizing such services without case management may present an extra deterrent that propels people into nursing homes, impoverishing themselves and becoming Medicaid recipients.

DEVELOPING CAPITATED SYSTEMS

Capitation is a longstanding approach to controlling health costs. It is exemplified in health maintenance organizations (HMOs), which charge patients a monthly fee that covers all hospital and outpatient expenses. Several demonstrations are underway, in fact, to test the effects of giving HMOs an average payment for each Medicare enrollee and making the provider responsible for all services ordinarily covered by Medicare. But the issue becomes more complicated for long-term care, which is not a Medicare benefit and which is not generally offered by a consolidated provider. Currently, a concept called the social health maintenance organization (S/HMO) is being tested in four locations. Here a consortia of physicians, hospitals, nursing homes, and home health providers have formed S/HMOs and, in exchange for a capitated fee, undertaken to provide all ordinary

Medicare-covered services plus additional long-term care coverage in nursing homes and in the community (Leutz et al., 1985). Although the long-term care benefits are somewhat limited in these programs, the experiment is of great interest, particularly because it tests the possibility of transferring some money from the acute sector to long-term care and still achieving efficiencies.

LONG-TERM CARE INSURANCE

Long-term care insurance presently can hardly be purchased, and existing policies are both expensive and limited in their coverage of nursing home costs. Most do not cover home health care and homemaking at all. Meiners (1984) has studied the feasibility of such insurance and described the major barriers to its development. For the insurance to be profitable to the underwriter and still be reasonably priced, sufficient numbers of relatively young and healthy persons must be persuaded to buy the protection. Furthermore, the long-term care available through the insurance must be clearly superior to what is available under Medicaid. Underwriters are also concerned about what they call "moral hazard," that is, claiming benefits unjustifiably. This seems a particular threat if desirable services like homemaking are included.

A study of retirees revealed an interest in purchasing long-term care insurance, particularly among those who had an experience with a nursing home through a relative (American Association of Retired Persons, 1984). Still, the technical problems remain unresolved. The insurance principle cannot be applied to a service that will eventually be needed by so many people, unless a large pool of people at low risk can be attracted; however, people seem reluctant to purchase such insurance far in advance. Some speculate about marketing a combination long-term care insurance and life insurance package. Some policy-makers speculate about the prospect of marketing long-term care policies to adult workers, with their parents as beneficiaries, and perhaps urging this benefit through the workplace. Either way, a greater pool of persons at low risk may be attracted.

ENCOURAGING PRIVATE SAVINGS FOR LONG-TERM CARE

Some authorities are enthusiastic about infusing more private money into payment for long-term care. They advocate increased incentives for saving and establishment of financial mechanisms to generate funds for care. Given research evidence that few people plan specifically for their long-term care needs (Kulys, 1983), some argue for information campaigns that would raise public anxiety about long-term care costs and encourage people to plan for incapacity before it occurs. For example, Bass (1986) developed a model for "life care planning" in which social workers would join with financial and legal planners to assist middle-class citizens in making long-range provisions for physical and/or cognitive incapacity. Bass views her approach as fostering quality as much as reducing demands on public funds. She even suggests—in our opinion, unrealistically—that foundations and private charitable groups should be solicited to sponsor individuals or families without money, so that even the poor could set up financial trusts for long-term care.

INCENTIVES FOR INCREASED FAMILY CARE

We saw in Chapter 2 that families already provide large amounts of care to their relatives. Nevertheless, considerable enthusiasm has been generated for programs that would induce families to give more care and for longer times. The proposals include direct payment and tax breaks to family caregivers (Arling and McAuley, 1983; Nelson, 1982), but none have been tested for cost-effectiveness. It is hard to imagine any financial inducement or tax incentive valuable enough to make most people leave the labor market and provide long-term care services. Such sacrifices are more likely made out of duty and affection. Monetary incentives might simply increase the cost of care without changing public behavior. Another possibility, of course, is that the promise of money would bring new family members into caregiving. Perhaps, however, we should be concerned about interrupting the self-selection that determines family help. Quinn and Tomita (1986) cite numerous case examples of financial exploitation and physical abuse occurring in situations where a caregiver is dependent on the pension or social security check of a frail elderly relative.

Up to now, the United States has not taken the position that adult offspring have legal responsibility for the care of their parents. Care of parents, and in particular, legally mandated financial responsibility, may be more than is reasonable to dictate. There may also be a hidden cost of such parent care. It is possible that some adults would deplete their own resources more quickly and have less reserve for their own care needs.

Efforts to add private dollars to the system do not necessarily decrease overall costs of long-term care and may, in fact, result in increases. Efforts to induce or require more care from adult children seem bound to save money, but volunteered care from citizens has hidden costs for the persons helping and for the labor force. Furthermore, the emphasis on family care is unflattering to both the elderly and their younger relatives. It is a paternalistic stance that implies the elderly should be taken care of by a relative regardless of their own preferences, seemingly removing the locus of decisionmaking from the older person. It also implies that relatives of the elderly need incentives to care for their parents, ignoring the visible fact that parents are receiving care from willing adult children and other relatives, many of whom are stretching themselves to the breaking point.

PREFERENCES

We repeatedly have noted that the preferences of older people should be honored as much as possible. We urge that their preferences guide whether they enter a facility and which one, and what services in facilities or in the community should be like. Preferences are, by definition, highly personal, but common patterns can guide development of long-term care programs. Unfortunately, available information about such preferences is only patchy.

A number of large surveys deal with opinions and preferences for health policy and other public policies for the elderly. Although long-term care is not the primary focus, each has suggested some relevant findings. A large Harris poll that compared the views of persons over 65 with those of the general population found that people of all ages held positive attitudes towards governmental assistance for income security and health care of the elderly even if it meant an increase in their personal taxes (Harris & Associates, 1975). Another large probability sample of about 1,000 persons over 18 and a smaller sample of physicians was undertaken to determine opinions about the health issues of the day. Respondents also approved government caring for the aged; 89% concurred that government should help when the aged have no other resources. But 58% agreed that aged parents' children should be financially responsible for their care even if they lived in a nursing home, 39% agreed that parents should be placed in a home if it could be afforded, and 34% agreed that aged parents should take care of themselves until they die. Persons over 65 were more likely to support the idea that the elderly should take care of themselves (50% agreed) and less likely to think adult children should be responsible for their care; 45% of those over 65 and 65% of those between 18 and 64 agreed with this premise (American Board of Family Practice, 1985).

The American Association of Retired Persons (AARP) (1984) conducted a national study of its members to determine their needs and preferences for insurance for nursing home and home health services. Most (80%) preferred home health services to nursing homes, and a large segment (40%) worried about having enough money to pay for either. Widespread confusion and considerable false security was found about Medicare coverage and coverage of private supplemental insurance (79% expected Medicare would pay for all or a part of a nursing home stay). Almost half the sample (41%) were aware of nursing homes because a friend or relative had recently been in one. This group was more likely to believe that they themselves would require extended stays in nursing homes at some time and that they themselves would need home health services at some times.

Baker (1983b) did 550 interviews with residents of Sun City, Arizona, a relatively affluent retirement community. Home health care and home-delivered meals were seen as the most attractive services to develop in Sun City, whereas congregate meals, day centers, and friendly visiting were seen as least attractive. If respondents could no longer live at home, life care communities were the most frequently chosen option by far (88%).

Other information on preferences comes from relatively small-scale studies or from tangential questions inserted in larger studies. Kulys (1983) reported that elderly persons in the Chicago area preferred not to enter a nursing home, but that most expected to do so if they needed care. Brody's (1981) study of families with three generations of adult women revealed that the granddaughter generation believed more strongly than the grand-mother generation that adult children should care for their parents, and that all the women preferred to pay for care or have someone purchase it than to have a daughter leave the workplace to provide it. Cicirelli's (1981) study of middle-aged and elderly adults in Lafayette, Indiana, reinforced the commit-ment between the generations but revealed a possible shift in public atti-tudes; younger adult children with younger parents were more accepting of services from governmental agencies and voluntary organizations. This finding was compatible with the larger AARP survey, which found that 62% found "going on welfare" to pay for nursing home or home health care acceptable, and that the younger respondents were more accepting of government help than the "old-old." Cicirelli's study also found some incongruence between the way the elderly and the middle-aged generation ranked help the elderly would require and expect from adult children. The elderly gave high rankings to protection, help in negotiating bureaucracy, and securing reading material. The adult-child generation gave high ranking to home health services and personal care, which were ranked low by the elderly. The area of greatest congruence was transportation, which was first on the middle-aged persons' lists and second on the elderly respondents' lists.

Various small studies (Knowles, 1975) have attempted to determine the preferences of people already living in nursing homes. The Coalition for Nursing Home Reform sponsored a study of residents' views about regula-tions (Spalding, 1985). Over 400 nursing home residents in 10 states partici-pated in a series of focus groups. They emphasized the importance of choice (on matters such as roommates, food, and routines), human kindness and responsiveness from aides and other personnel, and competent performance of staff.

A few studies have tried to determine the differing views of several parties to long-term care. A small study that asked nurses in hospitals, nurses in home health agencies, and elderly persons to react to a vignette with a judgment about whether the person described could best be cared for at home, in his son's home, or in a nursing home produced the following results: the home health nurses chose his own home, the hospital nurses chose the nursing home, and the elderly were divided. These differences occurred despite the fact that on objective indicators of the ability of the setting to meet different aspects of well-being (i.e., activity needs, diet needs, environment needs, health needs, medication needs, self-care needs, and social needs), all respondents judged that the nursing home would be the preferable setting (Grier, 1977). Kane, Bell, and Riegler (1986) examined the value preferences held by different groups for nursing home outcomes (such as physical well-being, comfort, social well-being, emotional well-being, cognitive ability, ADL abilities, and satisfaction, and definitive outcomes like death, discharge home, and discharge to hospital). The groups polled included nursing home residents, families of nursing home residents, regulators, nursing home administrators and personnel, and health professional students. Respondents were asked to rate the importance of improvements and declines in each of those areas to the residents, imagining residents with different mixes of physical and cognitive impairment. The respondents were able to enter into this exercise thoughtfully and tended to rate many areas as more important than the preservation of life; the ratings of family members of residents were somewhat atypical of the rest of the respondents.

What are we to make of this disparate material on preferences? Some findings are fairly universal. Older persons prefer to avoid nursing homes. They prefer not to disrupt the lives of their children, but their children are willing and see a duty to help their parents. The elderly seem willing to accept public welfare programs and the public seem correspondingly willing to be taxed to finance them. However, little information is available about the nature of preferences for specific program features, largely because little systematic information has been sought.

PART II
Evidence About Effective Long-Term Care

5

Effective Long-Term Care

Part II of this book examines reported evidence about the effects of long-term care programs. The following four chapters review information about effective long-term care programs in the community and in nursing homes, and about effective systems of long-term care.

We approached these reviews with some criteria for effective long-term care programs and effective community systems of long-term care. This brief chapter introduces the way we defined program effectiveness. Like everything else about long-term care, the development of criteria proved more complicated than we first expected.

DIFFICULTIES IN DEMONSTRATING EFFECTIVENESS

The nature of long-term care makes its precise definition difficult. Although the name suggests a process extending over a prolonged period, it is hard to tell at the outset just when that period has begun. Often the name is used to distinguish it from acute care, but this distinction fails on at least two grounds. First, the categories are not mutually exclusive; one can require acute care while receiving long-term care. Second, not all post-acute care is appropriately referred to as long-term care. If we use the concept of substitution, for example, much community care that occurs after hospitalization would more correctly be viewed as a substitute for acute care rather than for nursing home care.

Although functional impairment is a ticket to long-term care, no unanimity exists about the expectations of a long-term care program with regard to the functioning of its clientele. Tension between rehabilitation and custodial care, sometimes explicit and sometimes unrecognized, interferes with the establishment of unambiguous program goals. Funding distinctions highlight the arbitrary separation, producing distinctions such as day health care versus social day care, skilled nursing facilities versus intermediate facilities, home health aides versus homemakers. Some programs seem predicated on a belief that long-term care should always aspire to affect functional improvements, whereas others settle for making people more comfortable. A third view argues that community services have an intrinsic value in that they permit people to stay in their own homes regardless of any effect on functioning or comfort. For clients with senile dementia, the field is also divided about whether cognitive improvement or diminution of cognitive decline should be built into all, most, or very few programs. In our view, rehabilitation or functional improvement may at times be an appropriate long-term care goal, but not always. The decision comes from careful consideration of the client and informed judgment about what is possible and desired. Then the challenge is to match clients with appropriate programs.

At the point of discharge from an acute hospital, the decisions about appropriate programs are especially murky. At present, similar looking patients can be sent on seemingly different courses without a clear rationale beyond the availability of resources. For example, fractured hips and strokes are among the common reasons for admission of older persons to rehabilitation units, but they also are frequent reasons for admission to home health care or skilled nursing facilities. Why is one source of care chosen over another? What difference does it make where the patient is treated? Surprisingly we have few ready answers to such basic questions. Of course, we do know something about the price of services rendered in different locations, but even here our knowledge is superficial. We can measure the cost (or charges) for care given by the visit, the day, the hour, or sometimes even for an episode, but we rarely look at the total cost. A comprehensive picture should also include the costs of delays in recognizing complications. In fact, sometimes a program that acts expeditiously to identify problems seems more expensive because the client receives care to deal with the problems uncovered, adding immediate costs.

We cannot yet examine the true episodes of long-term care. Most management information systems do not permit aggregation over time and across providers. Usually the data systems are geared to the payment system and reflect the fragmentation of our funding. Thus patients moving back and forth between the hospital and nursing home are treated as though each move began a new event. Therefore, many statistics are misleading. For example, one is left with the impression that most nursing home stays are short when, in fact, many are simply interrupted by a hospitalization that leads to readmission to a nursing home if the patient survives.

Many of the most enthusiastic reports about the effectiveness of long-term care programs are based on a potential fallacy. Enthusiasts look at the population at risk and eligible for services and assume that, were it not for the innovation, all of those persons would have declined in function or have demanded care. This "there-but-for-the-grace of the-program" phenomenon occurs with alarming frequency. Given the enormous variation among those eligible to use a program, careful attention to the fate of control groups is virtually essential to understanding the effects of an intervention.

Long-term care interventions can be considered at increasing levels of generality. At the narrowest level, we can look at a unit of service—for example, a visit by a home health nurse, or a session of a training group for family caregivers, or a particular personal care service given to a nursing home resident on a given day. More usefully, we can move to the programmatic level, thereby looking at the effectiveness of a particular home health program, or day care program, or any other long-term care program.

But the effectiveness of long-term care in any given community depends on how programs are combined into a system adequate to meet community need, and how well the particular components of the system communicate and interact. At this system level, programs can be mixed and matched with considerable interchangeability and still achieve effective results.

These concerns caused us to approach specifying criteria for reviewing previous research with some caution. We strove to establish rules of evidence that focused on demonstrated effectiveness without being so stringent as to lose valuable information that might shed useful light on an innovation.

CRITERIA FOR EFFECTIVENESS

The smaller the unit of attention, the less meaningful information will be about overall effectiveness of long-term care. Therefore, in this book we do not consider the single unit of service—such as the visit, the interview, the individual bed bath or delivered meal, although these are certainly an appropriate focus for quality assurance efforts. Instead we deal with programs and systems. At the program level, we have amassed information about home care and day care (see Chapter 6), other community long-term care programs (see Chapter 7), long-term care in nursing homes (see Chapter 8), and the relationship between long-term and acute care (Chapter 9). The discussion of effective systems of care (included in Chapter 10) reviews efforts to improve care at the level of the community by combining services in new ways, altering incentives or communication patterns, or changing benefit structures.

In our review of programs, we were guided by the view that an effective program should have the following characteristics:

- a stated goal or goals;
- activities or program elements that theoretically would be expected to achieve the goal;

- targeting of the program to a particular population or populations deemed likely to benefit from the program;
- correspondence of both the goals and the program elements to the preferences of the people served;
- achievement of the stated goals;
- achievement of those goals efficiently;
- no unintended negative effects.

Defining the elements of an effective *system* of care is even more complex. Individual program components can be mixed and matched in various ways to achieve a satisfactory result. In reviewing materials about systems of care, we were guided by the belief that an effective community system should have these characteristics:

- it should offer a considerable range of services both in the community and in facilities;
- it should permit as much choice as possible to those who require service;
- its component services should be of acceptable quality, with all provider incentives directed toward maintaining and improving that quality;
- it should be organized in such a way that treatable problems causing dysfunction are likely to be identified and treated;
- it should be visible to potential users;
- it should be equitable in serving those with need;
- it should be equitable across generations—that is, its demands on family members who give care should be fair;
- it should be characterized by clear communication among organizations financing and/or providing service;
- it should be accountable to the public for the quality and accessibility of all services, both public and private.

Regarding the cost of care, which has been a major theme in public policy, we suggest that an effective system of long-term care should:

- keep government costs to a minimum;
- keep private costs to a minimum;
- maintain a reasonable balance between public and private costs;
- be accountable to the public for its *total* costs, public and private.

These criteria concerning cost spring from the premise that long-term care will inevitably require both public and private dollars, but that reductions of public expenditures cannot be celebrated if private costs soar out of hand. The cost of the system is the sum of public and private dollars spent on services given by nonprofit and for-profit organizations and practitioners. Policymakers should be accountable to the public for development of a system in which the overall costs are as streamlined as possible and in which public and private money is mingled in a way that fairly protects all citizens.

Although listing these criteria provides a helpful grounding, they still need elaboration, particularly in the context of the value-laden, political decisions that must be made about long-term care. Below we discuss some of the criteria that are particularly difficult to apply.

GOALS

It seems axiomatic that an effective program has clearly stated goals. In fact, however, many long-term care programs are vague about their goals or state numerous, and even somewhat conflicting, objectives. Perhaps this is not surprising. Formulating reasonable and appropriate goals for long-term care turns out to be a difficult conceptual task.

By its very definition, long-term care is directed to persons with problems in functioning. Broadly stated, a long-term care program could be directed at remedying the dysfunction, or at compensating for it—that is, providing services that make up for the disability and allow the client to proceed with as normal a life as possible. If long-term care is directed at improving or maintaining functioning, then its success can be measured by functional outcomes.

If long-term care is meant to compensate for irremediable impairment, measures of effectiveness are hard to define. At the least, those functional limitations should be accurately identified and the resultant needs adequately met. This logic leads to the expectation that an effective long-term care system will produce a measurable reduction in unmet need in the community. But unmet need is a difficult, rather subjective concept that usually requires professional judgment.

Another approach to determining how well needs are met is to check for the frequency of deleterious events thought to be associated with unmet need. Admission to a nursing home has been viewed as such an event and is often seen as a sign of inadequate long-term care in the community. This reasoning is faulty, however, on two scores. Entering a nursing home may be appropriate and positive rather than deleterious for some people. Moreover, long-term care should improve functioning or compensate for dysfunction among nursing home residents as well as among those living in their own homes. Other events—such as death or serious accident—are also ambiguous to interpret. Long-term care assuredly cannot prevent the former, and preventing the latter may be at the cost of severe social restrictions for the clientele.

Yet another approach to evaluating long-term care for chronic irremediable problems would be to measure such intangibles as happiness, social involvement, and meaningful activity. Here, too, a problem arises. If the long-term care is designed to compensate for functional impairment, rendering that impairment as little disruptive as possible, then long-term care is a maintenance function. Such maintenance is surely effective regardless of how happy, productive, or socially active the client is. The job of long-term care is to render the life as "normal" as possible; there will, then, be enormous variation in how those lives are led.

Often it is stated that long-term care should be delivered by the "least restrictive alternative." The idea is sound, but much judgment is indeed needed to decide what constitutes the least restriction. Conventional wisdom suggests that the nursing home is the most restrictive alternative, followed by other congregate settings such as board and care homes and adult foster homes, and that living in one's own home is least restrictive. However, a nursing home need not be unduly restrictive (rules can be changed), and it is possible that a person captive in a back bedroom or a five-floor walkup is in the most restrictive setting of all.

Finally, there is considerable debate about the appropriate focus of long-term care—that is, whether the goals should be directed toward the functionally impaired individual or toward a family constellation. We perceive the individual as the appropriate target of long-term care. Work with the family then becomes a strategy for providing that care. And, if family members suffer negative effects from giving care, these could be construed as unanticipated consequences of the program.

TARGETING

Health and social service programs typically are in danger of serving those less in need of the program than others who remain unserved or of claiming results that could have been accomplished without the program. This may be an even greater risk in long-term care because the clients who are most vulnerable are also most immobile and isolated. Similarly those caregivers who are most burdened are perhaps too burdened to get to a source of help. Those who find their way to meal programs, senior centers, and support groups may represent a less needy group.

All this suggests the need to construct a formula for seeking the most impaired. At some point, however, clients might be too impaired to benefit from a particular program, and, indeed, the most cost-effective use of service may be an additional increment to a person whose physical or social resources are already good. Without coming to closure on this thorny problem, we gave extra attention to programs that clearly defined both the target population they hoped to reach and the characteristics of the group actually reached.

NATURE OF EVIDENCE

The characteristics of an effective program, and criteria for proving that the program is effective, are, of course, different issues. Without getting bogged down in details of research design and analysis, we did value more highly studies with the following characteristics:

- *Comparable control groups are used.* Randomized designs were most impressive, but at the least, we sought descriptive evidence that the group receiving the program and the comparison group were comparable. Before-and-after comparisons were sometimes the best we could produce, but we viewed these with the most hesitation. Policies have been changing so rapidly in the last decade that such comparisons are especially dangerous.

- *An intervention that actually takes place.* Some well-known and ambitious long-term care studies were flawed because the program being tested never was fully implemented. In such cases either only a part of the sample received the service or the service did not occur with the intensity expected. In lesser-known studies—for example, small studies of support groups—the implementation frequently fell short of the plan. From such underdeveloped studies, it is possible to learn something about the challenges of implementing a program and perhaps what clients want, but usually information about direct program effects are limited.

- *Sufficient sample size to generalize.* We do report some studies with quite small samples—especially studies testing different therapeutic or environmental programs in nursing homes. The size of the sample made a particular difference if numerous subgroups were created and a large number of variables examined.

- *Appropriate and accurate measures.* Here we were concerned with whether any inaccuracies entered the study because of data collection or scaling methods. If costs were examined, we were interested in whether all relevant costs were included.

- *Length and completeness of follow-up.* As we suggested above, misleading information is sometimes produced because only a fragmentary portion of a client's experience is captured. Of course the appropriate spacing of follow-up depends on the goals of the program—it is appropriate to look for initial outcomes of posthospital programs rather quickly after discharge. We especially welcomed longitudinal studies that allowed us to look at the complete course of long-term care for those who use it. And studies were viewed as weakened if they lost large numbers of subjects during their course.

REVIEW PROCESS

In our review of evidence, we considered both our criteria of effectiveness and the methodological issues just outlined. For the most part, we do not report on studies without comparison groups, those with tiny samples, or those with other problems that made drawing conclusions difficult. In the chapters that follow, we group studies on similar topics together in tables to permit easy comparisons. Typically these tables include descriptive information about the program, its intended purpose, its activities, and its target population. Without getting bogged down in technical detail, the tables also include brief summaries of the research design. Both these considerations determine how findings can be interpreted. For convenience, we have grouped studies on a topic, say day care or respite care, but the variation among programs in the same general categories is impressive. We cannot aggregate information without comparable interventions, target populations, and study measures. We tend to use the same approach in our tables and discussion of each topical area, but the exact scheme varies sometimes when a particular subject necessitates distinct types of comparative analysis.

6

Home Care and Day Care

Home care and day care are the two community long-term care programs that come most readily to mind. Most authorities regard them as important planks in a long-term care system. Yet the experience with both these forms of long-term care is difficult to interpret and evaluate.

Strictly speaking, home care and day care are terms that describe the location of a program, rather than a program itself. The mix of possible personnel and services given at home or in day programs is enormous. Moreover, the goals of home care and day care vary widely, both for individual clients within programs and among programs with specific emphases. It is no more sensible to evaluate home care or day care across the board than to do so for hospital care or ambulatory care. Just as hospital care is not good for everyone, day care and home care must be addressed with specific clients in mind. To answer questions about effectiveness, we need to be able to describe program characteristics, populations served, and goals sought.

Unfortunately, much of the material about home care and day care describes interventions that are vague in substance and intent or, conversely, that ambitiously promise to be all things to all clientele. Also, home care and day care have often been tested as part of a larger package of long-term care benefits and programs. In this chapter, we review only the information we gathered about home care and day care as single programs. Chapter 10 presents evidence about coordinated *systems* of long-term care.

PROBLEMS OF EVALUATING HOME CARE

Home care is the most frequently and enthusiastically advocated component of community long-term care, and logically so. Most multifaceted community long-term care programs have at their core the delivery of a variety of services in the client's home. Given the mobility problems of the clientele and the need for services that facilitate life at home, this emphasis makes sense. Bringing services to people's homes, it is argued, prevents or postpones the need for them to relocate in institutions. It is also argued that, disregarding the cost of housing itself, home care is less expensive than care in nursing homes. Moreover, assuming that many people needing long-term care finance their own housing and board, the public cost of care at home should be cheaper overall than that of institutional care.

In this chapter, we explore knowledge about home care. Unfortunately, no definitive information is available, partly because of inherent difficulties in studying the effects of home care programs and partly because tests that have been set up are often extremely limited in their generalizability.

Definitional Problems

Home care could include all professional and paraprofessional long-term services that are provided in the recipient's own home. These embrace physician's services at one end of the continuum of cost and skill and housekeeping or chore services at the other. The services of registered nurses, licensed practical nurses, physical therapists, occupational therapists, speech therapists, nutritionists, social workers, and other mental health professionals might also be included. Even the services of volunteer or minimally paid companions might be considered long-term care at home.

The functions of home care also differ. They can include medical diagnosis and functional assessment; health care treatments and monitoring of regimens; health education; training and supervision of family caregivers; personal care for sustained and even indefinite periods; homemaking for sustained or indefinite periods; and terminal care. If the care is designed to give relief to family members, it may be called respite care. If it is designed to allow terminally ill persons to live comfortably and meaningfully at home, it may be called hospice care and carry with it a more diverse team of home care providers than is associated with a typical home health agency.

Even the concept of "home" can vary. Home might mean an isolated house in the country, a detached home in the suburbs, an efficiency apartment, a bedroom or apartment in a family member's home, or a unit in a building entirely occupied by frail elderly who use home services. Needless to say, the cost of delivering services at home would differ depending on the size and location of the home, the presence of others living in close proximity to help with care, and the prospects for economies of scale because the home is located in a complex with others needing care.

Home care, therefore, varies in its personnel mix, its service package, the populations served, and the sought-after outcomes of the program. Quite clearly the cost of these different packages varies. Studies of the effectiveness of home care are compromised if the nature of the intervention and its intended effects are unclear. Worse, the interventions and their purposes might vary from client to client, while the evaluation looks at all outcomes across all clientele without comparing subgroups.

Health Versus Social Home Care. Despite the diversity of home care, some crude distinctions can be made. The more common distinction is between home health care and homemaking/chore service. The former includes the services of nurses, physicians, and other technical personnel and, as defined by the Medicare benefit, personal care (bathing and toileting assistance, for example) done by home health aides under supervision of a nurse. Other services that do not involve professional personnel or hands-on care of the patient fall into the general homemaking/chore category. These would include housekeeping of all descriptions, meal preparation, and companionship and supervision. Clearly a different set of objectives and evaluative criteria could and should be applied to these two forms of home care.

Home Care as a Substitution. Another distinction can be made on the basis of whether home care is conceived as a substitute for other care and, if so, what services it seeks to replace. Some care is given at home as an efficient substitute for acute hospital, primary care, or rehabilitation regardless of the mix of professionals and paraprofessionals, hands-off and hands-on personnel involved. In such instances the choice is made to send someone home from hospital early, to treat a time-limited condition (e.g., a broken hip) at home instead of in the hospital or to initiate care at home to avoid a hospitalization entirely, and the appropriate health care and supportive services are arranged. The care will likely include both health and social services, both professional and paraprofessional providers. It is usually time-limited or episodic.

In contrast, some home care is given in order to allow the individual to continue to live in the community. If the older person's problem precludes maintaining a home without assistance, compensating services must be given in the home or relocation to a more sheltered group living situation would be needed. Similarly an older person may be unable to live in the home of a daughter or other relative without some outside assistance. Services thus required correspond to the rhythms of everyday life and include assistance with getting up and going to bed, day-to-day cleanliness and grooming, and food preparation and consumption. The care is likely to be heavily paraprofessional, but professional supervision and intermittent professional service might be expected.

Sometimes home care services might achieve both types of substitutability. For example, clients receiving care at home to permit them to remain there might also have a physician or nurse practitioner visit them there to provide primary care and monitor drug regimens. In all likelihood the latter services could also have been obtained by transporting the client to a clinic situation. It is possible to compare the benefits and costs of primary care at home to those of primary care in the clinic. Therefore, the client receives home care to enable the continuation of home life, and home care simultaneously functions as an alternative locus for a specific health service. The literature on home care is confusing and contradictory partly because this distinction is often ignored.

Chapter 4 introduced the problem of demonstrating that home care can substitute for nursing home care, a problem we shall return to in Chapter 10 in a review of systematic efforts to prevent or postpone nursing home admission. But not all home care can be categorized as substituting for one or more services somewhere else. Some home care can be seen as equivalent of hospital or nursing home care, but home care can also be justified in its own terms without reference to any substitutability. Once substitution is no longer an issue, we then are forced into an overdue focus on the improvements home care can make in the well-being of its clientele.

Difficulty of Defining Home Care Goals

Home care is too diverse to be measured by a single yardstick. In some instances, the patients are terminally ill, and expectations that the program will decrease morbidity and mortality would be highly inappropriate. In other cases, the home care is rehabilitative, and some functional improvement should, therefore, be expected. Much home care consists of personal services to compensate for functional impairment. The provision of home care could affect other aspects of health as well. Physical health may be improved or maintained by continued care and attention, for example, in prevention of skin breakdown in immobile persons. Home care can also affect morbidity and mortality through early detection and treatment of acute illness or drug reactions. On the other hand, home care may even result in a *decrease* of functional abilities if homemakers and home health aides assist with or perform activities formerly done by the client. (Such a decline in functioning may be more apparent than real if, at baseline, the client was performing the tasks only inadequately and with great difficulty.)

We found little discussion about what physical and functional gains should be expected from home care. But even less attention was given to the appropriate psychological and social effects. Should home care make people happy, less depressed, more secure? Should it enhance social activities and interaction? Or is it more reasonable to expect that home care clients be generally satisfied with the service and have fewer unmet needs?

An analogy from another service field might illustrate the issue. Most persons use the services of barbers and beauticians. Customers evaluating such services generally talk in terms of the outcome of primary concern, namely their appearance. Although the provider of service may be noteworthy for the manner of his or her work, his personality, or his ability to engage the customer in conversation, most people would not continue to patronize such an establishment if they did not leave feeling more attractive than when they entered. Indeed some studies have suggested that barbers, beauticians, and even bartenders serve as effective therapists for some of their customers, but that is not the primary service they are in business to provide and thus would not be the criterion on which their services should be evaluated.

The customer leaving a beauty shop feeling more attractive does not necessarily, or at least realistically, expect that the improvement in her appearance will improve her overall life experience. The choice of an appropriate measure of outcome is thus very important in evaluating a service fairly. In general, the more global the measure, the less appropriate it is likely to be in evaluating a specific service. However, the case of home care seems to present a special problem. The services are indeed diverse; their nature will depend in large measure on the individual client's needs. The establishment of a good personal relationship is often an important ingredient in the care process. It would be foolish and inefficient to argue too strenuously for attempting to separate the components of such care. One hardly wants a stream of "specialists" coming to the client's home to deliver services like companionship, homemaking, and personal care.

The outcomes of home care should thus be expressed in terms of enabling the client to remain at home, maximizing function, and making life more worthwhile. Each of these come with appropriate cautions. One does not wish to create stringent incentives that keep people in their homes when they really need more supervised care. Neither does one want a Dickensian situation in which the elderly client is deprived of needed services in the name of rehabilitation. For the psychological measures, one is likely on safer ground aspiring to client satisfaction with the services provided and the person providing them than with some such grandiose concept as life satisfaction.

Comparison Groups and Target Populations

Closely related to defining the service and its outcomes is the choice of comparison groups. Home care may be compared directly to some other locus of care: for example, hospital or nursing homes. Most often home care is hypothesized to have a desirable effect on the use of other health and social services, particularly hospitals, nursing homes, and ambulatory care. In such cases, a sample of patients who receive home care is compared to a group who do not, and the subsequent use of other services in the hospital, doctor's office, and/or nursing home is observed.

Each function of home care just described—i.e., home care as a cost-effective alternative for episodic or time-limited care, custodial home care to permit a client to live independently, and home care to improve functioning of the functionally impaired in the community—suggests different target groups and different comparisons to be made. Moreover, the service strategy, targeting, and potential outcomes would differ depending on the kind of home situation being facilitated—for example, a frail elder living alone in his own home, a frail elder with a spouse in their own home, or a frail elder being maintained in the home of a relative.

The most direct way to study the effect of home care on use of other services would entail a highly controlled experiment with a specified group of people. For example, an experiment could be designed that sent people with specific diagnoses and functional levels home from the hospital early, comparing their costs and results to a group who remained in the hospital. Similarly, categories of patients could be treated at home for acute problems that would otherwise require hospitalization and compared to those entering the hospital. A group of nursing home applicants whose functioning made them eligible for institutional care could be enlisted to try home care with appropriate services, and the two groups could be compared on morbidity, mortality, functional outcomes, service use, and costs. (Here measures of psychological and social well-being would also be appropriate because what is being tested is a large social change.) A few studies have experimentally tested the replacement of hospital care by home care for acute treatment, but these have usually been done outside the United States, where a more comprehensively organized health care system permits such targeted experiments (Gerson and Hughes, 1976; Gerson and Berry, 1976). Otherwise we could locate no studies where a defined group of users, who would otherwise receive their care elsewhere, were assigned to home care and the results compared.

Another way to study home care is to identify a group of frail elderly people who would seem to benefit from care at home and compare those offered such care to those who are not. In such a study, presumably the intensity and nature of services would evolve in response to need and the likely effects of the program would differ from client to client.

Yet another approach makes a new benefit available to the clientele and compares the outcomes of those given the benefit and those not offered it. Here, the study must take into account that some people in the experimental group who receive the benefit will not use it, whereas others who do not receive the benefit will get the service one way or another. The most obvious example of this type of study is the test of a homemaker benefit under Medicare that was launched in the early 1970s. Weissert's thorough analyses of this particular study (discussed below) took into account all possible patterns of use in the experimental and control group to extract information about the usefulness of the homemaking service. However, what was really being tested was the usefulness of a homemaking benefit, and a rather narrow one at that, since it could only be used when the criteria for Medicare home health had been met. In the furor created by the negative results of this study, many critics overlooked the fact that the study did not purport to test the general effects of homemaking for the frail elderly needing long-term care and that therefore the findings should not be applied to that purpose.

Finally, home care has almost invariably been included in the array of community-based long-term care benefits developed for the long-term care demonstrations reviewed in Chapter 10. In such instances, however, the home care (either home health care, homemaking, or both) is arranged or allocated by a case manager who serves as a gatekeeper to the services and is theoretically in a position to plan care, drawing on potentially interchangeable forms of services. For this reason, we cannot say that home care per se has been tested in the demonstrations.

EFFECTS OF HOME CARE

Descriptive Studies

Short of designing experiments to test the effects of home care, various investigators have gleaned valuable information about its likely effects by studying groups already receiving home care. Table 6-1 summarizes 13 such studies done since 1976. The studies presented there range considerably in sample size, focus, and scope, but each further specifies information about users of home care, the types of services they receive, and/or the outcomes of the cases.

Five studies present information on a fairly large scale, although the programs studied and the methods used differ considerably. In an early study, Emling (1976) looked at a sample of persons who used Michigan's statewide chore service plan, wherein the state purchased housekeeping and personal care for low-income persons using flexible program guidelines. Caregivers could be friends, neighbors, or nonlegally responsible relatives chosen by the client and approved by state caseworkers. This descriptive study showed that the program served an elderly, moderately impaired clientele and that the amount of service received varied with functional abilities but not with the client's diagnosis. The average service included six chores and took four hours a day. Laundry and shopping were by far the most frequently performed services.

Moving to the opposite end of the professionalization spectrum, the Veterans Administration study (1985) used operational statistics to describe the services of its 49 hospital-based home care teams. By definition each hospital program had a ceiling of eight professional personnel and was expected to cleave to a productivity standard of 50 patients and 350 visits per month. Three-quarters of the clients lived with family caregivers, and the team judged that one-fourth of those family members were themselves severely impaired. A special cost study at six sites showed that a score of 5

TABLE 6-1 Descriptive Studies of Home Care

Source	Program Description	Study Design	Findings
Brickner et al. (1976)	Hospital-based team of nurse, physician, and social worker provided health care and advocacy services and linked clients with agencies that provided friendly visiting and homemaking. Clients were referred by local agencies, churches, and welfare hotel managers in the Chelsea area of New York City. Begun in 1973, the program served 466 people, average age 80 and two-thirds living alone.	Researchers observed 47 home visits. They calculated time and cost and projected an average per visit cost to which they added estimates of food, rent, and the value of ancillary services. An expert physician panel determined whether clients were candidates for nursing homes and, if so, actual costs were compared to potential nursing home costs.	From a sample of 29 cases, 23 were candidates for nursing home care. A semiambulatory client receiving two hours per day of nursing care would cost $8,359 a year, about half of nursing home costs at 1975 rates; a bed-bound client with four hours per day of service would cost $12,079 in the community compared to $32,162 in nursing homes at 1975 rates.
Emling (1976)	Statewide chore service plan in Michigan that assisted SSI or potential SSI recipients in purchasing housekeeping or personal care. The providers were friends, neighbors, and nonlegally responsible relatives chosen by the client. A caseworker did the assessment, made a care plan, and negotiated pay. Maximum payment in 1976 was $270 per month.	A descriptive study with cases randomly drawn from caseworker files during a five-month period in 1975–76. The study profiles clients, providers, and costs, trying to relate the latter to client characteristics.	Clients were 75% female, owned their own home (62%), and were moderately impaired. Most frequent services were laundry (92%), shopping (87%), personal care (58%), and yardwork (12%). Most clients had a single provider, typically a female in her 40s, providing an average of six chores for four hours a day. The number of services needed and hours of services varied with functional level but not diagnosis.

Widmer, Brill, and
Schlosser (1978)

Visiting Nursing Service in
Bronx with full array of professional and paraprofes-
sional services (including
transportation) used grant
funds to make available services that were uncovered
by third parties and that patients could not afford; 420
patients were seen during
15-month period.

During a 15-month study
period all patients were assessed on admission and
discharge. They were classified on admission into three
functional groups: (1) needing help on household and
marketing activities (39%);
(2) needing help in one or
more ADLs or IADLs (28%);
and (3) entirely dependent
in one or more ADLs or
IADLs (33%). Through dia-
ries and monthly interviews
complete data were col-
lected on all health, housekeeping, and service costs
except drugs & hospital
stays to determine home
health needs when all cost
barriers were removed.

Average length-of-stay was 52.4
days, and 74% of patients had only
one admission to the home care program during the study period. Functional group was best predictor of
length-of-stay. Mean cost was $765
per admission but 10% of the population used 47% of the costs and
20% of the population used 67% of
the costs. Main cost differential in
heavy cost patients attributable to
home health aides, personal care,
and homemaking. Median total cost
per admission was $347 compared
to monthly average SNF costs of
$1380 and ICF costs of $857 at the
time.

TABLE 6-1 Continued

Source	Program Description	Study Design	Findings
Anderson, Patten, and Greenberg (1980)	11 nursing home facilities and seven home health agencies were selected for comparison of clientele. All were in three urban Minnesota counties. The nursing homes were a random sample by county, level of care, and ownership, excluding unusually small or atypical facilities. The home care agencies included three public nursing programs, three nonprofit agencies, and one proprietary agency.	The home care clientele were divided into three groups: (1) receiving nursing only; (2) receiving nursing, home health aide and perhaps homemaker services, and (3) receiving homemaker services only. The nursing home care and home care users were compared, using all 550 clients of the home care agencies and a random sample (70%) of the nursing home clients for an N of 450. Cross-sectional study used a detailed interview with all participants and a health assessment.	The home care group was more incapacitated than the ICF nursing home residents, who resembled the "homemaker only" home care users; SNF residents were similar to the home care group receiving home health aide/homemaking and nursing care. Mental functioning was poorer in nursing home group. Core services (i.e., case management, mental health, special education, personal care, and nursing services) were used proportionately more by SNF and ICF residents, and a high percentage of home care services were used by a small proportion of clientele; regardless of setting, physical functioning was best predictor of service use. A year later, 50% of home care clients no longer received services, 8% were known dead, and 8% were in nursing homes; 80% of nursing home residents still were receiving services, and 17% were dead. Life satisfaction was similar for both groups. Federal government bore two-thirds of cost of nursing home care and three-fourths of home care when Title XX was included in the latter.

| Inui et al. (1980) | Context was VA Hospital in Seattle with 305 acute beds, 12 specialty hospitals, and a hospital-based home care program begun in 1973. A nurse screening at discharge from medical and surgical wards over a five-month period was done to make an independent judgment of the need for home care in VA program. | 2,613 patients screened first for general program eligibility (e.g., geography) and then for nine criteria of VA for home care. Screening done through chart audit, interview of staff, and interview of patients. | More than half the 2,613 patients were ineligible for home care. Of the 1,063 remaining, 85% were judged inappropriate for the VA program. Of the 161 eligible persons judged to need home care, only 60 (43%) were referred to the hospital-home care program by the staff and only 58 of these were accepted. Thus in five months, 64% of patients appropriate for home care did not receive it. |
| Rosenfeld (1980) | Home health agencies in Massachusetts are licensed to serve specific geographic areas and vary in auspice, patient-staff ratios, staff size, and patient characteristics. The study used a sample of 45 of these agencies, all of which experienced the same state reimbursement system. | To learn what variables other than reimbursement influence agency behavior, a sample of 45 agencies and about 18,500 patients was used. Regression analysis was done to determine what client and agency factors were associated with outcomes, such as service intensity and duration (i.e., average number of RN and aide visits per patient, length and intensity of visits, and percent of caseload receiving intensive services). | The 45 agencies varied widely in type of patient (percentage of Medicare and/or Medicaid), comprehensiveness of service, and visits per case and intensity (i.e., ratio of visits over episode length) when age and income distribution in communities were controlled. Variation in service was due to characteristics of agencies rather than risk factors in communities (e.g., agencies with a higher percentage of Medicaid clientele had more intensive service and more use of aides). Availability of home health aides to the agency influenced service patterns more than percentage range of catchment area over 65. |

TABLE 6-1 Continued

Source	Program Description	Study Design	Findings
General Accounting Office (1981)	Medicare certified home health care.	Nurses did record review of intermediaries and of randomly selected cases in 37 home health agencies. Clients were visited when records were ambiguous; 85 physicians were interviewed regarding their roles in authorizing treatment plans; 150 beneficiaries were interviewed in their homes to see if informal care could have been used.	Record audit showed 27% of the visits provided were either not covered or questionable, usually because, in the opinion of the auditor, clients were not homebound. In other cases, the services were deemed too great. Of the 150 persons visited, 28% had a live-in partner willing to provide the care. Physicians took no active role in the program.
Hayslip et al. (1980)	A rural county in Maryland had six agencies giving home care, including a commission on aging, a department of social services, a meals on wheels program, hospital home care, and private home care. Two agencies offered all services (i.e., skilled and unskilled home health, transportation, telephone reassurance, in-	Two surveys were done: (1) interviews with about 300 randomly selected elderly country residents; and (2) questionnaires and follow-up interviews with the agencies.	Elderly most often mentioned heavy household tasks and social/community services as needs. The five most mentioned specific needs were personal transportation, medical transportation, lawn care, lifting, and grocery shopping. Points of dissatisfaction concerned lack of publicity about services, high costs, confusing service patterns, and inefficient delivery. Perceptions of service adequacy and needs varied by electoral dis-

	Description	Method	Findings
	home mental health, environmental maintenance) and two others offered most. The potential target population was low income (17% less than $600 a month) and two-fifths lived alone.		trict. Agencies perceived that they were meeting needs, but actually the targeting was to districts above the county's poverty level. Study suggested a mismatch between needs and services.
Kaye (1984)	Three programs under Title III-B of the Older Americans Act offered home care to the elderly, including social and health supports, homemaker/home health aide, and chore maintenance. The programs differed in size: small (less than 25 staff), medium (25–50 staff), and large (over 50).	A survey questionnaire was administered to 91 direct (e.g., homemakers) and indirect (e.g., administrators) providers. Program adequacy was gauged by measurement of the differences in scores between workers' perceptions of program capacity and program responsibility.	Respondents believed agency capacity and responsibility diverged and, except for satisfying daily needs of clients, programs met their responsibilities inadequately. Indirect staff were more critical than direct staff, and a majority of all respondents thought more time needed to be spent with clients. Program adequacy was seen greatest when assistance during evenings/weekends, long-term care needs, unexpected needs, emotional and medical needs were at issue.

TABLE 6-1 Continued

Source	Program Description	Study Design	Findings
McAuley and Arling (1984)	Not applicable.	A subsample of 524 persons 65+ from the 1979 State-wide Survey of Older Virginians was interviewed to examine the types of care received at home and factors explaining type and numbers of formal and informal services used.	Homemaker assistance was used by the highest proportion of the sample (about ⅓), followed by meal preparation (21%), continuous supervision (13%), personal care (12%), and nursing care (9%). ADL impairment was most closely related to receiving more types of care, but persons with more education, better social resources, and poorer mental health also received more forms of care.
Beland (1985)	Three home care programs in the province of Quebec were analyzed: two social-medical programs with homemakers, nurses, and social workers attached to a local community service center; and a medical program based in a department of health.	100 clients in each program were compared with a random sample from each of the three programs' catchment areas (N=350 to 400 per area); clients compared with those in catchment areas were at risk of nursing home because of living alone, inability to do housework, or more than three chronic illnesses. Measures included housing conditions, social isolation, use of services, functional status, and psychological well-being.	Clients in three programs had lower morale, more physical incapacity, and poorer self-rated health than high-risk nonusers; nonusers had small support networks and less often had supporters living in the home; clientele group made more applications for special housing than the controls.

124

Veterans Administration (1985)	As of 1985, the VA provides hospital-based home care in 49 programs systemwide. Each home care team has a ceiling of 8 personnel and a productivity standard of 50 patients and 350 visits per month. Home health uses professional multidisciplinary teams, including physician, and is designed to care for severely or terminally ill homebound people.	Statistical description of patients served systemwide; reviewed evaluations at two sites and performed cost studies at 6 sites; multiple regression used to predict the number of home visits as a function of patient characteristics, such as ADLs and diagnosis and program characteristics.	In 1984, 9,850 patients were in system, average age was 69, and almost 200,000 visits were made by 43 programs; three-quarters of patients lived with a spouse or family member and one-fourth of caregivers were judged to have severe or moderate limitations. Data from 6 sites showed average daily cost of $12.90. An ADL of 5 or 6 on the Katz scale and a diagnosis of cancer were main predictors of heavy service. Evaluation of 2 programs showed that after rehospitalization about 40% or more were discharged back to home care and about 35% died in hospital or went to nursing homes. Among those dying in hospital, most died within a few days of admission, suggesting the acuity levels of those maintained in home care.
Chappel (1985)	Home care is provided in Manitoba as a universal benefit. Need for care is determined by home care coordinators in the local office of the Department of Health and Social Services. Homemaking is provided directly by public employees, and professional services are either purchased from agencies or provided by direct public employees.	400 users of home care in 1980 randomly drawn from provincial records and compared to 400 non-users. Sample was stratified by sex.	Users were significantly more likely to be female, older, live in apartments, have more chronic illnesses, functional disabilities, and worse self-perceived health. Among the young elderly, users had fewer social supports; this distinction disappeared among the older clientele. Users were more likely than non-users to use other formal services and informal services.

or 6 on the Katz ADL scale was highly predictive of heavy cost clients. At two VA locations, the outcomes of home care clients after rehospitalization was studied. About 40% died in hospital, most within a few days, leading the authors to conclude that persons with severe and serious acute illnesses were being maintained by the program.

Anderson, Patten, and Greenberg (1980) compared persons using home care in three urban Minnesota counties with nursing home residents in the same locations, using a sample of all 550 home care clients and a randomly selected group of residents. Their snapshot showed that the persons receiving home care tended to be more impaired than those in ICFs, but the group in SNFs were the most impaired physically and cognitively. A high percentage of home care services were used by a small proportion of the clientele. A year later 50% of home care clients were still on the caseloads, only 8% were known to be in nursing homes, and 8% were known dead. In contrast, 80% of the nursing home population were still receiving nursing home care, and 17% had died. Although comparing nursing home users to home care users is risky (because they are likely to be incomparable), the researchers here were careful to describe groups according to their functional abilities.

Chappell's study (1985) made a different comparison, contrasting those who used home care programs to other community-dwelling elderly in the Canadian province of Manitoba (where all citizens may receive publicly subsidized home care regardless of their income). Users were older and had more functional disabilities and chronic illnesses. Users had fewer social supports, but this distinction disappeared among the oldest clientele. Those who used home care were likely to be heavy users of other health and social services *including* informal services from relatives and friends. Beland (1985) compared 300 clients of three home care programs in Quebec to a random sample of elders in the three programs catchment areas with similar results.

Studies by Widmer, Brill, and Schlosser (1978), and by McAuley and Arling (1984) provide further evidence about use of home care services. The study by Widmer and her colleagues was designed to discover what the utilization and costs would be if home care users had no financial barriers to service. Therefore, a home health agency used grant funds to finance any services uncovered by other sources and monitored costs over a 15-month period. Like other researchers, they found that utilization was highest among the most functionally impaired and that the heaviest costs were accounted for by a small proportion of the 420 clients studied. McAuley and Arling interviewed more than 500 elderly Virginians to examine and try to explain the types and volume of formal and informal services they received at home. Once again ADL impairment was strongly linked to receiving more types of care. Homemaker assistance was used by about one-third of the sample and assistance with meals by about one-fifth. Persons with more education and better social resources tended to receive more types of service than did persons with poorer mental health.

The study by Brickner and colleagues (1976) was done in a single hospital-based home care agency that received clients on referral from local agencies, welfare hotel managers, and churches in the Chelsea area of New York City. Although it was an uncontrolled study, the large caseload (466 people) and the advanced age of the clientele (average age 80 and two-thirds living alone) add interest. Efforts were made to estimate complete costs, including rent and food, for those staying at home. In a small sample of 29 cases reviewed by an expert panel of physicians, 23 were considered nursing home candidates. In 1975 dollars, the costs of those diverted from ICFs averaged about $8,360 a year, or half the ICF rate, and those diverted from SNFs about $12,000, compared to about $32,000 in a nursing home. Bed-bound SNF-level clients received about four hours per day of service on average.

The five remaining studies in Table 6-1 all pertain in one way or another to the ability of home care programs to target effectively or apply criteria consistently. For example, nurse auditors looking at records from 37 Medicare-certified home health agencies (General Accounting Office, 1981) found that 27% of the visits were inappropriate, that many other visits were at too high a level of service, and that family members would have been willing to give some of the service themselves. According to Medicare rules, therefore, the clientele were being overserved. In contrast, an independent audit of hospital discharges from the Seattle Veterans Administration found that only 43% of those who met criteria for VA home care were ever referred (Inui et al., 1980). Rosenfeld (1980) studied the behavior of 45 home health agencies in Massachusetts, analyzing 18,500 patient records. He found that service amount, intensity, and comprehensiveness varied according to external factors affecting agency reimbursement rather than the risk factors of the population in the catchment area. Hayslip and colleagues (1980) pointed up incongruities in the perceptions of elderly residents of a rural Maryland county compared to staff of the six agencies giving home care in the region. The agencies thought they were meeting the most extreme need, but actually they tended to give most service to neighborhoods above the poverty level. Areas of need as perceived by the public were personal transportation, medical transportation, lawn care, lifting, and grocery shopping. Finally, Kaye (1984) found that workers in home care agencies perceived that the programs inadequately met the needs of the clientele.

Taken together these studies suggest that home care tends to reach those with severe functional impairments, including some people more disabled than some nursing home residents; that within a home care program a small percentage of the clients will consume disproportionate resources; that those receiving formal home care services also receive informal care; and that homemaking services including laundry, shopping, and heavy household tasks are needed and valued by the users. The studies also provide fragmentary evidence that agencies often fail to target home care even according to the criteria of their own programs and that persons who might be appropriately referred for services may be overlooked. We now turn to experiments where those receiving some form of home care were compared to an appropriate control group who did not receive the service.

Evaluative Studies

Ours is not the only effort to aggregate studies of the effectiveness of home care. Hammond (1979) published an early synthesis of research, reporting primarily on work done before 1975 on home care as an alternative to acute hospital care. Although the author concluded that home care was substantially cheaper than hospital care, much of the evidence consisted of professional opinion about need for care and estimates of what the costs might have been had a different course been followed.

Hedrick and Inui (1986) did a more recent and stringent review of the effects of home care, concentrating on the 12 studies they could locate that met their criteria of an experimental or quasi-experimental design. (Their review centered on home care per se, rather than home care of the elderly.) They scored each study according to methodological rigor and then examined outcomes on six variables: mortality, physical function, nursing home use, hospital use, outpatient visits, and costs. The evidence prohibited any definitive statements about the effects of home care because results conflicted, the nature of the home care tested varied widely, too few studies with methodological rigor were located, and not all studies looked at all variables of interest.

After these cautions, Hedrick and Inui tentatively concluded that home care programs had no effect on mortality (9 of the 11 studies looking at mortality showed no effect), had little effect on nursing home use (four of eight studies looking at nursing home use, including the more rigorous experiments, showed no effect), had no effect on inpatient hospitalizations (7 of 10 studies looked at hospital use), or actually increased hospital bed days (2 of these 10 studies). Similarly, home care was associated with an increase of outpatient medical care. Only five studies dealt with overall costs, three finding no effect and two highly rated studies finding an increase in costs for those using home care. The effect on functional status was more mixed, with most finding no effect, one study finding a negative relationship, and one highly rated experiment finding a positive one. Hedrick and Inui's review excluded outcomes not examined by four or more studies; therefore, they do not report on satisfaction measures or other indicators of mental or social well-being.

In Table 6-2, we compare seven studies of the effects of home care, all of which were included in the Hedrick and Inui review. We omitted two studies done before 1975, both with small samples, and three later studies with either small samples, many subjects under age 65, or both. Five of the seven studies were true experiments, with patients randomly assigned to receive home care or usual services. One study (Hughes, Cordray, and Spiker, 1984) was a quasi-experiment where clients of a particular home care program were compared to persons receiving home-delivered meals. Finally, the Mitchell (1978) study, also a quasi-experiment, differed markedly because the group receiving home care at a Veterans Hospital was compared to persons entering the VA's own nursing home or community nursing homes. No effort was made to manipulate the destination, but rather any persons discharged from hospital to one of the three aftercare programs during a three-month period was enrolled and followed for three months.

The studies presented in Table 6-2 are heterogeneous in their interventions and target populations as well as their outcomes. Table 6-3 presents the contrasts more starkly for the six studies that compare home care users to others living in the community. The intervention included registered nurses (Katz et al., 1972), paraprofessionals (Nielson et al., 1972; Weissert et al., 1980b) and team approaches. Even these distinctions fail to exhaust the differences. For example, though both Nielson and Weissert examined the addition of paraprofessional personnel, only those with no need for skilled nursing service were eligible for homemakers and personal care attendants in the Neilson study. In contrast, the Weissert study tested the effectiveness of homemakers specifically for that population who met Medicare home care criteria and therefore were receiving nursing or other skilled services. Similarly, the team approaches included nurses aides with LPN and RN supervision by phone or in person as needed (Selmanoff et al., reported in Hedrick and Inui, 1986), a core nurse/social work team supplemented by a wide range of others as needed (Hughes, Cordray, and Spiker, 1984) and a highly skilled team of physician, geriatric nurse practitioner, and social worker (Groth-Juncker, 1982; Groth-Juncker and McCusker, 1983; Zimmer, Groth-Juncker, and McCusker, 1984, 1985). The latter program was designed with the expectation that physicians would make home visits often rather than as a rare exception.

What can we make of the results of these studies? More often than not, no significant differences were observed between the experimental group and control group on the outcomes studied. Slight advantages in mortality were found for home care users in two studies, and four of the six studies found attitudinal change in outcomes such as contentment, satisfaction, or perceived health of the patients. In one case, the greater satisfaction extended to family members. In the Hughes study, home care clients deteriorated in physical function. The picture on use of nursing homes and hospitals is mixed. On the whole, however, the results are discouraging to advocates who previously had argued that home care would prevent or postpone nursing home use.

TABLE 6-2 General Studies of the Effectiveness of Home Care

Source	Program Description	Study Design	Selected Findings
Katz et al. (1972)	Patients age 50+ discharged from chronic disease rehabilitation hospital received visits by Visiting Nurse Association.	Randomized controlled trial of 300 subjects equally divided between experimental and control groups. Two-year follow-up looking at physical function, mortality, nursing home, and hospital use.	Home care group had more hospital admissions than controls; other differences not significant.
Nielson et al. (1972)	Home aide service including housekeeping, meal planning, shopping, bathing, dressing, reading to, and assistance with writing was offered on discharge from Benjamin Rose Hospital in Cleveland to persons over 60 with no need of intensive nursing.	The sample of 100 persons was enrolled in the two weeks before hospital discharge and randomized into equal groups. Measures were done at baseline, two weeks post-discharge, and six months and one year after enrollment. The dependent variables were survival, contentment, and institutional placement.	Those with home health aides spent fewer days in nursing homes, homes for the aged, and mental hospitals, and had fewer admissions to institutions. No difference in hospital use. Self-reported contentment and contentment measured by scales were greater for experimental group. The service had most impact on contentment for patients with fractures and arthritis and most impact on institutionalization for those who had a live-in family caregiver. No significant differences were found for stroke patients or for males.

Selmanoff, Mitchell, Widlak, and Mossholder (1979). Reported in Hedrick & Inui (1986).	Nursing and personal care services from aide, LPN, and RN with maximum 12 hours a week aide service. RN and LPN visit and monitor by telephone as needed. Eligible persons needed to be 60+ and chronically disabled.	Randomization to experimental or control group with assessment at intake, four and six months after service started, and three months after termination.	Experimental group had a higher use of nursing homes and a lower mortality rate than the control group. No significant differences in functional status or use of hospitals.
Mitchell (1978).	Veterans Administration Home Care Program with team of MD, RN, dietician, social worker and, as required, PT & HHA.	Subjects were all patients leaving acute care in four VA hospitals and entering VA home care, a community nursing home, or a VA hospital-based nursing home for three months. $N=318$ (108 in home care). Programs compared by reassessment three months later or at discharge from after-care program.	Home care patients had improved functional status compared to VA nursing homes but not community nursing homes. Home care patients had fewer rehospitalizations than those in community nursing homes but not in VA nursing homes.

TABLE 6-2 Continued

Source	Program Description	Study Design	Selected Findings
Weissert et al. (1980b) Weissert, Wan, and Livieratos (1980)	Homemaking was made available as a Medicare benefit for persons meeting criteria for Medicare certified home care (prior 3-day hospitalization, rehabilitable, needing skilled service) in four cities—Providence; Lexington, KY; San Francisco; and Los Angeles. Homemaker providers not described.	After baseline assessment, eligible subjects were randomly assigned to homemaker benefit/no homemaker benefit. Subjects were reassessed every three months for one year. The study analyzed the costs and effects of intervention on variables such as physical and mental functioning, institutionalization, mortality, social activity, and contentment. Methodology included the use of a 3-stage analysis on the major criterion outcomes of physical functioning, institutionization, and death: The analysis compared (1) experimental and controls excluding missing/contaminated cases, (2) uses and non-uses of services, (3) all assigned experimentals and controls. N varied from 630 to 778 depending on analysis used.	Significant positive impacts were found on mortality and contentment. In the 3-stage analysis, mortality was the only consistent and significant outcome. Services did not affect physical functioning. When users and non-users were compared, users who were male, living with others, and severely dependent had higher levels of hospital use. Costs for the experimental group averaged $3,432 more than for controls, mostly because of the cost of the homemakers themselves.

Groth-Juncker (1982) Zimmer, Groth-Juncker, and McCusker (1984, 1985).	Home health care team of MD, geriatric nurse practitioner, and social worker delivered primary care to homebound seriously ill or terminally ill patients in Rochester, NY; a 24-hour on-call service was included; program financed by fee-for-service with regular mechanism for third-party payments, supplemented by grants (e.g., to pay the social workers).	Subjects were homebound, wanted to stay at home, had significant physical illness, and a caregiver to help. Before randomization sample was stratified into terminally ill/nonterminal; ability/inability to answer questionnaires; and being a member of a couple, both of whom were in the study. Measures at baseline, three months, and six months were: health utilization; health status; morale, patient, and caregiver satisfaction; mortality and place of death. N=167, 85 home care and 82 control.	Team patients had fewer hospitalizations, nursing home admissions, and outpatient visits than controls but more emergency room visits. Including costs of home care program, the overall costs of the team patients were less but not statistically so. No differences on functional status or morale, but patients and particularly patients' caregivers were more satisfied with health care received. Further analysis showed that the differences in cost and hospital use were all attributable to the 20% of the sample who were terminally ill.
Groth-Juncker and McCusker (1983)	Home health care team described above in Groth-Juncker, 1982; Zimmer, Groth-Juncker, and McCusker, 1984, 1985	Randomized trial described above. This study examined the first 100 deaths, comparing place of death for the 68 who had expressed preference to die at home and the 32 who had preferred to die away from home.	25 patients died at home, 33 in hospital, and 2 en route to hospital; the longer the period of home care and the more intervening hospital admissions, the more likely the patient was to die away from home; 72% of those who had preferred to die at home got their wish; the others changed their mind or caregivers succumbed to pressures of long illness; pain control not factor in place of death.

TABLE 6-2 Continued

Source	Program Description	Study Design	Selected Findings
Hughes, Cordray, and Spiker (1984)	Hospital-based programs of coordinated health and social services for homebound persons in Chicago area, age 60+, who did not require 24-hour supervision. Services included RN/social worker assessment, home health aide, homemaker/chore, physical therapy, podiatry, lab tests, telephone reassurance, volunteer visiting, and if patient could not travel, MD visits; patients were accepted for maintenance care without prior acute hospitalization.	Quasi-experiment with 122 experimental subjects served by program and control group of 123 clients of AOA Title III program in geographically contiguous area. OARS instrument used; nine month post-test; analysis of covariance used in pre- and post-design. Outcomes included institutionalization, perceived physical well-being, physical activities, receipt of community services, mortality, and costs.	Both experimental and control group members were very old and extremely impaired at baseline. Mortality rate identical for the two groups. Expanded home care associated with increased subjective perception of good health but decreased ADL capacity and increased use of community service. No difference in hospitalization and substantially greater nursing home use for controls (28 controls and 16 experimentals admitted in nine-month period); costs for experimental group were 19.6% higher than for controls; savings realized through less nursing home care and fewer home-delivered meals were offset by high costs of comprehensive home services. Costs for experimental group were skewed by a few high-cost users.

TABLE 6-3 Comparison of Six Home Care Experiments on Selected Parameters

	Experiment (Senior Author)					
Parameter	Katz	Neilson	Selmanoff	Weissert	Groth-Juncker	Hughes
Limited to post-hospital	Yes	Yes	Unspecified	Yes	No	No
Providers	Nurses	Homemakers, aides	Aides with RN and LPN backup	Homemakers	Team with MD and geriatric nurse practitioner included	Team
Targeting	50+, post-rehabilitation	Chronically ill but *not* needing skilled RN	Unspecified	Qualified for skilled home care under Medicare	Seriously and/or terminally ill	Homebound elderly
Sample size	Experimental = 150 Control = 150	Experimental = 50 Control = 50	Experimental = 64 Control = 60	Experimental = 424 Control = 354	Experimental = 82 Control = 76	Experimental = 122 Control = 123
Designed	Randomized	Randomized	Randomized	Randomized	Randomized	Quasi-experimental
Outcomes favoring home care	None	Nursing home use Contentment	Mortality	Mortality Contentment	Hospital use; out-patient department use; Satisfaction of patients and families	Nursing home use Perceived health
Outcomes favoring control group	Hospital use	None	Nursing home use	Cost	Emergency room	Physical function Cost
No significant difference	Mortality, physical function, nursing home use	Mortality, hospital use	Physical function, hospital use	Physical function, hospital use, nursing home use home use, costs	Mortality, physical function, morale, nursing	Mortality, hospital use

This is too small and contradictory a body of experimental work to permit definitive statements. It would be tempting to try to explain troublesome findings; for example, one could argue that the decline in functioning for home care users in the Hughes study was the natural and beneficial result of providing services to those who had previously performed the tasks only poorly and with difficulty and suffering. Sometimes the authors, or later revisionist critics, undertake such explanations. However, advocates tend to be suspicious only of findings that fail to support home care, while accepting the favorable ones. It is probably safer to regard the whole body of evidence as slight indeed.

Table 6-4 presents still more studies of home care. Unlike the experiments just discussed, these nine studies were directed toward narrower questions about the details of home care delivery. They are helpful in examining the art of home care rather than its overall effectiveness. Some of the studies addressed persons under 65 as well as the elderly. Five of the studies explored the merits of reorganizing home care in some way. For example, Lee and Stein (1980) studied the effects of combining the categories of homemaker and home health aide into one job category jointly supervised by a voluntary public health agency and a county welfare department. Albeit an uncontrolled study affecting a small number of clients in a rural area, the results suggested that economies could be achieved by this sensible step. Sparer and colleagues (1983) studied home dialysis programs that trained home health aides to assist with Medicare covered dialysis, compared to randomly selected control programs. This intervention did increase the frequency of home dialysis in the experimental programs, but no differences were found in mortality, hospitalization, or costs. The costs of the home health aides made home dialysis comparable to hospital dialysis in half the experimental facilities.

Jette and his colleagues (1981) did an interesting study in the context of a Massachusetts home care corporation to test whether homemaker services could be "unbundled." In unbundling, the affective and instrumental aspects of the service were separated, and the latter further divided into tasks such as laundry, meals, and cleaning. Concrete services were contracted from private vendors, including cleaners and restaurants, while home companions took care of the affective goals of home care. New clients were randomly assigned to the experimental condition or usual service. No differences were seen in satisfaction or dependability of service, though the experimental group received about 25 minutes more per month in case manager time to arrange the service. This small experiment ($N=44$) is illustrative of the kind of practical questions that can profitably be examined in the context of an operational home care program.

Two of the studies deal directly with a nursing intervention. In an English county where homemaking was already available, Gibbins et al. (1982) piloted an intensive home nursing service for the very seriously ill. Com-

TABLE 6-4 Studies of Specific Aspects of Home Care Effectiveness

Source	Program Description	Study Design	Findings
Lyons and Steele (1977)	Six-week classroom program and six-week on-the-job training combined with classes to train low-income seniors as home health aides for the elderly in Florida.	55 persons who had graduated from the program were mailed questionnaire (with 65% response rate). No comparison group.	Program trainees did *not* get as much employment as they desired nor did they meet earnings expectations. Of 31 who indicated any employment, the average amount of work was 73 hours in the previous month.
Schlenker (1980)	Home Health Grant Program provided grant for development and expansion of home health services. Agencies typically used them to develop skilled nursing and home health aides in unserved or underserved areas. 47 of the 56 agencies receiving grants in 1976 were in designated preference areas based on high percentage of elderly or indigent. Grants were for one or one and one-half years and ranged from $10,000 to $230,000.	56 grants were studied to see if they resulted in more service and to determine ratio of visits to dollars of grant expenditures. Regression analysis to see what factors were associated with successful programs. A matched control group of agencies not receiving grants was used to compare increases in visits in experimental and control programs.	Increase in total visits was about 30% greater for grantees than control agencies; Visiting Nurse Association status was the most important program variable associated with the more productive grantees; grantees in preference areas were less successful than in nonpreference areas, and this was associated in turn with low prevalence of visiting nurse agencies in preference areas.

TABLE 6-4 Studies of Specific Aspects of Home Care Effectiveness

Source	Program Description	Study Design	Findings
Lee and Stein (1980)	The homemaker program at a county welfare department and the home health aide program at a voluntary public health nursing agency jointly set up a demonstration of a homemaker/home health aide to serve clients who would otherwise have had aide service from both agencies; homemakers helped with meds and range of motion exercises.	No control group. Some before-and-after comparison of costs of clients who had previously received service from both agencies.	49 clients served; average age, 75; average frequency, three days a week; after five months, 25 still received services, 10 had goals accomplished, 4 went to nursing homes, and 4 were referred to other agencies. Authors claimed an average saving of $33.86 per client per month compared to receiving both services because the generic worker was paid less than the home health aide and spent less time per week than the sum of the two services.
Jette et al. (1981)	At one of Massachusetts' home care corporations, affective and instrumental services (e.g., housekeeping, laundry, and meal preparation) were separated, and the latter contracted to private vendors, including restaurants and laundries, while companions were hired for the former.	Subjects were 22 new clients needing four or more hours of service per week (N=22); controls were randomly assigned from current clients; evaluation measured client satisfaction after 2–4 months of service, and costs were calculated.	No significant differences between groups in satisfaction over amount of service, worker dependability, concern for client needs, and quality of performance. The experimental group rated their companions highly. The experimental group received an average of 25 minutes more per month in case manager time to coordinate and supervise service.

Gibbins et al. (1982)	A health district in England pilots an intensive nursing care service in addition to existing home helps to keep people at home. Referrals from MDs were reassessed by nurse in consultation with physician; 23 patients received intensive nursing service of 21 or more hours per week; 5 patients received intensive home help as well.	Three groups were followed: 24 people accepted to project; 24 referred but not accepted because too ill or insufficiently dependent; and a control group of 11 hospital patients matched for age and diagnosis. At three months and six months, these groups were compared on ADLs, medications, communication, and temperament.	In six months the program provided 2,500 hours of intensive nursing and 2,560 hours of intensive home help; recipients preferred this to hospital treatment. In only five cases were community costs higher than hospital costs, and had hospital capital cost been included only one case would have been higher.
Sparer et al. (1983)	Home health aides were trained and paid to assist Medicare patients with home dialysis. Family members could also assist, but at half the pay rate. Eight facilities trained aides and eight were controls. N receiving home dialysis at each facility ranged from 45 to 500.	Comparisons were made to see if the incentive increased those accepting home dialysis, did not adversely affect quality of care, and resulted in overall savings.	Frequency of home dialysis increased 160% in two years for experimental facilities and 30% for controls. No differences in hospitalization rates and mortality rates. Cost results mixed, but paying for dialysis aides did bring home dialysis to comparable cost of hospital dialysis in half the experimental facilities.

TABLE 6-4 Studies of Specific Aspects of Home Care Effectiveness

Source	Program Description	Study Design	Findings
Bass and Rowland (1983)	Two home care corporations were studied, one in urban Boston (with 1,400 clients) and one in suburban Boston (630 clients). Services provided were homemaking, shopping, laundry, cleaning, grooming, bathing, meal preparation as ordered by case managers.	A random sample was drawn from the two home care corporations (total N=750). Descriptive data and client satisfaction data were collected through a mailed questionnaire (43% return) and a subset of 200 telephone interviews.	Average age of sample was 78 with 69% in 70–80 age category; 84% were female; 87% lived alone; 57% unable to leave home without help and 16% homebound. Satisfaction was high—42% considered services good and only 4% called them poor; about one-third said they would stop living independently without the services, but 35% said they would try to do the work themselves; two-thirds had received services for 18 months or more—average number of homemakers per client was four and case managers, two; 70% thought the homemaker showed concern for their well-being, and the same percent viewed the homemaker as a friend; 90% said they would file a claim if service was bad. The most valuable services tended to be light cleaning, laundry, changing linen, shopping, bed making, and errands; 76% thought they had the right amount of service and 22% would have liked more; degree of confinement was highly related to service need.

Sager (1983a)	Targets for this study were persons discharged from six Massachusetts hospitals to nursing homes.	Fifty SNF patients were interviewed and assessed regarding their needs at home; family members interviewed regarding their opinions of needs and willingness to supply services; professionals also asked to produce care plans. The costs of the *hypothetical* plans made by the various respondent groups were compared to the costs of present care in the nursing home.	Average cost of institutional care was less than hypothesized home care costs in most cases. Professionals, however, disagreed on plans and when most costly plans were excluded the home care plans became more comparable. Home care most likely to be cost-effective when nursing home care was expensive. Family and patient plans would be less expensive to provide than professionals' plans. The 18 professionals differed, particularly in personal care and homemaking prescriptions. Those who saw the patients prescribed more service than those who just reviewed assessment data. Families and patients sought less paid help then professionals.
Lind (1984)	Clients ready for discharge from VNA received one of two follow-up interventions: monthly monitoring visits from RNs or monthly telephone reassurance by volunteers who referred clients to RNs as needed. N=261.	Random assignment was made to the two interventions. One-year follow-up on mortality, rehospitalization, and return to regular VNA service. Only 50% of sample was 65+.	No statistically significant differences but monitored group had less rehospitalization and fewer hospital days than the telephone group; more of the monitored group was returned to active nursing. The subgroup of patients that returned to the hospital or to regular VNA service after 1–2 monitoring visits had longer lengths of stay and higher mortality rates than the other patients.

pared to matched controls, the care of patients in the program seemed less expensive and the clients definitely preferred to stay at home. Not all those getting intensive home nursing also needed intensive homemaking because family sometimes provided that service. Lind (1984) experimented with two kinds of follow-up for patients discharged from a Visiting Nurse Association: monthly telephone reassurance from volunteers (who referred to RNs if it seemed needed) and monthly monitoring by RNs. No significant differences were found on mortality, rehospitalization, or return to regular VNA services. Unfortunately, no central group that received any follow-up at all was included.

Two quite different studies examined preferences and values related to home care. Bass and Rowland (1983) studied a large random sample of clients of two Massachusetts home care corporations. Satisfaction with the services was high. Interestingly, about one-third stated they would stop living independently without the home care services, but a similar proportion said they would try to do the work themselves. It would be intriguing to better understand the differences between those two groups, but one is still left to interpret the policy implications. The knowledge that a third of the sample would have tried to do the homemaking themselves if the service were withdrawn should not be used to suggest that they were inappropriately receiving care. The study sample was extremely frail (almost 70% were between 70 and 80, 57% were unable to leave home without help, and 16% were completely homebound). The other study of values was in the hypothetical realm (Sager, 1983a). Patients about to leave the hospital were assessed regarding their home care needs by members of different disciplines. The clients and their families were also asked their views of the needs, and the latter were asked how much service they would provide. Professionals differed in the care plans they devised, and, on the whole, families and clients produced plans that would be less expensive to implement than those of the professionals.

The last two studies are rather different. Schlenker (1980) looked at the value of federal grants awarded to stimulate the development of home care in unserved or underserved areas. On the whole grantee agencies did increase visits more than control agencies, but the most important factor associated with productivity was status as a visiting nursing agency. Finally, Lyons and Steele (1977) did a follow-up of a program to train low-income persons as home health aides for Florida seniors. The disappointing result was that trainees were unable to establish viable careers in the home health field.

A major national demonstration linking expanded home care for the elderly to employment of welfare recipients began in 1982 (Orr, Williams, and Bell, 1984). This multi-state demonstration project—the AFDC Homemaker-Home Health Aide Demonstration—trained AFDC recipients as home health aides and assigned them to low-income seniors at risk of

nursing home admission. On the one hand, the study te~~s~~
recipients could move to economic independence throu~~gh~~
other hand, it tested whether seniors receiving an ex~~p~~
aide and homemaking benefit would have reduced a~~d~~
homes. Both the AFDC recipients and the elderly
randomized into experimental and control groups, making this doub~~le~~ ~~~~
quite rigorous. Results of this study are not yet available, but early specula-
tion suggests that the effects will be positive for the AFDC recipients but
minimal for the elderly.

After a comprehensive search and using generous inclusion rules, we
identified relatively few empirical studies of home care for the elderly.
Undoubtedly more studies are needed, including more of the practical kind
that asks questions about how to make home care better or more efficient.
The paucity of that latter kind of study may reflect our slowness to accept
home care in principle and our continuing preoccupation with first proving
that it can substitute for nursing home care.

Home care is the centerpiece of all the demonstration projects that
attempt to show that an array of community services, mediated by a case
manager, can substitute for nursing home care. Some of the most thoughtful
study has been devoted to that question, which we shall return to in Chapter
10.

PROBLEMS IN EVALUATING DAY CARE

Adult day care presents evaluation problems similar to home care. The
intervention is diffuse, designed to serve varying populations and achieve
miscellaneous goals. For example, day care is sometimes expected to meet
specific rehabilitation goals or at least to improve or maintain overall
functioning; at other times it is expected to enhance social involvement or
alleviate depression. Respite for caregivers is also a goal, at times even
including sufficient relief to allow a family member to remain employed. But
despite all these objectives, day care is even less developed than home care in
the United States, and the evidence of its effects is even scanter.

For our purposes, adult day care is long-term care services provided in an
outpatient setting to which clients are transported. Usually the transportation is an integral part of the program, though sometimes clients and
families arrange it themselves. Under many arrangements clients may spend
an inordinate proportion of the day being transported to and from day care.

Like home care, adult day care is often separated into medically oriented
"day health programs" and programs loosely called "social day care."
Adult day care differs from nursing home care in that it is offered only for a
limited time during the day. It differs from senior centers in that the
activities are prescribed for the participant on the basis of an initial assess-

nt. Providers include hospitals, nursing homes, social agencies, and freestanding day care centers established by voluntary groups such as churches.

The boundaries between day health and social day care are imprecise. Some day services provided in hospitals also entail meals and recreational activities, whereas day care under social services auspices can include varying degrees of health services and personal care. Day care programming is a "black box" that has been filled in many ways. However, adult day care covered by Medicaid usually must meet staffing specifications that put it squarely in the health camp.

Views about day care in the United States have been influenced by programs in Great Britain. There, the day hospital is an integral part of geriatric services in most regions of the country. Typically a hospital-based geriatrician has a number of inpatient beds for geriatric assessment and short- and long-term rehabilitation. In this context, a day hospital program allows patients to be brought to the hospital during the day for further diagnosis and observation, and to receive therapies. The day hospital also permits discharge from hospital to the day program as an intermediate step. Although the British day hospital has not been rigorously evaluated, it is viewed with an enthusiasm that has been contagious to visitors from abroad. In Britain, separate psychogeriatric day hospitals have been developed that combine diagnostic work and skilled custodial care. Social day care is also available in England under the management of local social services authorities.

The British day hospital model unfortunately translates poorly into the United States context. When superimposed on a well-staffed geriatric unit with medical and other therapists available, the day hospital has a potential for integration with acute medical care that is diminished if the adult day health programs are freestanding or located in nursing homes. Day health care centers in the United States, similar to the British example, tend to serve clients for an abbreviated day and a limited number of days per week, but they seldom are tied to clear therapeutic goals or provision of medical care. Furthermore, in the United States, day care programs tend to merge the demented into regular programs, thereby surely diminishing the pleasure of the experience for both the cognitively impaired and the cognitively intact.

Choosing the appropriate outcomes for day care is particularly challenging. If the intervention is tailored to the individual client, some goal attainment measures might be used. Functional measures are most appropriate in a rehabilitation context. Measures of psychological and social well-being may at times be reasonable. More so than with home care, day care is expected to have a direct impact on family caregivers. However, we located no studies where the caregiver's work experience was measured directly, and when family factors were examined, they were usually considered as factors associated with successful day care rather than as outcomes in themselves. Some studies discussed below described "closed cases" as outcomes, hinting that a discharge from day care to the community is a positive result. However, given the repeated theme of consumer dissatisfaction with day care, such a result may represent mere dropout.

Using information generated in the 1970s, Palmer (1983) reviewed day care in the United States. He judged that Massachusetts then had the largest systematic program, which began receiving Medicaid coverage in 1975 and was serving more than 800 clients at 45 sites by 1979. Program guidelines required a 1:6 staff-to-patient ratio, a 2-person minimum staff, and a registered nurse 4 hours a day. Palmer cited 1978 data that showed about 360 new admissions that year, 52% from hospitals or nursing homes and 50% impaired in four of eight ADL categories. Forty percent lived alone. In Massachusetts adult day care was used in conjunction with home health or homemaking services by about half the clientele. In 1978, 37% of the discharges went to institutions and 42% went home. However, the latter figure does not connote improvement in all cases. Some were discharged because of anxiety about travel in winter, some were disruptive in the program, and some ran out of Medicaid and could not afford private coverage. Of the 42% discharged to the community, 40% were referred to home health, 10% to mental health clinics, and 5% to congregate housing.

EFFECTS OF DAY CARE PROGRAMS

Descriptive Studies

Table 6-5 summarizes 11 descriptive studies of day care. Four of the studies examined program-specific data, and the remainder presented data on clients themselves. Two of the latter studies attempted to identify factors associated with dropping out of day care.

Weissert (1975) did one of the earliest examinations of day care programs. Limited to ten programs, the study developed distinctions between health-oriented day care and other, more socially oriented programs. The per diem costs of the programs exceeded nursing home costs, so, to be a cost-effective substitute, the day care would need to be offered only a few times a week. Similarly, Hannan and O'Donnell (1984) examined a small number of day care programs in New York State, dividing them into health-oriented programs, supportive programs, and a mixed group.

Weiler, Fine, and Reid (1982) looked specifically at the Adult Day Health Care programs in California, polling a variety of providers and knowledgeable citizens to find out why the programs expanded at such a disappointing pace after they became eligible for Medicaid funding in 1978. The authors indicted the stringent requirements for countywide planning, licensure, high staffing levels, and frequent reporting as culprits. In particular, reimbursement policies did not allow for the likelihood of running under capacity at

TABLE 6-5 Descriptive Studies of Adult Day Care

Source	Program Description	Study Design	Findings
Weissert (1975)	Ten adult day care programs; selection universe unclear but programs were meant to vary in affiliation, size, location, ethnicity of clientele, and single site versus multisite programs.	Comparative descriptive study of ten adult day care centers to develop models of day care and to consider cost-effectiveness.	Author derived a two-fold classification: a physical rehabilitation model and a social model, the latter having a potpourri of interventions. The programs studied varied in every respect including history, admission criteria, intake procedures, staffing patterns, services rendered, sources of support, and costs. The author suggested that the health model may serve persons who would otherwise be in institutions. Day care was more expensive than institutional care on a per diem basis and, therefore, would be likely to be cost-effective only if used sparingly and if other community services were used sparingly too.
Chappell (1982) Chappell (1984) Strain and Chappell (1980)	A provincially funded adult day care (ADC) program, begun in Manitoba in 1979, provided planned and supervised recreation and	No controls. 126 clients, 50+, were measured at the beginning of ADC, at four months, and at one year on variables such as physical,	Changes in functional and mental disability reached statistical significance only in the period between the fourth month and final interviews, whereas changes in life satisfaction

	socialization for clients on a 1 to 2 day-per-week basis. Objectives include relief to the family, prevention of premature institutionalization, minimization of the incidence of emotional and physical disability, early detection and assessment of illness.	mental, social functioning; life satisfaction; services utilization. Further analysis attempted to determine factors which, upon admission to ADC (e.g., demographics, physical and mental condition, utilization of the program), predicted improvement or deterioration in mental and physical functioning.	and social integration occurred mainly in the first four months of the program. ADC had the most positive impact on physical functioning for those who live alone or with few relatives; on mental functioning, for those who were still married.
Weiler, Fine, and Reid (1982)	Nonprofit adult day health care (ADHC) programs reimbursable by Medicaid in California. A law passed in 1978 covered day care but required a countywide plan for licensing of all programs and stringent staffing and reporting requirements. Five years later only 25 programs were in place statewide serving about 1,000 people with an 18% closure rate over the period. Of 58 counties, 47 had no adult day health programs and 37 had no plan.	Study focused on problems of implementation, surveying four groups: adult day health care (ADHC) administrators, ADHC potential providers, staff to ADHC planning counsels, and knowledgeable persons in counties with no planning counsels. No consumer survey was done.	Reimbursement policies deterred development of ADHC, insistence on countywide planning was dysfunctional, start-up grants would have been helpful; unpredictable daily census made planning difficult; reimbursement policies did not allow for client vacation or for payment for nursing home residents being weaned from institution.

TABLE 6-5 Continued

Source	Program Description	Study Design	Findings
Arling, Harkins, and Romaniuk (1984)	Ten adult day centers in Virginia. All programs offered transportation, noon meals, personal care, reality orientation, ADL supervision, and recreation. Some provided occupational and physical therapy.	116 clients were interviewed (40% of total). Clients were compared to persons screened in the preadmission program and approved for nursing home care, and to persons screened in the preadmission program and found ineligible for nursing home care.	Day care clients and other two groups were similar in age, sex, race, marital status, and number of living children. They were significantly less likely to live alone or with nonrelatives, were more educated, had higher incomes. Mental status and self-reported health was similar for all groups, but day care clients had much less hospital use and significantly greater vision and hearing problems than both nursing home group screening groups, and significantly greater ADL dependency than those accepted for nursing homes. Findings do not support authors' summary that nursing home applicants are so similar to day care users that many of them might be better served by day care.
Cohen (1984)	A 1982 grant for Adult Residential Day Care allowed Mountain States Health Corporation in Boise, ID to train unemployed community residents to provide adult	Descriptive information on clients and their providers.	40 unemployed persons were trained as caregivers, but three-quarters dropped out. The project was difficult to implement; 36 clients were served but it took a year to get a caseload of 8 and 1½ years to get

day care in their own homes. A geriatric nurse practitioner/social work team selected and trained providers, selected users, and acted as case managers for the clients. Eligible clients were age 70+, living alone, had complex care needs, diagnosis of depression, two admissions to hospital in the year, noncompliance with medications, and were lifeline clients, and/or "borderline ICF eligible."

12. The program underestimated the number of persons meeting the criteria who "refused to leave home for day care." Over 60% of the clientele ended up being served *in the client's home* instead of in day care.

Hannan and O'Donnell (1984)

Fifteen day care programs in New York state compared; further selection criteria unclear.

Day care programs were surveyed for information on their clientele (demography and impairments); 1980 cost data from Medicaid statistics were used; comparison data on characteristics of residents of ICFs were taken from New York State Health Department. For analysis, day care programs were divided into health-oriented programs, supportive programs, and mixed.

The health-oriented programs had much higher hourly costs (an average of $9.19 compared to $2.74 in the supportive programs), with transportation contributing more than one-fourth of the costs. The clients of the supportive and the mixed programs had higher levels of impairment than ICF residents and higher proportions of public-pay clients.

TABLE 6-5 Continued

Source	Program Description	Study Design	Findings
Mace and Rabins (1984)	Adult day care centers nationally that served one or more clients with senile dementia.	980 centers on a 1983 list (believed complete) were polled, and 444 (45%) responded that they served demented clients; 78% of that group returned usable questionnaires asking them about their clientele, programs, and outcomes. Data provided by programs were estimates only, and many findings are aggregated by program rather than client.	The 346 centers served an estimated 10,000–15,000 clients, 2,000–3,000 demented. Most centers served a mixture of demented and nondemented. No relationship between percentage of demented clients and average length of stay. Centers serving greater proportions of demented were open longer hours less likely to make home visits, more likely to have groups for families, had more impaired demented clients, and reported costs near the mean ($20 a day) compared to higher or lower costs in facilities with a lower proportion of demented. Easier access to physicians encouraged centers to admit demented clients. Respondents believed they had beneficial effects on the functioning of the day care clients.
Morales-Martinez, Carpenter, and Williamson (1984)	A geriatric day hospital at City Hospital in Edinburgh, Scotland, serves persons 65+ in a defined geographic area with a population of 20,000 age 65+. The 30-	All persons admitted to day hospital in the six months from August 1981 to January 1982 were included in the study and followed until July 1982, making a mini-	One-third of the patients were referred from the acute geriatric assessment ward, and almost all the rest from GPs; 22% were one-time attendees who were dropped from follow-up analyses. Of the 260 remain-

Reference	Setting	Sample / Method	Findings
	place day hospital is located close to the admission ward of the hospital. Referrals are encouraged from general practitioners and families. Complete medical and therapeutic services are available, and most patients are transported by ambulance.	mum of six months follow-up. (N=334, including 239 females and 95 males.)	ing patients; about 70% attended weekly and 24% twice weekly; 104 were short-term attenders (2–6 times), 56 were medium-attenders (7 or more), 63 were in the current caseload at the beginning of the study, and 37 were planned as "chronic attenders" until death or rehospitalization. At the end of the study period, 63% of short-termers, 41% of medium-termers, and 52% of the current caseload had been discharged home; mortality ranged from 14% of short-termers to 22% of the current attenders, and long-term institutional case ranged from 13% of the short-termers to 16% of the medium termers. Of the 37 chronic attenders, 5 died and 6 went into long-term placement; only 7 people from the other categories become chronic attenders.
Barresi and McConnell (1984)	A day care center in a rural Ohio county.	An impaired group of day care attendees (N=35) was compared to an impaired group in the community (N=93) who did not attend day care, using a modified OARS instrument.	Day care attendees were more likely to be female, without spouse (widowed, divorced, or never married), living with others, with higher incomes, cognitively impaired, and emotionally undisturbed.

TABLE 6-5 Continued

Source	Program Description	Study Design	Findings
Rinehart (1984)	New York Service Program for Older People, Inc., a freestanding mental health clinic, utilizes an activity therapy model in its ADC program, incorporating creative arts therapy, socialization, verbal therapy, etc. Most persons enrolled in the program have prior psychiatric hospitalization.	The author reviewed patient characteristics to determine if any were disproportionately related to patterns of attendance. No parametric tests were used. The variables were sex, age, ethnicity, income, living arrangement, home care, psychiatric diagnosis, psychiatric hospitalization history. The subjects were the 70 participants enrolled between September 1980 and December 1983.	The only characteristics that appeared related to low attendence were living alone and receiving home care services. Only 29% of those participating more than 12 months received home care services in contrast to 66% who participated for less than three months.
Wallace (1984)	A study of the records of 177 participants of a local adult day care center to determine the characteristics of those who leave the program before treatment goals are reached. The participants were 50+, had an average of 2.1 medical problems and 1.3 psychological problems. Most had been referred to ADC for reasons of socialization or caregiver respite.	35 factors, taken from client records, were entered into a stepwise regression analysis to determine the characteristics related to program attrition. These factors included sex, age, attendance, medical problems, referral reasons, supporting systems, living arrangements, source of funding, reasons for termination.	The significant variables, in order of impact, were lack of external funding, sex (female), number of days scheduled (the greater the number of days, the higher the attendance). Also, those participants who had been referred to the program in order to prevent institutionalization or to relieve caregiver stress remained in the program longer.

| Gilleard (1985) | Four psychogeriatric day hospitals in Scotland (two urban and two rural) linked to psychiatric hospitals. | 129 first-time referrals between July 1981 and July 1982 who had a family supporter living with them or visiting at least three times a week were included. Outcomes examined in six months. Sample reduced to 69 by then because of death or missing data. Analysis done to predict what factors related to the family caregiver, the day care service, or the client predicted service status outcome (i.e., still attending day care, ceased attending but living at home, or living in an institution). | Small sample, sample loss, and lack of theoretical framework make findings questionable. Major self-care impairment, a high level of professional care, and poor premorbid relationship of patient and family caregiver independently contributed to entry in an LTC facility; low level of self-care impairment, low professional input, and good premorbid relationship predicted leaving day care and staying home; poor health care and staying home; absence of anticipated disadvantages of staying home, continence in the dependent person, and family help were associated with staying in day care, and the reverse (good health in the supporter, absence of anticipated disadvantages in the day hospital, an incontinent patient, and lack of other family help) were associated with keeping the person at home. Levels of strain and distress in supporters were not associated with the outcomes. |

153

the outset of the program. They did not poll consumers nor entertain the possibility that the product was inadequately meeting consumer's needs.

Proponents of California's law expected many more than 1,000 Medicaid day health care users by the time the program was five years old, but the basis for the estimates of the likely need were unclear and seemingly excessive.

In an appendix on that topic, Weiler and his colleagues stated that originally planners assumed that as many as 31 places per 1,000 persons over 65 might be needed (based on at least one person outside a nursing home of equal impairment to those inside and a formula of 1.6 persons served per ADHC place). Using more conservative estimations that only 25% of the target group of persons at risk of nursing home admission would be willing to use day care, Capitman (1982) suggested a ratio of 7.75 places per 1,000 persons over 65. By comparison, Great Britain advances lower ratios for health oriented day care, namely 2 places of day hospital per 1,000 in the population over age 65 and 2 to 3 psychogeriatric day care places for the demented. The California experience involved "thinking big" and then finding that counties were not implementing programs and that those that were implemented were underutilized.

The final study of programs concentrated on those day care programs in the United States that served one or more persons with senile dementia. Mace and Rabins (1984) polled a sample of almost 400 such programs. The information gathered is somewhat limited by the reliance on imprecise information from the employees who filled out the questionnaire. It did suggest that most day care serving the demented does so in programs integrated with other clients and that the respondents believed they were achieving therapeutic gains.

The descriptive studies using client data were largely inconclusive. A Virginia study compared day care users to applicants for nursing homes who were screened by the state's preadmission screening program, dividing the latter into those approved for placement and those denied. The day care group was more educated, more well-to-do, and less impaired than both comparison groups, especially those approved for nursing homes (Arling, Harkins, and Romaniuk, 1984). Similarly, a comparison of impaired elderly who attended and did not attend a day care program in an Ohio county found that the day care attendees were more likely to be younger, live with others, have no spouse or confidante, have more income, and be more disoriented, but have fewer emotional disturbances (Barresi and McConnell, 1984). Looking at psychogeriatric day hospitals in Scotland, Gilleard (1985) tried to determine client, caregiver, and programmatic characteristics associated with whether the client remained in day care, left day care but remained in the community, or went to an institution. In this example, interpreting the results as a positive or negative reflection on day care is impossible. In contrast, the analysis by Morales-Martinez, Carpenter, and

Williamson (1984) presented a year's worth of follow-up data from a well-established geriatric day hospital in Edinburgh. It illustrated how a stable service might look when the day care is well integrated with health care. Many clients were served with relatively few visits and short lengths of stays, and, at any given time, the group of clients expected to attend indefinitely remained a manageable size. The biggest samples come from the Manitoba studies where day care clientele were followed longitudinally (Chappell, 1982, 1984). The greatest gains in concomitant reduction in use of other health services seem to have occurred within the first months of day care, with fewer further gains at the one-year followup.

Demoralizing results come from an Idaho demonstration project that trained unemployed persons to give adult day care in their homes (Cohen, 1984). The rationale was that seniors would get individualized attention in private homes, and close, rewarding relationships would ensue. In fact, the authors stated they were "taken off guard" by the unwillingness of the seniors who met their eligibility criteria to leave their own homes for day care. Eventually, most of the caregivers came to the home of the older person, so the day care became converted to home care or home companionship.

Two studies looked specifically at factors associated with poor attendance patterns. In a psychogeriatric setting, Rinehart (1984) found an association between poor attendance and both living alone and receiving home care service. Wallace (1984) looked for characteristics associated with leaving the program before treatment goals were reached; in rank order, the important variables were lack of third-party payment, sex (female), and number of days scheduled (those scheduled for a higher number of days were more likely to remain in the program). Other suggestive ideas about program attendance come from a less research-oriented report on a single program in Virginia followed through its three-year history (Hackman, 1978). Daily attendance averaged about 40 persons although the quota was 60. The author generalized the following lessons: Transportation was crucial; clients living alone had nobody to get them ready for the bus; a special bus was needed; most clients were wary and reluctant at the outset; a medical examination at admission was important; and more community education about day care was needed.

Studies of Effectiveness

Table 6-6 shows eight experiments and quasi-experiments examining the effects of day care. Only two of the studies included (Weissert et al., 1980a; Cummings et al., 1980) were randomized experiments, and the latter included subjects under 65. Two were basically before-and-after studies where the clients served as their own controls (Oster and Kibat, 1975; Chappell, 1984). Gurland and Mann (1982) compared their sample to

TABLE 6-6 Experiments or Quasi-Experiments on Adult Day Care

Source	Description of Program or Study	Study Design	Selected Findings
Oster and Kibat (1975)	The Stroke Day Care Center, instituted in 1972 by St. Martin Place Hospital, Madison Heights, MI, provided comprehensive day care to patients with stroke or related disabilities. Services included rehabilitative medical care, cardiology, neurology, physical and occupational therapy, speech therapy, social services, nutrition, transportation. The major goal of the demonstration was to test the feasibility of lowering the costs of patient stroke care.	Data on 108 day care patients treated over a 1½ year period (1972–73) were compared to the hospital records of all stroke patients one year before the project began, using the Center's admission criteria. The patients ranged in age from 25 to 81, with an average age of 47.	There appeared to be a slight decrease in the length of hospitalization and hospital care costs for the day care patients, but it was not statistically significant. Note: Mean age was 47.
Rathbone-McCuan et al. (1975) Described in Weiler and Rathbone-McCuan (1978).	Adult day care program based on Levindale Home for the Aged in Baltimore. Day care was organized according to a therapeutic model.	Day care users were compared to three comparison groups: a community apartment group, a social agency clientele group, and a group of institutional residents. Improvement or maintenance of functioning was the major outcome variable.	Authors reported that day care clients compared favorably to comparison groups on maintenance or improvement of functioning and that costs were overwhelmingly less. Study is flawed because comparison groups were uncomparable on need for improvement, and much judgment was used.

Study	Description	Results
Weiler, Kim, and Pickard (1976)	Freestanding day care programs (called Centers for Creative Living) sponsored by the local health department in Lexington, KY. Care given according to a therapeutic model.	31 clients of the day care program were compared to 35 control group clients on the waiting list for day care.	Participants improved or maintained physical and mental health compared to the controls, but the controls had greater ADL and IADL independence (66% of the controls improved in functioning compared to 36% of the day care group).
Cummings et al. (1980)	A rehabilitaton program based in a hospital targeted at persons with strokes, amputations, and other disabilities (but not recent spinal cord injuries), with third-party coverage and a responsible person living in the home; intensive program with five-days-per-week attendance and a wide range of therapies offered (including physical and occupational therapy, psychological services, radiology, speech therapy, chemotherapy, nuclear medicine). Clientele not limited to elderly.	96 patients were enrolled in the study and randomized to day care or inpatient rehabilitation. Outcomes measured included ADL, IADL, cognitive functioning, acceptance of disability, psychological well-being, and cost.	Experimental group made more use of intraprogram services, did better in locomotion and transfers (but not other ADLs), and required more assistance from families. No difference found in medical status, mental status, psychological well-being, adjustment to disability, or IADL. Absolute costs of day care were greater before adjustments based on "research costs" and occupancy rate of day care; after adjustment, day care was less expensive.

TABLE 6-6 Continued

Source	Description of Program or Study	Study Design	Selected Findings
Weissert et al. (1980a)	Four nonrandomly selected day care programs (White Plains and Syracuse, NY; Lexington, KY; San Francisco, CA) were analyzed in this study. The programs (1975–77) had health care and therapeutic capabilities, providing nursing, podiatry, patient activities, social services, personal care, nutrition, meals, transportation, physical therapy, eye and hearing exams. Clients were eligible for skilled services under Medicare. Most were referred from community service agencies and hospitals.	Medicare recipients were randomly assigned to day care coverage or control group, and assessed at baseline as well as quarterly in a 12-month period. Instruments include Katz's ADL Scale, a mental status questionnaire, a contentment and a social activity scale. Data were collected on costs and service use from sources such as Medicare billing records and client interviews. Analysis controlled for background variables and a multi-stage comparison was made between controls and experimentals.	The only significant difference was a positive impact on mortality. When baseline differences were controlled there was no significant impact on ADL function or institutionalization. Hospital and nursing home costs were lower for the experimentals, but when day care costs were added, the experimentals averaged $2,692 more per year than the controls. For a significant portion of the day care group, day care appeared to serve as an additional rather than substitutional benefit.

Capitman (1982)	The California Adult Day Health Program supported, through Medi-Cal benefits, 24 ADHC centers in 11 counties (1982). The centers were staffed with medical, nursing, and social service personnel to provide a comprehensive package of health maintenance, personal care, and psychosocial services. The program was designed to substitute for institutional care as well as prevent the need for such care. Participants averaged 12–13 days of ADHC attendance per month.	A single sample test-retest design involving 297 ADCH participants (April 1980–March 1981) was used to measure factors such as functional change, delivery of services, mortality rates, institutional diversion; consumers and families were polled for satisfaction. The cost of the same care at home was estimated and comparisons drawn.	More then 87% of the sample, whose members had severe impairments, maintained or improved their level of ADL and psychosocial functioning. The mortality rate was 12% (12-month period). Participants gave the program an overwhelming positive rating; caregivers viewed it as a source of respite, a support for home care efforts, and an opportunity for involvement in the health care system. The estimated cost to deliver the same services at home was about $700, more than twice the monthly ADHC costs per client.
Gurland and Mann (1982)	Participants at two-day treatment centers in New York were compared with ICF/SNF patients to determine if equivalently frail older people are treated as effectively in day facilities as in nursing homes. The programs were attached to nursing homes and specialized in rehabilitative therapists and medical services. Similar but more extensive comparisons were made in London.	In New York, 63 subjects, 21 from each of three settings (day treatment, ICF, SNF) were matched by level of ADL dependence and intellectual impairment. Extremely impaired elders were excluded. Measurement scales from the Comprehensive Assessment and Referral Evaluation (CARE) were used. Subjects were reassessed nine months later (1979). Similar comparisons in London included day centers as well as hospitals.	In New York, fewer day treatment center patients than nursing home residents declined in ADL functioning (18% vs. 44%); this was also the case in intellectual functioning (15% vs. 34%). Results were not significant due to the small sample size but at least suggest that day treatment is at least as effective as nursing home care for those with moderate disabilities. Differences in mortality rates were also not significant. In London there were similar findings, although results were more uneven across settings.

TABLE 6-6 Continued

Source	Description of Program or Study	Study Design	Selected Findings
Chappell (1982, 1984)	A provincially funded adult day care program, begun in Manitoba in 1979, provides planned and supervised recreation and socialization for clients on a 1- to 2-days-per-week basis. Objectives include relief to family members, prevention of premature institutionalization, minimization of the incidence of emotional and physical disability, early detection and assessment of illness.	Manitoba Health Services Commission records were reviewed on 360 ADC participants at one year prior to and one year following admission to the program. Comparisons included the analysis of total medical services and types of services/medical visits.	Significantly more participants showed a decrease in total health services, although the change per individual was not large. Types of visits showing a significant decrease were physician office visits, consultations, laboratory services, miscellaneous category. Such changes may reflect increased monitoring and socialization at ADC, although the lack of controls make this speculative.

nursing home users. Oster and Kibat made comparisons to hospital patients, Rathbone-McCuan and her colleagues (reported in Weiler and Rathbone-McCuan, 1978) compared the day care to three community samples, and Weiler, Kim and Pickard (1976) used those on the waiting list for day care as the comparison group. With the exception of the Manitoba program described by Chappell, all the day care studied was oriented toward providing health-related service.

Capitman's study (1982) examined almost 300 users of the California adult day health care centers discussed previously. He reported improvement in ADL and psychosocial functioning, and overwhelming satisfaction with the program from consumers and their family caregivers. He estimated that giving such services at home would have cost twice as much. The Manitoba study went beyond estimates to review Health Services Commission records for a group of 360 day care clients one year before entering the program and one year following entry. Using these complete records of health care utilization they found that participants showed a significant decrease in the use of total health services, particularly physician office visits and consultations, and laboratory costs in the year following admission to day care. Both studies using institutional controls found differences favoring the experimental group, but none reached statistical significance. Among the quasi-experiments with community controls, Rathbone-McCuan and colleagues (1975, reported in Weiler and Rathbone-McCuan, 1978) found that the day care clients improved or maintained functioning better and cost less than the controls, but the study leaves methodological questions. The Weiler, Kim, and Pickard (1976) study found that the 31 day care clients compared favorably in physical and mental health to the waiting list controls but that the control group had greater ADL and IADL independence.

The study by Weissert and his colleagues (1980b) is the major experiment in day care done in the United States. It was conducted under the same experimental Medicare authority as the Weissert homemaking studies discussed earlier in the chapter. Therefore, clients needed to meet the Medicare requirements for skilled care before being randomized to the day care benefit, and costs were calculated only in terms of Medicare costs. The average number of days of attendance in day care was 70 for the study year, but one-fourth of those assigned the day care benefit did not use it at all. Day care participants used less inpatient hospital services than controls and had fewer nursing home days and nursing home admissions, but after controlling for baseline characteristics, the differences were not significant. The experimental group experienced lower nursing home and hospital costs, but when costs of day care were added, the day care group averaged almost $2,700 more per year than the controls. Only about one-fifth of the controls used nursing home services during the study year, leaving the author to conclude that day care was an additional benefit rather than a substitute for nursing homes.

Because day care has so many advocates and the Weissert study was so disappointing, it has been sharply criticized. Weiler (1980) complained that it compared those assigned the benefit to those not assigned the benefit despite a non-use rate of 25%. He added that Medicaid costs should have been examined as well as Medicare costs, since most publicly purchased nursing home care falls under that program. Other critics (Zawadski, 1980; Klapfish, 1980) complained that the four day care sites were more expensive than the average program in the country.

A randomized experiment testing the effect of day care in reducing nursing home use is underway in four Veterans Administration Hospitals (Hedrick, 1985). Until these results become available, the Weissert study remains the major experiment. In some ways, it is unfortunate that the most rigorous study of day care carried with it all the constraints of a Medicare demonstration. Still the lack of clarity about day care goals would have made any test rather difficult. And the cumulative information about day care, at least in the United States, suggests that the formula has not yet been found that makes day care attractive to the large number of potential users. It seems that those who do stay with the programs are enthusiastic, but many fall by the wayside. The inconveniences of transportation, the difficulty in getting mobilized, and perhaps even a preference for privacy and companionship of one's choice probably all help account for the resistance. The expense in relation to the perceived benefit is probably also a factor for those without coverage by third parties, but experiences like that in California or Idaho suggest that financial coverage is not sufficient to attract clientele.

It is surely inappropriate to insist that clients adapt to day care services (especially as they seem expensive). Rather the evidence seems to suggest that day care programs need retooling, including greater consideration of desirable programs for specific target groups, and perhaps, for the health-oriented programs at least, a clearer integration into an overall health care and rehabilitation plan.

In summary, both home care and day care are attractive programs conceptually. Both offer a mechanism to address a strong client preference—staying in the community. They remain relatively untested and vaguely defined. In different contexts, they address a varied set of objectives from rehabilitation to respite care. As part of a total community long-term care strategy they need to be carefully focused and well targeted. Moreover, presently available evidence makes day care a much less certain investment than home care.

7

Other Community Long-Term Care Services

This chapter reviews evidence about services (other than home care and day care) that have been organized as part of community long-term care efforts. Ten kinds of services have prompted enough research and discussion to generate at least a simple summary table:

- Congregate and home delivered meals,
- Adult foster care,
- Respite care,
- Supportive programs for family caregivers,
- Volunteer programs,
- Geriatric assessment services/units,
- Hospice,
- Mental health programs for the elderly,
- Protective social services,
- Housing and home maintenance/repair.

Several other programs—notably transportation, telephone reassurance, and emergency alarm systems—are also components of long-term care, but we could uncover even less evidence about their effects.

As a classification system, this listing is miserably deficient. The topics overlap and defy precise definition. Some modify, refine, or are contained within home care, the subject of the last chapter. For example, hospice and respite care are often provided by home care personnel. Some, such as supportive programs for family caregivers and mental health programs, can be offered to people living in long-term care facilities as well as in the community. Some entries on the list technically fall outside long-term care, such as protective social services, mental health programs, and geriatric assessment units, which fall under acute care. Although geriatric assessment units are best categorized as part of health care because the intervention is brief and occurs in an acute setting, in our view, an adequate functional and health assessment that includes physical functioning is a prerequisite for an effective long-term care system. Similarly, housing in the sense of bricks and mortar is not long-term care, but services provided within congregate housing, programs to equip or modify housing for the disabled, or even programs facilitating home-sharing are usually considered long-term care. Hospice is organized as a Medicare benefit, thus putting it in the orbit of the acute care sector, yet the services are that peculiar blend of long-term health, personal care and social services that is the quintessence of long-term care.

In fact, our list is a reflection of the piecework and patchwork of long-term care. It also illustrates the confusing programmatic boundaries of long-term care services. Most of the ten services are numbered among the community programs that may be financed through Medicaid waivers for community care to prevent nursing home use. In particular, home delivered meals, adult foster care, respite care, and home modification join home nursing, homemaking, and adult day care as services sometimes offered under waivers. Transportation, another potentially waivered service, has inspired almost no relevant research to determine its contribution (Bell and Revis, 1983).

Case management could have been added to the list. It too is permitted under Medicaid waivers, and some form of case management or coordination of services has formed a part of almost every waiver application. We reserve our discussion of case management until Chapter 10, where we discuss systematic approaches to improving long-term care for a client group or a community. This organization is not entirely arbitrary. We view case management as a promising and perhaps an essential mechanism to govern access to long-term care services rather than a service in its own right.

CONGREGATE AND HOME-DELIVERED MEALS

Functional impairment may interfere with purchasing, preparing, or even eating meals. Home-delivered meals are one solution to the first two problems. (Alternatively, a homemaker could prepare one or more daily meals while in the home.) Congregate meals—that is, meals taken at a central place—typically serve a less frail population and offer social activities as well as nutritionally sound noon meals.

As presently organized under Older Americans Act funds, congregate meals probably should not be considered long-term care. The population served is rarely functionally impaired. Referring to research done in the 1970s and earlier, Tobin (1978) pointed out that meal programs that seek out an especially impaired group may lose their hardier clientele. Therefore a program that totes up a large number of "meals served" may be less well targeted to the severely impaired than one serving fewer meals.

A review of nutrition policy for the elderly done at the Aging Health Policy Center at University of California at San Francisco (Nestle, Lee, and Fullarton, 1983) concluded squarely that most elderly persons who are malnourished do not participate in congregate meal programs. The study called for improved outreach, low-cost transportation, and expanded home-delivered meals. Newer data from a series of interviews with 700 representative clients at meal sites in metropolitan Cleveland suggest that congregate meal sites may now be serving a more disabled group than in the early days of the Older Americans Act (Harel, 1985). The average age of users was 72, the group definitely was poor, and considerable disability was noted. Black clients were significantly more disabled than whites in three areas: sense of personal security, health and functional status, and knowledge of or access to benefits and resources. Yet, even recognizing that some meal sites serve persons with substantial physical and cognitive impairment, one suspects that most people who can transport themselves to a noon meal can surely prepare a meal at home.

Perhaps congregate meals could be considered a preventive service in long-term care. To establish preventive efficacy, we would need to show that some combination of the nutritional supplements, the companionship, the effort mobilized to go to meal sites, and the educational and recreational programming helps older persons maintain functional abilities and independence. Nobody has begun to test this premise, let alone determine which aspect of the program, if any, has the desirable preventive effect. In contrast to congregate meals, home-delivered meals are clearly used as part of long-term care plans.

Surprisingly little study of meal programs has been done, either to refine and improve the service or to establish its efficacy in meeting established goals. Table 7-1 presents three studies of meal programs. One study was a small-scale quasi-experiment conducted at two congregate meal sites in Colorado over a five day period (Harrill et al., 1980). Nutritional outcomes favored the experimental group, but the magnitude and meaning of the differences are unclear. The second series of studies, by the New York City Department for the Aging (1982), polled a 25% random sample of its home-delivered meal clients. The four resultant reports presented descriptive data about clientele, their needs, and their use of other services. In contrast to Harel's study of congregate meal users, few differences were found between black and white clients in New York City, but, if anything, the white group proved somewhat more disabled. The authors concluded that the clients had unmet needs for many services other than meals.

TABLE 7-1 Congregate and Home-Delivered Meals Programs

Source	Description of Program or Study	Study Design	Selected Findings
Harrill et al. (1980)	A study measuring the nutritional impact of Title III-C congregate meals on elderly participants at two meal sites in Larimer County, CO.	In a quasi-experimental design, 59 participants and 32 nonparticipants of similar socioeconomic status were compared on nutrient intake and selected biochemical measurements after noon meals were served over a 5-day period. Measurements included laboratory evaluations and 24-hour dietary recalls.	Although nutrient intake levels were generally acceptable for both groups, participants had higher mean intake levels for energy and several nutrients. A small but larger percentage of nonparticipants had low serum protein values, and the mean calcium, iron, thiamin, and riboflabin intakes of nonparticipating women were less than the recommended daily requirements.
New York City Department for the Aging (1982) Meyer, Engler, and Lepis (1982) Engler and Meyer (1982)	In FY 1981 the New York City Department for the Aging, through the Older Americans Act Title III-C and the Community Services for the Elderly programs, provided home-delivered	In 1981, one hour in-home interviews were conducted with a random sample of 25% of the program's participants (N=1006). In addition to findings on characteristics such as client social	Participants appeared to be in social and economic need: The rate of SSI and Medicaid coverage was about twice that of the overall New York City population. About 90% were unable to prepare their own meals. 92% were satisfied with the program.

Engler (1983)	meals for 8,000 persons 60+ and homebound.	and health status, data were collected on participant satisfaction.	Areas in which there was the most dissatisfaction were (1) food not hot enough (26% of those surveyed), (2) food not delivered on time (17%), (3) portions too small (14%). 83% rejected the proposal of weekly delivery of frozen meals for storage and reheating. The majority (58%) had not been visited at all by someone in the program.
Kirschner et al. (1983)	A nationwide study of Title III-C congregate and home-delivered meal services. Conducted in two waves (1976 and 1982), it presents descriptive analyses of participants and operations, and evaluative analyses in areas such as nutritional impact and effects on social interaction.	In 1982, interviews were conducted at a sample of 70 sites representing providers in 29 states. 350 staff members and about 3,500 participants or nonparticipants (from locales adjacent to the programs) were interviewed. 34 of the sites had also been visited in 1976–77.	Three-fourths of the congregate meal participants could be considered priority recipients by virtue of their older age, low income, minority status, isolation; they tended to be worse off than non-participants. Home-delivered meal participants were older, poorer, and in worse health than congregate participants. The services enhanced dietary intake, especially calcium intake. The value of social contact was ranked highly by participants. Nutritional educational activities had no impact on dietary intakes away from the sites.

Satisfaction with the service was high, but a common core of complaints was also identified.

Finally, Kirschner and colleagues (1983) did a national study of both congregate and home-delivered meals at 70 sites in 29 states, interviewing participants and nonparticipants living in the same neighborhoods. These investigators found that the participants at congregate meals were older, more isolated, and poorer than nonparticipants. As expected, home-delivered meal recipients were older, poorer, and in worse health than those who used the congregate programs. The participants in the congregate programs valued the social contact highly. However, nutritional educational activities had no impact on what people ate away from the meal site.

ADULT FOSTER CARE

Foster care, a staple in public policy for care of dependent children, is a relatively new concept for adults. An adult foster home is a private home where a small number of people receive room and board in a family-like setting. Such homes are not certified care facilities and, though they are licensed in a few states, are not expected to adhere to rigid health standards. They have no care staff and are limited in the amount and type of personal care or monitoring of health regimens that can be done. On the positive side, foster care settings should permit residents much more personal freedom than is possible in a nursing home.

Adult foster care, known under a variety of names, was pioneered as an aftercare strategy for psychiatric patients. As an option in long-term care for the elderly, it is little developed, with only a slim research base to support its use. Table 7-2 reports five studies of adult foster care. The two studies with the largest samples—those of Linn and colleagues and those of Sherwood and colleagues—were directed toward mental health patients and younger adults as much as the elderly, leaving only three studies with small sample sizes geared exclusively toward the experience of the frail elderly.

The major randomized experiment involved almost 600 male psychiatric patients from five cooperating Veterans Administration hospitals (Linn et al., 1977; Linn, Klett, and Cafey, 1980). Compared to the controls who remained in the hospital, the social functioning of those in foster homes was significantly better. Fewer boarders and more children in the home were associated with better outcomes. High levels of supervision by foster caretakers and intensive follow-up by social workers had a negative effect on schizophrenic patients but not on others.

The Pennsylvania Domiciliary Care Program offered supplemental payments for SSI recipients over age 18 to finance care in small homes (1 to 3 residents) or group homes (4-13 residents). These facilities provided 24-hour supervision and some personal care as well as room and board. The evaluation of the program compared clients of domiciliary care with matched controls for three categories of patients: aged, mentally retarded, and mentally ill (Sherwood and Morris, 1981, 1983; Ruchlin and Morris, 1983). The intervention had positive effects upon receipt of needed service, satisfaction with the living arrangements, and integration into community life for all the groups. For the aged group, however, it had no significant impact on functioning. For the group that had previously lived in institutions the rates of entering institutions were lower and the program was particularly cost-saving.

The Niagara program (Kraus et al., 1977) was a smaller-scale Canadian effort. Twenty-one foster home residents were compared to an equal-sized control group in homes for the aged, matched by age, sex, and length of time since admission. The foster care residents were comparable to the controls on satisfaction and mental outlook.

Two hospital-based foster care programs, both started in 1979, have been the subject of considerable systematic research. The Johns Hopkins University Hospital's Department of Social Work demonstrated foster care as a discharge planning option for persons eligible for ICF-level care. Oktay and her colleagues designed a quasi-experiment in which consenting persons eligible for the program were randomized to receive foster care or be in the control group. The model tested used a social worker and nurse practitioner to recruit and train foster caregivers and to monitor the program in the field. An early report on program implementation (Oktay and Volland, 1981) indicated some disappointments. Contrary to expectation, many ICF-eligible persons preferred to enter nursing homes than to risk foster care. In addition, family members often seemed resistant to foster care as an option, an attitude exacerbated because most of the clients were white and the available foster care families were black. Many of the hospital dischargees had already determined that they would enter a facility before they were approached for the study, and this decision, once taken, is hard to undo. For those who did enter the study and remained in their assigned category for a year, the experimental group did as well as the nursing home control group in functional status and goal attainment, and costs appeared to be about 17% below nursing home costs. The foster home group did better on objective functional measures (ADL, IADL, and mental status), but, disquietingly, seemed to have less social interaction and less subjective life satisfaction than the controls.

Queens Medical Center in Honolulu conducted a program similar to the Johns Hopkins demonstration (Braun and Rose, 1986; Vandivort, Kurren, and Braun, 1984). It also used a social worker and nurse team to select and train foster care providers and follow clients in the field, and was similarly open to ICF-eligible hospital dischargees. The program faced more ethnic diversity than the Baltimore project, with Filipinos predominating among the foster caregivers. The evaluation was limited to 40 participants who had

TABLE 7-2 Studies on the Effectiveness of Foster Homes for the Elderly

Source	Description of Program or Study	Study Design	Selected Findings
Kraus et al. (1977)	The Niagara Program of Foster Homes for the Elderly places persons who are 60+ and not in need of nursing care in homes designed to help them remain as independent as possible. Residents are encouraged to engage in hobbies and to participate in the recreation programs of homes for the aged.	A quasi-experimental design in which 21 foster home residents, matched with 21 controls from homes for the aged on the basis of age, sex, years since admission, were compared on factors such as moves, health care received, patterns of social life, mental outlook. Residents were interviewed by nurses. Statistical tests not used.	HA residents gave "health reasons" for their admission to a home, while FH residents gave "social reasons" (e.g., lonesome, pressured by family). Foster life style generally involved participation in household chores, considerable contact with outside, watching TV, with little socializing within the residence; HA residents tended to socialize with residents, participate in home activities. Residents were comparable on satisfaction, mental outlook.
Linn et al. (1977) Linn, Klett, and Caffey (1980)	In 1970, five VA hospitals participated in a cooperative study to evaluate foster care placement for male patients with a psychiatric diagnosis. Most of the homes (73%) were in urban areas, with a male caretaker present (79%), and were shared with other veterans from the	572 subjects, with a mean age of 47, were randomly assigned to foster care (experimentals) or continued hospitalization (controls). Four scales measuring social dysfunction, mood, activity, and overall adjustment were administered prior to foster care preparation, upon	Four months after placement, the experimentals were significantly better off than the controls on scores of social functioning and adjustment. Improved outcome was related to more children in the home, fewer boarders, smaller number of persons in the home. Too much stimulation in the environment, too much supervision by caretakers, and more intensive

	same hospital. Follow-up supervision was provided by hospital social work staff.	placement and four months after. Subsequent analysis (1980) also studied the relationship of foster home characteristics to improved social functioning.	follow-up by social work staff had adverse impacts on schizophrenic patients but not others.
Sherwood and Morris (1981, 1983) Ruchlin and Morris (1983)	Initiated in 1976 under the aegis of the state Office of Aging, the Pennsylvania Domiciliary Care Program offers supplementary payments for residents aged 18+, in approved domiciliary facilities (small homes from 1 to 3 clients and group homes from 4 to 13 clients). Residents must be eligible for SSI, incapable of independent living, and not requiring services obtained only in LTC facilities. The facilities provide 24-hour supervision, personal care, and household services.	Experimentals and matched controls in the subcategories of aged, mental health clients, mentally retarded were measured at baseline and after 10 months of residency. Clinical assessment and self-report data were collected in the areas of receipt of needed services, quality of living conditions, integration into community life, functional status, institutional days, cost/benefits.	Generally positive impacts upon needed services (e.g., escort, counseling, transportation), living situation (e.g., privacy, environment satisfaction), integration (e.g., extent of outside friends, interest in family visiting). No significant impact on physical functioning for the aged. Significant impact on institutional days for those who had entered from an institutional setting. 90% of program saving came from lower rates of institutionalization.

TABLE 7-2 Studies on the Effectiveness of Foster Homes for the Elderly

Source	Description of Program or Study	Study Design	Selected Findings
Oktay and Volland (1981) Oktay (1984)	The Community Care Program, begun in 1979 by the Johns Hopkins Department of Social Work, is staffed by a social worker and a nurse practitioner. It selects and trains foster home caregivers and provides ongoing monitoring and service to both patient and caregiver. Program is targeted to hospital discharges.	112 volunteers from those determined acceptable for community care out of a potential pool of 445 patients were randomly assigned to the Community Care Program (experimentals) or to nursing homes (controls). Groups were compared on pre- and post-tests, including mental status, life satisfaction, social interaction, ADLs, IADLs, and morale. The groups were also compared on attainment of treatment goals and on direct and indirect costs.	For those who remained in the assigned treatments for 12 months, there were no significant differences in functional status and attitude; experimentals tended to improve on objective measures (ADL, IALD, MSQ) while controls did better on subjective (health and life satisfaction). The experimentals appeared to experience less social interaction than the controls. There was no significant difference regarding goal attainment. Community care costs were about 17% below nursing home costs.

| Braun and Rose (1986) Vandivort, Kurren, and Braun (1984) | In 1979, the Social Work Department of Queen's Medical Center, Honolulu, began foster family care for elders eligible for nursing home care. Foster families were screened and trained; a social worker and registered nurse helped place and develop treatment plans to assure quality of care. Foster families' fees were based on the patients' ADL score. | A quasi-experimental design in which 40 pairs of participants and nursing home residents (matched on age, ADLs, extent of disease, at least six months in program) were compared on outcomes of physical functioning, self-reported and caregiver observation of well-being, costs. | Foster care patients improved more, but not significantly more, than their controls on a total of 12 ADL items. Between-group comparisons at follow-up showed no significant differences in self-reported well-being; on caregiver observations, foster patients were significantly more likely to say they liked the setting, to interact more frequently with children, to have a nickname and a task. Differences in costs represented a savings for private foster patients of about 42%, and for Medicaid patients, 57%. |
| Mor, Sherwood, and Gutkin (1986) | A national survey of residential care home (RCH) programs and a five-state survey of RCHs and their elderly residents. Information collected included types of services required by the programs, RCH characteristics (structural, provider, homelike environment, regulatory and fiscal, attitudinal), casemix of RCH homes, and resident characteristics. | An initial screening survey, followed by detailed questionnaires (1979–80) identified and collected data on 118 state RCH programs serving the elderly. In addition, structured interviews were conducted with owners/staff and residents of a purposive, random sample of eight programs in five states. | There were 118 RCH programs regulating 29,282 facilities serving the elderly with a total of 371,734 beds. In the subsample group, 13% of residents were rated as having a poor fit between their needs and the home environment; 44.3% had an adequate fit; and 42.5% a good fit. Match adequacy was strongly related to resident's reported satisfaction and negatively related to functional impairment, incontinence, or high personal care needs. |

been in foster care at least six months. They were compared to a nursing home group matched on age, ADL, and extent of disease. The foster care group maintained significantly greater ADL abilities and expressed more satisfaction with their settings. No differences were found in self-reported well-being, but researchers observed more social interaction in the foster care group. The cost calculations overwhelmingly favored foster care.

Additional evaluative data on adult foster care were presented in the Mor, Sherwood, and Gutkin study that was cited in Chapter 3 (1986). Residents appeared to have positive feelings about their homes. Only about 28% of the residents surveyed felt negative or ambivalent about living in a foster home, and these feelings may have been influenced by unrelated factors such as rejection and role loss. Also, in an independent judgment of the adequacy of the environment for the residents, the authors concluded that only 13% of the residents could be rated as having a poor fit between their needs and their environment. One additional and interesting finding arose from the residential care home survey. Although a strong suit of the residential care home is its potential for personal freedom and homelike environment, very few homes allowed residents to drink alcohol or lock their rooms from the inside.

Drawing conclusions from this body of research is rather difficult. Both the Baltimore and Hawaii studies were highly selective in the groups ultimately compared, with substantial dropout among foster care users along the way. The social acceptability of foster care also seemed a problem, and the results on the social variables did not uniformly favor foster care, as one might have expected. On the other hand, the program is clearly less expensive than nursing home care, and surely has potential to serve as a less restrictive environment.

At least one state has developed substantial experience with adult foster care. In Oregon, adult foster care (by definition, a facility serving five or fewer people) is an integral component of the state's long-term care program. A deliberate effort was made to stimulate that part of the service sector in the mid-1970s when Oregon's community care efforts were generally expanded. At first used to divert persons from nursing homes, the total group of adult foster care users tripled between 1976 and 1986, and the Medicaid adult foster care clientele had increased from 900 in 1981 to 1800 in 1986. As part of this expansion, a private market for adult foster care has also taken hold in Oregon (Ladd, 1986). Typically, elderly persons enter foster care from hospitals and receive home-based services in the foster care setting. In Oregon, where adult foster care has developed on a large scale, the program seems to have achieved social respectability and is a preferred alternative to long-term care facilities.

A final question, concerning the place of foster care in the long-term care continuum, is raised by the Mor, Sherwood, and Gutkin survey. In discussing their findings on the case mix of residential care homes—that older residents of family-type residential homes appeared to be less healthy and more disabled than the residents of the larger, more regulation-conscious homes under department of health programs—the authors questioned the wisdom of the possible use of such owner-occupied homes as an outlet for the spillover effect of Medicare's DRGs. Increasing provider burdens could lead to poor care, which would be difficult to police in such decentralized settings.

RESPITE CARE

Respite care represents a pattern of accommodation to informal support rather than a specific program. It can refer to care given at home, in a nursing home, or even in a hospital. The characteristic feature is that the care enables family members to get relief from their own caregiving responsibilities (Henkleman-Kelly, 1983; Yocum, 1982). Although the focus is thus on the family caregivers, one presumes some advantages accrue to the clients being served. Similarly, home care, day care, and other services not formally designated as "respite," surely carry advantages for family caregivers as well.

Table 7-3 summarizes six studies of respite care. None used experimental or even quasi-experimental designs. Each concentrated on cataloging the perceived advantages of the program or describing what happened to program participants, but in no case was there a comparison group who did not receive respite care. As befits an ill-defined category, the programs studied were a hodgepodge. One study reported on nine persons receiving hospital-based respite care in Great Britain (Packwood, 1980), four examined respite provided in the home, and two looked at respite in long-term care facilities.

The three community programs were themselves disparate. The Wilder Caregiver Support program in Minnesota provided weekly respite for the specific purpose of allowing caregivers to attend a weekly two-hour support group (Patten, 1984). Thus, the respite tested differed markedly from relief that might have allowed caregivers to do what they pleased. Furthermore, the effects reported were as much effects of the support group as of the respite care. Similarly, a respite program in Marin County, California, represented a self help effort on the part of the wives of chronically disabled men (many with senile dementia) who organized themselves and got a small grant to finance the salary of a full-time nurse. Respite arrangements included four hours per week of home care and an extended weekend of out-of-home respite. (The latter was a camping outing that both wives and husbands attended. The wives relaxed while the husbands received care). Participants in this effort were extremely satisfied, but the evaluation cannot distinguish the effect of respite from the empowerment associated with organizing the program (Crossman, London, and Barry, 1981).

TABLE 7-3 Studies on the Effects on Respite Programs

Source	Program Description	Method	Selected Findings
Howells (1980)	A non-Medicaid facility in New York State gives respite for periods of up to six weeks for intermediate- and skilled-level patients. Four single rooms are designated as respite beds, and a staff member is assigned as program coordinator. The services provided are identical to those for the LTC residents.	Descriptive statistics were collected on 45 clients who used the program from 1979–80. Data collected included age, sex, DMS-1 score (rated level of care), length of stay, costs, participant satisfaction.	The average DMS-1 score for the participants was 161, just below the SNF starting point; 18 admissions were eligible for SNF care, 25 for ICF care, and 8 for lower-level care. Personnel costs were over 80% of the costs identified with the program, although no new personnel were required for the program. All 45 of the participants were satisfied with the program; 11% returned for a second admission. Other positive impacts included the arrangement of home health services for 11% and changes in the medical regimens of clients using multiple medications.

Study	Sample	Method	Findings
Packwood (1980)	Twenty-two chronically ill persons in Middlesex, U.K., most 75+, were admitted to medical wards or geriatric departments for two-week periods to provide holiday relief to their caregivers. Only persons who were currently receiving public health services were selected; priority was determined by the care receivers' degree of dependence and the amount of stress upon the family.	Nine patients were interviewed, along with their family caregivers and 17 hospital staff members.	Six patients had no objections to the program. Reasons included the opportunity to experience skilled nursing expertise and hospital care, and the variety or change of pace provided by the hospital experience. Three disliked the program for reasons such as separation from family, boredom, insufficient help with ADLs. All family members found the experience positive; reasons included the break from responsibility and the opportunity to renew other family relationships. Staff expressed concern that the patients might discharge themselves while their families were on vacation.
Crossman, London, and Barry (1981)	Caregiver wives of chronically disabled men in Marin County, California, obtained a grant (1979–81) to implement a respite program providing four hours of home care per week, extended out-of-home respite (1–4 full days), and community education. Home care was provided by one full time nurse, dividing her services among 10–15 family caregivers.	Client satisfaction survey and observations of authors.	Observed positive impact upon self-esteem, particularly due to developing and obtaining the foundation grant. All caregivers found the service valuable, with comments emphasizing the value of "being able to get out of the house," "peace, quiet, and rest," the nurses' visits raising the mood of the care receiver.

TABLE 7-3 Continued

Source	Program Description	Method	Selected Findings
Nurick (1983)	The Foundation Long-Term Care Project provided respite care over an 18-month period (1980–81) at six SNF/ICF facilities throughout New York State. Respite was provided 134 times at an average of 18 days per client. In the majority of cases, care was provided for purposes of vacation or relief (72%) to private-paying patients (66%).	Structured questionnaires and phone interviews were used to gather data from clients and family at the point of admission and one month following the service. In addition, follow-up data were gathered on 15 clients who were institutionalized within one month following the study.	Seventy-eight percent of the patients were very satisfied with the program; 2% were not satisfied; 83% would use it again. One month following the service, caregivers rated the patient's condition as the same (51%), better (19%), or worse (17%); 33% of caregivers said they would have considered institutional placement if respite were not available. Twelve percent of the patients were institutionalized within one month of the service, suggesting that respite is either a last effort by caregivers or that it breaks down barriers to institutionalization.

Patten (1984)	The Wilder Caregiver Support Program in Minneapolis, MN, founded in 1980, provides respite assistance to informal caregivers, allowing them to attend weekly 2-hour support groups. The groups are designed to help extended the caregivers' support networks, to provide mutual support, education/training, and socialization.	Structured questionnaires were mailed to all former and current participants in the program; the analyzed data represented 66% (86) of the participants.	Out of 16 areas of concern, the six areas with the highest proportion of caregivers reporting "a great deal of impact" were: having someone to talk to (68%), learning how other caregivers cope (66%), learning about services and resources (63%), feeling cared for by others (54%), taking your mind off your problems (43%), getting out of the house (42%). The three areas where caregivers felt no impact were: helping the care receiver become less dependent on you (42%), helping other caregivers find friends (32%), getting more recognition for one's worth (32%).
Netting and Kennedy (1985)	Project RENEW, under the auspices of The Greater Knoxville Senior Citizen Home Aide Service, trains and uses volunteers to provide time-limited (3–4 hours) companionship and supervision for frail elderly persons while family members are absent.	Descriptive and qualitative data presented on the volunteers, including their background, activities most often engaged in, and problems encountered. Family characteristics and reasons for using/not using the service were presented; instruments were used to measure the family's level of burden and client functioning.	Activities most engaged in by volunteers were talking and watching TV with clients; problems encountered were unpredictable and required "flexibility." A major difficulty with primary caregivers were their feelings of guilt at leaving older relatives even for brief periods of time. Erratic changes in family households (e.g., level of functioning) made it difficult to assign and schedule volunteers. Respite on Sunday mornings was a popular time.

Project RENEW, funded by the Levi Strauss Foundation, was housed in a large nonprofit homemaking agency in Knoxville, Tennessee. The grant allowed the agency to recruit, train, and supervise volunteer companions, who received expenses only, to provide in-home respite. Although originally a more ambitious evaluation had been contemplated, findings were limited to information about launching such an effort (Netting and Kennedy, 1985). To the surprise of the planners, many caregivers were uncomfortable leaving their relative with the respite worker even for brief periods of time. The program was difficult to schedule, but respite services on Sunday mornings (probably to facilitate church attendance) were particularly popular.

Both studies of institutional respite were in New York State. Howells (1980) reported the experience of a non-Medicaid facility that reserved four single rooms for respite purposes. The 45 frail elderly persons using the program in the study year reported high satisfaction. The respite admission was also used to stabilize medical regimens and arrange home-based services. Finally, Nurick (1983) reported on a demonstration done at six New York nursing homes. Data were collected for 134 episodes of respite, both at the time of the service and one month after discharge. Again the patients and their caregivers were largely satisfied, and a third of the caregivers indicated that they would have considered permanent institutional care had respite not been available. Twelve percent of the patients entered an institution within a month of the respite care.

This body of research must be considered preliminary. Not only are no comparisons offered, but the goals of respite are somewhat unclear, and the characteristics of the users and the outcomes achieved also vague. Certainly, this evidence provides no clues about whether a respite benefit should be financed, or the likely costs of various options. No home-based respite that allows an extended vacation has been tested, and no basis exists for comparing home respite to institutional respite because the two forms have been offered for such different durations and purposes. Furthermore, some confusion has been introduced by a tendency to call all short-term nursing home use for those who live in the community "respite care." Some such admissions may, in fact, be short-term trial placements to allow a prospective nursing home resident to become familiar with the setting. Such trials might also be a way to strengthen a natural "marketplace," allowing persons considering a long-term stay an easy opportunity to try one or more places before committing themselves.

SUPPORTIVE PROGRAMS FOR FAMILY CAREGIVERS

Conventional wisdom asserts, probably correctly, that caregiving is a lonely task for many family caregivers, that caregivers tend to be overwhelmed by the demands, and that they could be bolstered and sustained by programs designed to increase their knowledge and competence, and bring them into contact with persons in similar predicaments. Social work, nursing, and gerontological literature describe support groups offered to family caregivers (Henkleman-Kelly, 1983; Crossman, London, and Barry, 1981; Sonberg and Emrich, 1982). Such groups have become a program staple for many health and social service agencies. Some become self-sustaining, often organized as "clubs" of people faced with common disabilities like stroke, Alzheimer's disease, arthritis, Parkinson's disease, and so on. Like self-help or support groups in other fields, the efforts range from small, self-selected group therapies to something resembling a large-scale social movement. Evaluation seldom occurs.

The 1984 reauthorization of the Older Americans Act specifically mandated that Area Agencies on Aging undertake efforts to educate and support caregivers, especially those caring for victims of senile dementia.

Such efforts largely take the form of support groups. Other approaches to family caregivers are aimed at changing incentives to make caregiving easier. Tax breaks and service credit banks, for example, have been suggested. However, we located no empirical studies of efforts to change the conditions and inducements for family caregiving. To date, the proposals in this area are highly theoretical. Given the high volume of family care already in place, it is by no means certain that an untapped reservoir remains in wait for the right incentives to be invented.

Table 7-4 presents some data on efforts to support family caregivers. Two of the studies (Fox and Lithwick, 1978; Glosser and Wexler, 1985) illustrate the general quality of information available about support groups. Both asked participants to evaluate the worth of a closed-ended group with a fixed number of sessions. Such "studies" yield information about what the participants liked best and least but provide no data about how the group changed anyone's behavior.

The other two studies were more substantive. Indeed the programs they studied combined supportive and counseling efforts for families with actual services to the disabled relative. Both efforts were developed by the Community Service Society of New York. The Natural Supports Program (Buschman and Sainer, 1981; Zimmer and Sainer, 1981) was designed largely to describe how families can best be supported. The effort had two parts: (1) provision of home care and individual counseling to support family members' work; and (2) provision of educational and supportive group programs for caregivers. From interviewing about 90 families, the investigators learned that home care was the most valued service and that the individual counseling was directed mainly at helping families understand aging and dependency and resolve interpersonal conflicts. According to participants in group sessions in four communities, members thought that learning about resources was their most important need.

The Family Support Program was conducted by the Community Service Society of New York between 1976 and 1979 (Frankfather, Smith, and

TABLE 7-4 Studies on the Effects of Programs Supporting Family Caregivers

Source	Description of Program or Study	Study Design	Selected Findings
Fox and Lithwick (1978)	Social workers at a nursing home led six group sessions for adult children of confused parents, including topics such as the physiological and psychological aspects of senility, institutional aspects of care, coping with stress, and the stigma of having an institutionalized parent.	Open-ended questionnaires at the end of each session and a final group session on the helpfulness of the program were used to evaluate the program.	Topics especially helpful to the participants were information on the physical and psychological aspects of cognitive dysfunction and the aging process, a session allowing participants to air complaints/praise for the institution. Issues of coping and guilt dominated all sessions.
Glosser and Wexler (1985)	Eight weekly educational/support group sessions were provided to relatives of patients with dementia from a 400-bed hospital. The sessions, led by a neuropsychologist and geriatric social worker, covered areas such as skills for behavior management, interpersonal problems, information on dementia, support.	64 out of a possible 104 participants rated the sessions on a five-point scale of 17 items.	Items most highly rated were "finding out how others were dealing with their problems," "meeting people with similar problems," "sharing feelings," "information about medical aspects," "support from other members." Problems in "allocating caregiving duties" and other family conflicts were topics least effectively addressed by the sessions.

Buschman and Sainer (1981) Zimmer and Sainer (1981)	The Natural Supports Program, initiated in 1976 by the Community Service Society of New York, consisted of two components: (1) provision of services such as home care and counseling to supplement individual family caregiving efforts; (2) provision of educational and supportive group programs for caregivers. The project was designed to determine how family caregiving can be enhanced and supported.	Findings on the individual families were based on research interviews with 92 families; group data were gathered from 266 questionnaires returned by group participants in four communities.	Individual Families: home care was by far the most frequently requested service; counseling service related mainly to increased dependency, understanding aging, interpersonal conflicts. Requests for service were extremely modest. Caregiver involvement changed rather than diminished with services. Groups: Participants stated that learning about resources was their most important need.
Frankfather, Smith, and Caro (1981)	The Family Support Program (FSP), sponsored by the Community Service Society of New York from 1976 to 1979, was a service demonstration and research project designed to assist families in maintaining their disabled elderly at home. Basic caregiving responsibility remained explicitly with the families; program staff assisted in planning/ obtaining such services as homemaking, counseling, entitlement advocacy.	An exploratory-longitudinal design, in which interviews with and observations of families took place upon the families entry to the program and at yearly intervals. The study's emphasis was upon the performance of the family as a service provider and its relationship to formal services rather than upon client outcomes. A Functioning of Independent Living Scale was used to measure disabilities.	Services: *Homemaking* was the primary service requested by families (83%)—the study highlighted the problems in procuring long-term, responsible, companiable personnel. *Entitlement advocacy* was requested by 33%—problems included reluctance to spend down, fear of forced care, intrusiveness of bureaucracy. *Counseling*, received by 42%, was often not labeled or understood as such by clients. Only a small substitution of family care occurred. Families and clients did not understand options when they negotiated care plans.

Caro, 1981). This project used grant funds to assist family members who wished to facilitate home care for a disabled elderly relative who would have been functionally eligible for a nursing home. Care plans were developed jointly by program case managers, clients, and family members. The plans delineated the responsibilities of family members and the program, which could purchase a wide range of services up to a maximum per client. Although it proved impossible to test the program through a randomized experiment, a longitudinal design was adopted whereby interviews with and observations of each family took place upon entry into the program and at annual intervals. The resultant monograph is rich in detail about the process of developing such a program. Unfortunately, despite the program's emphasis on mutual care planning, the study showed that families and clients did not fully understand the care options open to them or their price. Moreover, the case managers, who were social workers from the agency, tended to recommend a familiar array of services.

Before a steady stream of information about programs to support family caregivers can be expected, some clarity about program goals is necessary. As it is, even the intended beneficiary is unclear. Are such programs added to existing community care to make life easier for family caregivers, or are they expected to reduce the amounts of formal service used?

Are the benefits expected to be felt further downstream in reduced institutional admissions for those receiving family care? Or is the idea that assistance to families will ultimately mean that the caregivers themselves will need less long-term care services later on. Theoretically, the latter effect could be possible if help for caregivers were associated with less physical, financial, emotional, and social strain on those giving care and, therefore, left more reserve for their own needs at some future point. Our tendency to lump all family caregivers together (whether they are adult children or spouses) and to focus on expenditures for the primary client (with the emphasis on public expenditures at that) prohibits even tentative conclusions on this topic. Furthermore, we lack long-term follow-up of family caregivers after death or institutional admission of the disabled relative.

Certainly educational and supportive groups for family caregivers should not be viewed in the same category as efforts to change the incentives for family care or to add services to make family care easier. To prove their worth, support groups will need to eliminate selection bias. Evaluations must go beyond immediate ratings of the participants to examine longer-range effects compared to control groups. Programs that change incentives for caregivers will benefit from clearer social agreement about whether the individual or the family is the appropriate unit of a long-term care plan, and the extent to which family members are to be held responsible as service providers of the first resort.

VOLUNTEER PROGRAMS

Volunteering is a way of life in the United States. Many long-term care programs are directly sponsored by sectarian organizations and civic groups, and many others depend on the efforts of volunteers. Certainly the amount of volunteer service is substantial, both for community programs, such as meals-on-wheels and friendly visiting, and in nonprofit nursing homes. In this book, we make no effort to review studies on the way volunteers of all ages contribute to long-term care programs in the community and in nursing homes.

Rather our focus is on programs where seniors serve as volunteers (Worthy, Eisman, and Wood, 1982). Here we see a dual focus for such programs: volunterism itself may have a positive impact upon the elderly volunteers; it may also, if targeted to the disabled, provide valuable long-term care services. The evaluative information presented here is limited to programs sponsored by ACTION, the federal agency responsible for the Foster Grandparent Program, the RSVP program (Retired Senior Volunteers), and the Senior Companion Program. Strictly speaking, only the Senior Companion Program, which provides a stipend to persons over age 60 who fulfill roles in programs for the frail elderly, often as home aides and friendly visitors, is a long-term care program. The other programs fall into the category of preventing long-term care in the sense that the voluntary activity may help sustain the functional abilities and independence of those who volunteer.

The five evaluations of ACTION programs, summarized in Table 7-5, provide some tantalizing preliminary data to suggest that such volunteer work may indeed benefit the volunteer. The first two (ACTION, 1984a, 1984b) were uncontrolled studies suggesting that persons over 60 can reliably and capably perform important human service roles with youth and receive good performance ratings from both the clientele and the professional workers. The remaining three studies used some type of control groups to assess the effect on volunteers and recipients of service. A three-year study comparing Foster Grandparents to those on the waiting lists for volunteer positions showed that the mental health and social resources of the volunteers (using the OARS instrument) improved or remained stable over time, whereas those of the controls declined—although this is not surprising given selection bias in the use of volunteers. The control group also experienced a mortality rate that was twice as high (ACTION, 1984c). In another study (ACTION 1985a), three groups of RSVP volunteers were assessed annually with the OARS instrument for three years, and their well-being was compared to that of the representative population of Cleveland that had been studied by the General Accounting Office (1977). Controlling for baseline differences, the volunteers deteriorated less in a one-year period on all five dimensions topped by the OARS instrument.

TABLE 7-5 Studies on the Effects of Volunteer Programs for the Elderly

Source	Description of Program or Study	Study Design	Selected Findings
ACTION (1984a)	The demonstration project, "FGP/RSVP Head Start" (1981) used Foster Grandparents and Retired Senior Volunteers to provide programmatic and managerial/administrative services in eight Head Start projects.	686 questionnaires were sent to FGP and RSVP project directors, Head Start directors and teachers, FGP and RSVP volunteers. 402 returned and completed questionnaires were analyzed for descriptive and evaluative data.	83%–94% of the volunteers were rated as excellent or good by the Head Start teachers; 80%–98% of the volunteers found their work personally meaningful and/or valuable to the program. Over 50% of the teachers found the volunteers more committed, reliable, and enthusiastic than volunteers in general; 10%–13% rated them as unsatisfactory.
ACTION (1984b)	A study of the impact of Foster Grandparents on juvenile offenders at three Georgia Youth Development Centers. The volunteers counseled, tutored, and spent time in other supportive ways with their assigned youth.	A nonrandom design in which 62 youths with foster grandparents and 42 youths waiting for grandparents were measured at baseline and at 2–15 months following (1982–83). The Coopersmith self-esteem and self-anchoring scales were used to measure outcomes. Analysis of covariance was used to control for baseline differences.	97% of the participating youths stated that their Foster Grandparent was helpful; 42% stated Foster Grandparents made a difference by discussing things with them, 29% by helping them. Participant youths had higher post-test scores on outcome (p<.07), especially in the first six months.

ACTION (1984c)	The Foster Grandparent Program, begun in 1966 under HEW and OEO, matches older Americans with children who have exceptional needs. Volunteers provide health, education, and social services in settings such as hospitals, schools, mental retardation centers, day care centers. Benefits include a stipend, transportation, meals, and annual physical exam.	From a stratified random national sample of 14 projects, 471 participants and controls (taken from program waiting lists) were measured in three phases over three years (1980 to 1983). The principal measurement instrument was OARS.	The overall functioning, the mental health, and social resources of the experimentals improved or were maintained over time, while those of the controls declined. The mortality rate of the experimentals was half that of the controls. The economic resources of experimentals were greater than those of the controls, but remained stable while those of the controls increased.
ACTION (1985a)	The Retired Senior Volunteer Program, administered by ACTION (PL 93-113, Title II) recruits and places volunteers, 60+, in community services such as senior centers, schools and libraries, nursing homes and hospitals, nutrition centers. Volunteers receive no stipend.	Data were collected from three subgroups of volunteers in three rounds, approximately 12 months apart. Subjects were measured on social, mental, physical, economic, and ADL dimensions (OARS) and compared with data from GAO study of the well-being of the elderly in Cleveland.	Compared to the aged population as a whole and the Cleveland population, volunteers were healthier, better educated, younger, and more affluent. Controlling for baseline differences, volunteers were found to have deteriorated less in a one-year period than the Cleveland elderly population on all five dimensions.

TABLE 7-5 Continued

Source	Description of Program or Study	Study Design	Selected Findings
ACTION (1985b)	The Senior Companion Program, authorized by Congress in 1973 and funded by AOA, provides stipends to elderly, 60+, engaged in part-time employment in supportive services to adults, often as senior health aides.	A national sample of 631 persons from six sites, representing four subsets (senior companions, clients, companions, and clients on the program's waiting list), was measured in three rounds between 1979 and 1984. Companions and clients on the waiting list who subsequently entered the program were compared to those still on the list. OARS was used as the measurement instrument.	Companions: The proportion of entering Companions rated as good or excellent on the economic scale improved from 0 to 50%, while the controls remained stable. Entering Companions significantly increased in mental health functioning while controls decreased. Clients: In comparison to controls, clients had less decline in social resources, areas of serious functional impairment, adjustment to health limitations.

A similarly designed study compared senior home companions and their clients to persons on the respective waiting lists for companion positions or for service. Both the companions and the clients compared favorably on some dimensions to the waiting lists. The companions showed gains in economic well-being and mental health compared to the controls, and the clients showed less decline in social resources or functional abilities (ACTION, 1985b). Presently a multi-site national randomized experiment is underway in which both companions and clientele are being randomly assigned for participation; outcomes of both groups are being evaluated by Research Triangle, Inc.

Pending the results of the randomized trial, we must allow for the possibility that earlier studies compared incomparable groups. Nevertheless, the evidence all points in a favorable direction, suggesting that the volunteer role enhances well-being and functioning among the elderly who choose it, and that such volunteers can also make contributions that are valuable to client groups of all ages.

GERIATRIC ASSESSMENT UNITS

The essence of care of the dependent elderly is the response to a person's multiple interactive problems, which may extend beyond the biomedical to affect other functional domains. Ironically, however, an appropriate assessment of health conditions is harder to arrange and/or finance than a socially oriented assessment. The geriatric assessment units considered in this section are programs that provide a comprehensive, multidimensional assessment of functioning and potential for improvement, including physical health and cognitive functioning, as well as psychological and social functioning. Such assessments may be done on an outpatient basis or in specialized inpatient settings. They usually are done by multidisciplinary teams; they sometimes include short-term therapeutic trials as part of the diagnostic efforts or to stabilize the patient at as high a functional level as possible. Like the day hospital, the geriatric assessment unit is a well-developed concept in Great Britain.

Although few geriatric assessment units have been developed in the United States, this intervention has been studied enough to prove its worth (Rubenstein, Rhee, and Kane, 1982). At the least, it has been demonstrated that systematic geriatric assessment can identify problems that ordinary medical care fails to pinpoint. In the last decade, numerous articles have highlighted organized programs of general geriatric or psychogeriatric assessment. Table 7-6 summarizes 11 studies with more than usual data about the problems identified through the program; four are descriptive studies and seven provide considerable before and after comparisons.

TABLE 7-6 Uncontrolled Studies of Geriatric Assessment Programs

Source	Description of Program	Findings
Descriptive Studies:		
Cheah and Beard (1980)	Patients admitted to a medical geriatric unit received psychogeriatric assessment via chart review. No specifics.	Of 241 charts reviewed, 119 new diagnoses of organic syndrom and 65 of dysphoria/depression were identified.
Currie et al. (1981)	Home assessments by MDs including ADL (no specifics); referrals from MDs, relatives, social service, mental health, and public health.	Thirty-six "significant new diagnoses" were found among 50 patients already evaluated in regular care, most commonly dementia and depression. Adjustment of medication schedule produced "beneficial effect."
Hogan and Cape (1984)	Persons referred for admission to a long-term care hospital received a medical evaluation and sometimes a review by rehabilitative services (no specifics).	Among 188 admissions 65 new diagnoses were found (37 treatable, 13 major); 21% discharged to community; 38% in community at follow-up nine months later.
Lichtenstein and Winograd (1984)	Referrals came from medical and family practice services of acute teaching hospital. Assessment included review of medical record, history and physical exam, mental status exam, ADLs, consultation with nurses regarding functional level.	Fifty new diagnoses found among 71 patients (17 psychiatric diagnoses); 62% of patients had recommended medication change; 18 patients headed for SNF changed course (14 home); in addition, another 17 went home.
Before-After Studies:		
Poliquin and Straker (1977)	History, physical exam, psychological testing, brain scan, ECG, EEG, audiometry, vision testing, pneumonaphalogram and CT scan when indicated administered to persons aged 60+ with acute psychiatric illness.	Fourteen new medical diagnoses and 12 exacerbations were found among 47 patients. Full remission of psychiatric problems in 11 patients, partial in 24.

Study	Description	Results
Sloane (1980)	Indigent patients from emergency room needing nursing home care were assessed by multidisciplinary team (no specifics). Pfeiffer MSQ, Katz ADL administered.	No significant change in Pfeiffer SPMSQ. Clinical improvement described in 8 of 29 patients. ADL differences not reported.
Reifler et al. (1981)	Elderly persons with signs of confusion and memory loss, often headed for nursing home, received multi-disciplinary evaluation including medical evaluation (for reversible causes of organic brain syndrome); psychiatric evaluation (diagnostic, family dynamics); social work home visit (social structure, family stress, home environment); architect (individual's abilities and desires, actual living situation); nurse/OT (ADLs).	Twenty of 82 patients showed objective evidence of improvement corroborated by patient and family.
Applegate et al. (1983)	Subjects were acute hospital patients likely to need nursing home care, with significant functional impairment, not chronically confused, not terminal, clinically stable. Assessment included: medical (undetected disease, mental status, medication): nursing (motivation, skin care, continence, ability to manage medications). PT (ROM, mobility endurance, gait); OT (ADL and IADL); psychologists/psychiatrics (orientation, memory, motivation, depression); social service (need for and availability of family and social support); nutritionist (diet and ability to plan menus); speech and audiology.	Ninety-one treatable conditions were diagnosed in 100 patients. Mobility scores improved in 58 of 87 patients; none deteriorated. Medications were reduced from 4.3 to 3.5 per person. Improvements in IADLs 13% to 51%; little deterioration. Forty-two percent of depressed patients improved. Eleven percent of patients improved motivation. Sixteen percent improved ability to handle own medication.

TABLE 7-6 Continued

Source	Description of Program	Findings
Larson et al. (1984)	Subjects were referrals from MDs and clinics, patients 60+ with global mental impairment. Assessment included: history, physical, neurological exam, including mini-mental state and dementia rating scale. Lab work including SMA-12, CBC, thyroid function, VDRL, B12, folate, CT scan, chest x-ray, and ECG.	Fifteen of 107 patients had potentially reversible dementia. Outcome assessment on 77 patients: 25 showed definite improvement in dementia and/or other medical conditions, 16 had cognitive improvement, 20 other medical.
Barker et al. (1985)	Targets were patients 70+ in six hospitals, with two or more of: living alone, 80+, low income, mental impairment, significant physical disability. Assessment included review of diagnoses, treatments, nursing and social problems, living environment, ADLs, mental and behavioral status, medications, aids and devices.	Decline of 21% in alternative care census compared to baseline period (after correcting for additional nursing home beds).
Liem, Chernoff, and Carter (1986)	Elderly VA hospital patients at risk of institutionalization received inpatient interdisciplinary team assessment (OT, PT, pharmacy, diet, psychology, speech therapy, and psychiatry led by a core team of MD, rehab nurse, and social worker). (No further specifics.)	Improvement in independent ADL (2% to 42%), walking (22% to 67%), continent (47% to 74%), alert (21% to 48%).

In general, all four descriptive studies showed that the assessments were worthwhile in generating new diagnoses. Psychiatric diagnoses such as depression and senile dementia were among the most often overlooked. Although these studies were uncontrolled, it appeared that the assessment units produced more than additional labels; they also altered the clinical or social course. For example, Hogan and Cape (1984) said that more than half their discovered diagnoses were treatable, Currie and colleagues (1981) indicated that adjusting medication schedules produced "beneficial effects," and Lichtenstein and Winograd (1984) claimed that patients destined to enter skilled nursing facilities changed direction and went home.

The before and after studies ranged in their claims for improvement, but the differences were a matter of degree. All the authors pointed to some beneficial results. Among the most positive were Applegate and colleagues (1983), who showed that mobility scores improved in 58 of 87 patients, that 42% of depressed patients improved, and that, given simplification of medication regimens, 16% improved in their ability to manage their own medications. Liem, Chernoff, and Carter (1986) pointed to dramatic improvements in ADLs and continence. Larson and colleagues (1984) found 15 of 107 patients had potentially reversible dementias. Barker and colleagues (1985) claimed a decline in the population of alternative care at the participating hospitals, after correcting for the development of additional nursing home beds during the study period.

Most impressive were the eight controlled studies of geriatric assessment, especially the four randomized clinical trials, summarized in Table 7-7. Schuman and his colleagues (1978) assessed the impact of a new geriatric program in a chronic hospital by making crude comparisons of those returning home in the year before and after the inauguration of the new program. Lefton, Bonstelle, and Frengley (1983) compared patients discharged from a hospital's geriatric unit to matched controls discharged from other medical wards, finding twice as much improvement in ADL and continence and half as much nursing home placement in the experimental group. Campion, Jette, and Berkman (1983), who compared the results of patients age 75 and over in an experimental ward with a geriatric consultation team and two control wards, reported less optimistic results. Perhaps the lack of positive outcomes is a reflection of the consultation model, where the assessment team had no direct power to implement its recommendations. Gayton and colleagues (1985) similarly found no effects from the work of a geriatric consultative team on an experimental floor of a Montreal hospital.

All five randomized trials reported significant positive effects. A Danish study randomly assigned persons over 75 living at home to receive a visit from a social worker who administered a structured health questionnaire, followed by advice and referral as needed. The experimental subjects enjoyed several benefits including improved mortality rates (Hendriksen,

TABLE 7-7 Experimental Studies of Effects of Geriatric Assessment Programs

Source	Description of Program or Study	Study Design	Findings
Quasi-Experiments: Schuman et al. (1978)	Targets were patients referred to chronic care hospital (a) requiring subacute-medical care, (b) suffering from terminal disease, or (c) needing rehabilitation. Assessment gave multidisciplinary team care (no specifics).	Comparison of patient group with referrals to chronic hospital in prior year and those referred to other services in same year.	More study patients returned home. Improvement in ADL comparable to rehab service.
Campion, Jette, and Berkman (1983)	Consulting team in teaching hospital. Only on referral from attending staff. Assessment included: physical functioning; depression screen; MSQ; review of medications and active medical problems.	All patients 75+ admitted to one teaching medical service of an acute hospital were compared to patients on two other wards.	Fewer patients on the consultation floor went home.
Lefton, Bonstelle, and Frengley (1983)	Acute hospital patients, age 70+, with rehabilitation potential, were refered for inpatient multi-dimensional assessment. (No specifics.)	Dischargees from geriatric unit were matched to general medical ward dischargees and compared.	More patients in geriatric ward went home. More patients improved in ADLs, ambulation, and continence.

Gayton et al. (1985)	Patients age 69+ admitted from emergency room to two medical wards in a Montreal hospital received services of a geriatric team (including geriatricians, geriatric nurse consultants, PT, OT, and activity counsellor). The team, MDs and nurse were consultative and spent 20% to 40% of their time on the two wards. The other team members provided direct care. Patients seen by team were identified by informal contact with regular ward staff.	Patients age 65+ on two experimental floors who received geriatric consultation team services were compared to patients on two other floors. Follow-up done six months later. Analysis of covariance adjusted findings based on age, sex, and ADL scores at admission.	No differences between experimental and control group in ADL, IADL, mental status, length of time in hospital, discharge destination, or consumption of medical services after discharge.
Experiments: Tulloch and Moore (1979)	Medical evaluation and vulnerability screening for health and social problems were done for persons 70+ on registration rolls of a group general medical practice in Oxford, England.	A random sample of patients of the general practice received the special medical/social evaluation and was compared to controls in the same practice.	Experimental group uncovered one new problem per patient from screening and another from on-demand care; screened group had more hospital admissions but fewer hospital days; higher referral risk to community agencies; no difference in prevalence of socio-economic problems or physical disabilities.
Hendricksen, Lund, and Stromgard (1984)	Persons age 75+ living at home in a suburb of Copenhagen received an evaluation of social functioning and health problems. The assessor provided no follow-up care but did give advice and referral.	Persons 75+ in the target community were randomized to experimental or control group.	Intervention group had fewer hospital days, lower mortality, more home help, lower direct costs.

TABLE 7-7 Continued

Source	Description of Program or Study	Study Design	Findings
Rubenstein et al. (1984)	Male veterans discharged from acute hospital and destined for nursing homes entered inpatient geriatric assessment unit (GEU). Multi-disciplinary team evaluation included medical, psychosocial, and functional evaluations. Short-term treatment done.	Patients 65+ from acute hospital wards were screened for study criteria. After informed consent and baseline evaluation, they were randomized to the GEU or control group.	GEU patients had lower mortality, more discharged home, more improved ADL, IADL, MSQ (Mental Status Questionnaire), and morale scores at 12 months, lower rehospitalization and nursing home admission rates, and lower direct costs.
Vetter, Jones, and Victor (1984)	Patients 70+ in one urban and one rural practice in Wales received one extra visit for a special assessment from a health visitor (i.e., a public health nurse with extra training on social programs).	Randomization to the experimental or the control group.	Urban experimental group had lower mortality; no difference in physical disability, anxiety, view of life, or use of district nurse in either; urban groups had more use of home help.
Allen et al. (1986) Becker et al. (1986)	Patients 75+ admitted to inpatient wards of the Durham VA Hospital received an assessment by a geriatric consultation team including a physician, clinical nurse specialist, and social worker within 48 hours of admission. The assessment and recommendations were placed in the medical record. The team made regular rounds and additional recommendations were added to the record.	One hundred eighty-five patients were randomized to the experimental group or a control group, which received an initial assessment and a problem list in the medical record. The team's recommendations for the control group were filed elsewhere and no follow-up was done.	In the experimental group, compliance with the team's recommendations was high (71%) and only 27% of the team's concealed recommendations for the control group were followed. However, the intervention had no effect on the rate of hospital-acquired complications, which was 38% for both groups.

Lund, and Stromgard, 1984). Two British studies were done in the context of primary medical care; in both cases, patients randomized to receive special assessments showed positive results (Tulloch and Moore, 1979; Vetter, Jones, and Victor, 1984). A randomized trial of a geriatric consultation team in the Durham Veterans Administration Hospital showed positive effects in changing the behavior of physicians to comply with the team's recommendations (Allen et al., 1986), but no difference between experimental and control groups in rates of hospital-acquired complications (Becker et al., 1986).

Finally, the only randomized experiment thus far reported in the United States for a distinct geriatric assessment unit showed dramatic positive effects (Rubenstein et al., 1984). Patients at a Veterans Administration hospital who had completed their acute care and were eligible for discharge to nursing homes were randomized to an additional stay in an inpatient geriatric evaluation unit. A year later, the experimental group had lower mortality, greater ADL, IADL, and cognitive improvement, better morale and lower rates of rehospitalization and admission to nursing homes. As documented in other descriptive studies, treatable problems were identified and remedied, and at the same time the number of drugs per patient and per diagnosis declined.

Taken together, systematic geriatric assessment seems to be well worthwhile, if it is carefully targeted. It has proved especially useful if it is directed toward those whose functional and medical status renders them eligible for nursing home care, and if those responsible for the assessment have the authority to follow up on their findings. Many of those at greatest risk come directly from acute care hospitalization. The details of geriatric assessment batteries, however, have been poorly specified, and it is far from clear what multidisciplinary personnel or procedure is needed to do the job. Several of the best done studies suggest substantial benefits from modest additions in service. Nor is it clear when an inpatient rather than an outpatient program patient is needed. Because geriatric assessment programs seem so promising, it is all the more important that the procedures used be described in a way that permits replication.

HOSPICE

Hospice may be considered a variant of long-term care, although its funding strongly suggests that for policy purposes it is pursued as an alternative to expensive hospital care rather than nursing home care. It can be delivered in several forms. Customarily hospices are divided into hospital-based units, (including some freestanding programs) and home care. Hospices can also be classified as organized programs and adapted programs; the former are officially designated as hospices and the latter provide the equivalent services for the terminally ill without the name.

Despite variations on the theme, hospices are characterized by the following features: (1) the patient's disease state has been diagnosed as terminal, usually with a prognosis of six months or less, and emphasis is placed on palliative treatment, i.e., aggressive efforts to prolong life have been abandoned; (2) the patient and family are treated as an integrated unit of need; (3) services are provided by an interdisciplinary team with inpatient and home care components coordinated; (4) services are available (but not necessarily provided) to the patient and family on a continuous 24-hour, 7-days-a-week basis; and (5) pain control and psychological well-being are prominent goals.

The hospice movement was imported to the United States with enthusiasm after initial encouraging reports of pioneering work at St. Christopher's in London and, later, at the Royal Victoria Hospital in Montreal. The initial extravagant claims may partially be explained by the hyperbole associated with new movements and by the need to promote innovative concepts by promising dramatic effects. At the same time, hospice was more than an innovation in care; it was a general reformation in the approach toward dying persons. It embodied a refutation of the cold, professional, highly technical, and austere approach typified by a modern scientific hospital. Instead, the hospice promised humanistic care with concomitant improvements in the quality of the last months and weeks of the patients' lives.

The hospice also had its own technology. It developed new methods of pain control that erased "the memory of pain" while using psychoactive medications as little as possible to avoid impairing cognition. At the same time, environmental changes were introduced to reduce psychological stress and increase social involvement. The expected outcomes, therefore, included reduction in pain and discomfort, reduction in negative side-effects of drug therapy, improved emotional well-being, and greater satisfaction. Moreover, the beneficiaries were also to include the families of the dying patients. Through direct and indirect help from the hospice staff during the course of the terminal illness and the period of initial bereavement, the hospice was expected to alleviate stress for family. All this was to be achieved at lower cost than the usual way of death.

Lubitz and Prihoda (1984) provided a financial justification for hospice care in their analysis of the use of health care services and Medicare expenditures in the last two years of life. Using a 1978 cohort, they estimated that the 5.9% of Medicare beneficiaries who died accounted for 27.9% of expenditures during the two-year period. Moreover, 46% of the costs of the last year of life were spent in the last 60 days. An Ohio study using Medicare Part A and Blue Cross hospital insurance claims suggested that hospice might curb the high costs of dying. Terminal cancer patients served by a home-based hospice were compared to those treated conventionally. The hospice patients used 50% less hospital care and ten times more home care with associated cost savings (Brooks and Smyth-Staruch, 1984).

Driven by the hopes of cost savings as well as the urging of advocates for humane death, Congress introduced legislation in 1982 to cover hospice under Medicare for persons of all ages. At that point, a strict definition was developed for hospices seeking Medicare reimbursement. They are required to include nursing care, medical social services, physician services, counseling services, short-term inpatient care, medical appliances and supplies, homemaker/home health aide services, and rehabilitation therapy. Nurses and homemaker/home health aides can be reimbursed for around the clock coverage to keep a patient at home during a crisis. Up to five consecutive respite days at one time are reimbursable. Bereavement counseling for survivors is required but not reimbursed. Core services (namely, nursing, medical social services, physician services, and counseling) are to be furnished directly by hospice employees and cannot be contracted, but a hospice can enter into agreements with other entities for inpatient care. Five percent of services are to be furnished by volunteers, and hospices have to document that the volunteers achieved cost savings. Drugs and biological treatments have to be furnished, with a 5% coinsurance not to exceed a fixed amount per prescription. A hospice is required to provide at least 80% of its patient days of care outside the hospital.

To receive care from a Medicare-certified hospice, the patient's doctor must certify that the life expectancy is six months or less, the patient must elect the benefit and waive other types of acute care. The patient is only allowed to exit hospice twice to receive ordinary care. Clearly legalistic trappings have been added to a humanistically oriented, creative intervention.

For reimbursement purposes, four levels of hospice have been established: routine home care, continuous home care, inpatient respite care, and general inpatient care. But because Medicare payment rates for hospice care are often lower than those for regular home health care visits, many agencies have opted to provide a hospice-like service without seeking an official designation. Terminal patients cared for in this manner cannot be reimbursed for much of their home care under Medicare without a special hospice waiver.

In evaluating hospice, it seems most appropriate to examine effectiveness per se. Although the pressures for data on which to base public policy call for *cost*-effectiveness analyses, one must first establish whether a new therapy is effective. Such tests of efficacy should be based on the best models of care available. Once efficacy is established, one can then study how to maintain the performance level while reducing cost. Experience has shown that the cost question is largely established by external events anyway. Certainly once hospices became covered as a Medicare benefit, the question became how much hospice care could be provided for the price paid.

Only two major evaluations of hospice care have been reported, both outside the Medicare-certified benefit. The National Hospice Study used a quasi-experimental design to compare hospital-based and home-based hospice with conventional care in 40 sites across the country, 26 of which were funded with special Medicare demonstration waivers (Greer et al., 1986). The second study, done by investigators at the University of California at Los Angeles, was a randomized controlled trial of an inpatient and home-based hospice operated by a Veterans Administration Hospital (Kane et al., 1984).

When the results of these two evaluations were made public, considerable controversy was created, especially because the findings in the two studies, summarized in Table 7-8, were consistent. Basically, they reported that hospice care was not generally better than conventional care, but it was no worse. Each study found some instances in which the experimental group did better than the control group, but for most of the variables examined, no differences were found. Where significant differences occurred, they tended to be in levels of satisfaction expressed by patients or their families,

TABLE 7-8 Summary of Hospice Effects Demonstrated in Two Major Studies

Measure	UCLA Study[a]	National Hospice Study[b]	
		Hospital Based	Home Care
Patient Variables			
Pain and Symptoms	−	+?	−
Karnofsky Performance Status/ ADL	−	−	−
Quality of Life Index	0	−	−
Satisfaction	+	−	−
Anxiety	−	0	0
Depression	−	0	0
Caregiver Variables			
A. Prior to Death			
Anxiety	+?	−	−
Depression	−	−	−
Satisfaction	+?	+	+
B. Bereavement			
Anxiety	−	−	−
Depression	−	−	−
Satisfaction	0	+	+
Morbidity	−	−	−

Key: + significant benefit; − no significant benefit; 0 not examined; ? weak or mixed effect.
[a]Based on Kane et al. (1984) and Kane et al. (1986).
[b]Based on Greer et al. (1986).

rather than in pain control, affect, or symptoms (Greer et al., 1986; Kane et al., 1984, 1985a, 1985b, 1986). The National Hospice Study found that the cost of home-based hospice care was cheaper than conventional care (Birnbaum and Kidder, 1984). The UCLA study, which looked at a hospice where hospital-based care predominated, found no differences in cost.

What should be made of these data? The hospice evaluations scrupulously examined multiple outcomes, including pain control, affect, and satisfaction for both patients and their families. The only differences attributable to hospice were in satisfaction, an outcome that some critics do not recognize as a legitimate difference. Yet, perhaps it is enough success for a service provided to terminally ill persons if it allows them to experience more satisfactory care in their last days (Rainey et al., 1984). This question raises a basic dilemma for policy-makers. In general, there has been a discomfort in accepting satisfaction as a sufficient outcome for service. We tend to expect differences in other more professionally recognized parameters. Partly because we fear the placebo effect of a new service, particularly one that has been introduced with such fanfare, and partly because consumer satisfaction is compatible with technically poor care, we have been conditioned to be dissatisfied with satisfaction as the sole measure of success. However, in the case of hospice, the therapy is intended not to delay mortality, but to improve the quality of available time. In this instance, perhaps satisfaction is the truest test of all.

Two more observations can be made. First, it is possible that the two hospices showed so little effect because standard care had already incorporated some of the pain control and humanistic measures originally introduced by hospices. If that is so, hospice may have had its effect before it was evaluated. Second, an orthodoxy in hospice has developed as a result of Medicare reimbursement rules, but no body of evidence is available to support the advantages of that particular model of staffing and eligibility.

MENTAL HEALTH PROGRAMS

Mental health programs have undergone considerable upheaval in the United States since the initiation of community mental health centers (CMHCs) and the gradual shrinking of the state mental hospital (Kramer, 1986). The fledgling centers have become responsible for comprehensive mental health services to elderly patients. Many critics claim that outreach to the elderly is severely lacking and that persons over 65 tend to receive much less psychotherapy or skilled outpatient attention than is warranted by the prevalence of depression, anxiety, alcohol problems, and other mental disorders among the elderly population (General Accounting Office, 1982a). Certainly the experience of the geriatric assessment units described earlier was that psychiatric diagnoses tended to be overlooked. Similarly,

Waxman, Carner, and Berkenstock (1984) found that physicians in geriatric practices also failed to uncover mental health problems.

We identified little research on the effectiveness of mental health services for the elderly. This deficit pertains to information about how to more effectively screen older populations to identify treatable mental health problems, how to organize services to better reach the frail elderly and their families in the community, and, of course, the effectiveness of various psychological individual, family, and group treatments with the old.

Table 7-9 presents some limited information about mental health programs, particularly for the elderly living in the community. The first part of the table lists some studies that examined how well community mental health centers reached the elderly, and the second part of the table includes studies of mental health interventions directed at individual clients. Arbitrarily, we have reserved discussion about the outreach of community mental health centers to nursing homes and mental health therapies in nursing homes to the next chapter, which deals with the effectiveness of various health programs in long-term care facilities.

Taken together the few studies of community mental health programs suggested that exacerbations of physical illnesses and other life events (moving, for example) can trigger a mental health crisis. Winograd and Mirassou (1983) did an age-specific analysis of a crisis intervention service, however, and found low rates of self-referral and family referral for elderly persons. Estes and Wood (1984) and Flemming et al., (1984a, 1984b) documented the drop in service to the elderly as a result of changing funding policies in the early 1980s. Both studies relied on interviews with agency personnel in various communities, so that the responses may have been somewhat self-serving. Nevertheless, the two studies (one involving eight states and one, 41 states) suggested a general shrinking of the capacity to serve the elderly, as well as poor and infrequent communication between Area Agencies on Aging (AAAs) and community mental health centers. Little information is available about the positive effects that might be expected from a vigorous effort to provide timely mental health services to the elderly, although a Toronto service (Wasylenki et al., 1984) claims that mental health consultation to community providers such as public health nurses led to improved family supports and accounted for a low rate of institutional admission among the persons served.

Three reviews of therapeutic mental health efforts with the elderly present rather damaging cumulative information. Merriam (1980) looked at 19 studies of reminiscence therapy, a popular approach with the elderly. Most of the studies had tiny, nonrandom samples and lacked control groups. Moreover, the interventions tended to be vaguely delineated and hard to distinguish from other mental health strategies. A larger-scale review done at Columbia University's Long-Term Care Gerontology Center looked at a large number of studies of the effectiveness of individual and group psy-

TABLE 7-9 Studies on the Effectiveness of Mental Health Programs/Treatment for the Elderly

Source	Description of Program or Study	Study Design	Selected Findings
Community Mental Health Programs: Winograd and Mirassou (1983)	A crisis intervention service, begun in 1980 under the auspices of the Milwaukee County Mental Health Complex, provides 24-hour mental health emergency services to all ages, including a crisis hotline and a mobile unit staffed with a multidisciplinary team of mental health professionals.	4,685 hotline calls and 528 mobile crisis visits in 1981 were analyzed to present age-specific data on demographics, precipitating events, client characteristics, and outcomes.	The most common precipitating event for the elderly was ADL dysfunction; severe depression was not a major precipitating event. Psychiatric problems of elderly clients appeared uncritical when compared with problems of danger to self, usually for a medical or ADL dysfunction. Rates of self-referral and family referral were lower for elderly clients.
Estes and Wood (1984)	A preliminary assessment of the impact of block grants, initiated by the 1981 Omnibus Budget Reconciliation Act, upon community mental health centers.	Administrators at 23 private, nonprofit CMHCs and 12 public CMHCs were interviewed by telephone (1983) as part of a larger 8-state survey of nine types of service agencies in 32 urban areas.	35% of CMHCs reported changes in Medicaid policies involving cost caps, reductions in services covered, increased copayments. 42% reported a reduction in full-time staff; 31% a reduction in service capacity. 71% experienced reduced federal funding; state and local funds appear not to be replacing such losses.

TABLE 7-9 Continued

Source	Description of Program or Study	Study Design	Selected Findings
Flemming et al. (1984a, 1984b)	A study of the impact of Alcohol, Drug Abuse, and Mental Health Services block grant program (part of the 1981 Omnibus Budget and Reconciliation Act) on the delivery of mental health services to elderly persons.	In 1983, 223 community mental health clinics (a 36% response rate representing 41 states) responded to a mailed survey requesting data on the impact of the block grant, aging programs, client population, funding, and staff. 11 CMHCs and 11 local AAAs were visited to provide in-depth information.	48% of CMHCs reported adverse effects due to the block grant; between 1981 and 1983 there has been a decrease in the CMHCs with aging programs (64%–55%); the aged remain underserved as only 6% of CMHC clients. AAAs and CMHCs have little contact or routine interaction with each other.
Wasylenki et al. (1984)	A community psychogeriatric service, begun in Toronto in 1979 and funded by the Ontario Ministry of Health, uses psychiatrists and clinical specialists in psychiatric nursing to provide client-centered case consultation and administrative consultation to community providers such as visiting home nurses.	Consultees for the first 100 client cases were interviewed six months following the provision of consultation regarding client outcomes and satisfaction with the program.	In 79% of the cases a precipitating life event led to the consultation: in 30% of the cases it was a move; in 22%, development of physical illness. 82% of the consultees were satisfied with the consultation. Authors speculated that consultation emphasizing social support modification (e.g., increase family involvement) may have led to a low institutionalization rate (19%).

Mental Health Interventions: Merriam (1980)	A review of 19 studies (1970–80) on reminiscence, with emphasis on its conceptualization, its relationship to other cognitive and affective activities, and its adaptive value in later adulthood.	The author critiqued research designs and looked for congruence in the way reminiscence was defined and associated with adjustment and aging.	Findings as to whether or not reminiscence correlates with adjustment in older age appeared equivocal. Studies differed in defining reminiscence and failed to differentiate it from other mental processes. Most studies used small, non-random samples.
Bennett et al. (n.d.)	A review and critical analysis of the 1970–80 research literature on individual and group psychotherapy and psychosocial programs for the elderly (e.g., reminiscence, life crisis, reality, resocialization, and remotivation therapy).	Studies were reviewed in terms of sample characteristics (e.g., size, age), program characteristics (goals, content, role of therapist, duration and frequency of treatment), research design, and outcomes.	The studies typically reported positive outcomes but conclusions were most often impressionistic rather than based upon controlled design, e.g., only two of nine studies on group therapy used experimental designs. When an experimental design was used, findings appeared to be mixed. Most studies failed to address the question, "What specific therapies are effective for what type of client?"
Zarit and Anthony (1986)	A critical review of the research literature on the effectiveness of institutional and community interventions/treatments for the demented elderly.	Studies on interventions such as behavioral modification, individual and group psychotherapy, reality orientation, critical life review, and environmental changes were reviewed regarding adequacy of research design.	Findings tended to be equivocal, and research designs were plagued by problems such as lack of controls, self-selection in sampling, non-objective measurements, poor conceptualization of outcomes. Few studies measured long-term effects.

chotherapy and psycho-social programs for the elderly conducted between 1970 and 1980 (Bennett et al., n.d.). The studies tended to report positive results, but most were based on small samples and no controls. When controls were used, the results became more mixed. Zarit and Anthony (1986) reviewed studies of the effectiveness of therapeutic efforts for persons with senile dementia and found a similar lack of rigor in the studies.

ADULT PROTECTIVE SERVICES/GUARDIANSHIP

Long-term care users are, by definition, functionally impaired. To some degree, almost all would have difficulty protecting themselves from physical attacks, and the dependency inherent in needing care means that many have little redress against a caregiver (either in the family or in a paid position) who withholds care, treats them in a denigrating manner, exploits them financially, or engages in outright physical abuse. "Elder abuse" has crept into the lexicon, joining child abuse and spousal abuse as a social problem requiring urgent attention.

Considerable effort has been devoted to classifying elder abuse and determining its incidence and prevalence. Estimates continue to vary widely, as was noted in a Project Share review of studies on abuse of older people (Langley, 1981). In 1986, Quinn and Tomita produced a detailed monograph on abuse of the elderly, which contains an extensive bibliography of previous work. They too chronicle the confusion in terms; the propensity to mingle physical abuse, psychological abuse, neglect, and even "self-neglect" in the data bases; and the inaccuracy of the statistics. On the other hand, they present a weighty volume of clinical anecdotes that attest to the frequency of what anyone would consider serious financial exploitation and physical maltreatment.

Conceptual confusion about elder abuse centers around those persons who are cognitively impaired. While it may be true that persons with senile dementia are particularly likely to become victims of abuse, that case has not been irrefutably made. It is true, however, that persons with substantial cognitive impairment will be unable to make decisions in their own interests. Legal vehicles for alternative decision-making, and programs to protect persons without family who are able or willing to fill the role responsibly, are therefore needed. Adult protective services, guardianship programs, and conservatorship programs all have developed to fill the role of responsible person. They *may* be used when abuse is present or suspected, but cognitive impairment is the trigger rather than maltreatment.

The research literature about the effects of programs in this area is extraordinarily skimpy. Projects funded to improve detection of abuse have concentrated on assessment methodology (Daiches, 1984) and have not developed and tested any batteries that have proved themselves sufficiently sensitive and specific to identify cases. Work is presently being done to develop a classification system for elder abuse, but again no tested typology has emerged. Many states have developed laws requiring mandatory reporting of elder abuse. A review of the 16 such statutes enacted by the end of 1982 showed that most states were unable to generate meaningful statistics from the reports and that protective social services to investigate the reports and work to remedy the substantiated cases fell far short of the need (Salend et al., 1984). We have not yet developed a literature that would suggest what intervention strategies are most effective to prevent elder abuse, to identify it, or to protect its victims from further abuse. Callahan (1982) even questioned whether labeling problems as elder abuse might do more harm than good.

Guardianship and conservatorship practices have received little systematic study (White and Steinberg, 1984). A few descriptive studies exist that cast doubt on whether the rights of the elderly are adequately protected during incompetency hearings and whether the court monitors the subsequent guardianship adequately. Peters, Schmidt, and Miller (1985) studied 42 competency cases adjudicated in Tallahassee between 1977 and 1982. In all instances, without question the courts opted against the limited guardianship mechanism, preferring to grant full guardianship even when the ward clearly retained some function. Most disturbing, monitoring of the guardianships was almost nonexistent. Furthermore, relatives seemed most willing to be involved as guardians when a substantial inheritance was at stake.

The most prominent study of adult protective services was shocking in its findings, all the more so because the study used a strong experimental design. Essentially, persons in need of protective service from participating agencies were identified, enrolled in the study, and randomly assigned to receive specialized, intensive services from caseworkers at Benjamin Rose Institute in Cleveland. The services included medical, legal, and homemaker/health aide services and appropriate placement in facilities. Social workers worked directly with clients and their families to alleviate stress and provide support. Meanwhile, the control group received only those protective services that were normally available in the community. At the end of the experimental year, the group receiving intensive protective services had higher rates of nursing home use, higher death rates, and no better scores on measures of mental and physical functioning or contentment than the control group (Blenkner, Bloom, and Nielson, 1971).

Many commentators have questioned these findings, and a recent reexamination of the raw data concluded that the study design was fatally flawed (Dunkle et al., 1983). These latter investigators argued that the study was too imprecise about the nature of the services received by the experimental group, that it exaggerated the importance of mortality and institutional placement as outcomes on which to base the success or failure of the study, and that an original plan to have two separate experimental groups, one receiving financial assistance, was scuttled and the two experimental subgroups inappropriately combined. Although we agree that admission to a nursing home may not be a clear negative outcome for victims of abuse, none of the objections to the study dilute the force of the negative findings, especially on mortality. At the very least, it seems that we need to know more about how to go about giving deluxe protective services to produce positive effects. Unfortunately, no further experiments in adult protective services have been reported, making the one, rather old study more influential than it might otherwise be.

HOUSING/HOME MAINTENANCE

Long-term care and housing are intertwined in a variety of ways:

1. Without an adequate, safe shelter, a frail elderly person is at risk for long-term care. Programs that build houses and/or make them available at affordable rents, or that assist with home maintenance, repair, or security, minimize the risk of the elderly residents' needing long-term care in institutions.
2. A specially designed or equipped home may enable a functionally impaired person to remain independent longer and to require fewer supportive efforts from family and friends. Therefore, programs that equip or modify existing homes to produce a better environment for functioning might be considered a long-term care service.
3. The nature and location of the home influences the amount, type, and cost of service needed for a functionally impaired tenant. If the elderly are well housed in accessible locations, services can be more easily targeted. These include meal service in a common dining room, home health services, emergency surveillance, and even health clinics.
4. A home is an asset that many older persons enjoy. If it has sufficient space, it is possible that home-sharing arrangements might be developed that allow a functionally impaired person some mixture of income, service, or security in exchange for room and board.

The bricks-and-mortar part of housing falls outside long-term care per se; yet an effective housing policy can provide a framework for more effective long-term care delivery. At the other end of the continuum, programs that arrange and/or finance home modifications or repair specifically to meet longterm care needs, or programs to promote home-sharing, might definitely be considered long-term care programs. Indeed, home modifications are permitted under Medicaid waivers. The arena of services within housing developments is a gray area that requires joint planning of housing and long-term care authorities. The space to permit congregate meals and social or health programs in public housing or housing subsidized by federal dollars is, of course, a matter of housing policy. Setting expectations for housing managers and training them about aging also falls to housing departments. Yet, many programs brought to housing units might well be considered long-term care. Once again, the key issue seems to be making sure that the service is organized and effective rather than establishing its jurisdiction label as housing or something else.

Table 7-10 reviews evidence on the effects of programs in this amorphous area of housing and long-term care. Two general references presented descriptive information about the clientele in housing programs and their overall satisfaction. Urban Systems (1976) studied a sample of tenants of housing projects, finding, among other things, that residents preferred having kitchens and were dissatisfied with one-room units. Struyk and Soldo (1980) examined home and neighborhood preservation programs, finding that renters were more likely to be served than owners.

The next four studies deal with services in housing. Brody, Kleban, and Liebowitz (1975) used a quasi-experimental design to look at the effects of congregate housing administered by the Philadelphia Geriatric Center. Compared to those who had applied for housing but moved elsewhere, and those who had applied but remained in their original housing, the experimental group had the greatest satisfaction with their apartment and living arrangement, the most social contacts, the greatest enjoyment of life, and the least desire to move. Of special interest were the group who stayed rooted to their home and who seemed the worst off. The authors speculated on whether a phenomenon of immobilization exists that needs attention. Lawton (1980) seems to bear this out in his study of persons who were rehoused in congregate housing for the elderly of various types. Although those who moved tended to be more functionally impaired than those who stayed, they also had higher morale, were more satisfied with their housing, and were more involved in social activities. Harel and Harel (1978) compared elderly residents of age-integrated and age-segregated public housing, finding that the former used more home health services but had better residential stability and survival over a four year period.

Sherwood and her colleagues (1981) presented a detailed quasi-experimental study of a congregate housing program—a low-income, federally subsidized, medically oriented project for the physically impaired and elderly. It was located adjacent to a hospital and had on-site health programs available. Compared to matched controls, the experimental group had a significantly lower rate of long-term care institutional use over a five-year period and a better four-year mortality rate. They were also more satisfied with their housing. The experimental group was likely to use more hospital care than the control, but the cost-benefit ratio, when examined over a three-year horizon, still favored the experimental group. Of particu-

TABLE 7-10 Studies on the Effects of Housing Programs

Source	Description of Program or Study	Study Design	Selected Findings
General: Urban Systems Research & Engineering (1976)	A descriptive and analytical study of congregate housing, including the characteristics and needs of residents, the types of programs offered, and their impact upon elderly residents' needs. Congregate housing is operationally defined as age-segregated housing for those 62+ with at least an on-site meal program.	A random, stratified sample of 27 housing projects was selected, representing all regions of the United States and differing in range of rent levels, type of services, and building size. Methods included interviewing residents and applicants, interviewing personnel, and studying records.	Findings on program impact included: Residents at all sites uniformly evaluated the services and design features of congregate facilities positively; knowing that services were there, if needed, was important; 2-meal-per-day food services, a medium-high level of medical service, and housekeeping (at least bi-weekly) were the services most preferred. Residents were dissatisfied with 1-room units and preferred having kitchens. Programs tended to increase rather than decrease resident contact with the community.
Struyk and Soldo (1980)	A critical review of existing housing and neighborhood preservation programs as they impact upon the elderly, including Public Housing, Section 202, Section 312, CDBG rehab loans and grants, housing allowances, housing improvement and stock preservation, Section 8.	Using available data, the authors evaluated programs in terms of six criteria: efficient targeting, housing improvement, equal opportunity, preservation of housing stock, cost minimization, and administrative simplicity. The authors drew upon HUD reports and the works of other program analysts.	The elderly were represented among recipients of subsidized housing in proportion to other income-eligible households; since elderly households had fewer persons in them, the per capita subsidy rates were higher for the elderly than for others; the elderly outside of metro areas were underserved by HUD programs. Elderly renters were overserved, while elderly homeowners receive no direct subsidies. Section 8 had high or high/moderate ratings on all six criteria; other programs had mixed ratings.

Services in Housing: Brody, Kleban, and Liebowitz (1975)	Intermediate Housing for the Elderly, under the auspices of the Philadelphia Geriatric Center, provided self-contained apartments with private bedrooms, kitchens, and sharing living rooms. Features included special designs to assure safety, a telephone "hot-line" to the center from each house, optional housekeeping, and provision of frozen meals.	A quasi-experimental design in which residents were compared at admission (baseline) and at six months with two control groups: those who had applied and moved elsewhere and those who had applied but had not moved. The three groups were similar at baseline regarding the four study variables: overall satisfaction with apartment and living arrangement, desire to move, enjoyment of life, social contact.	On all four variables the experimentals had more positive scores than the control groups. Problems of dissatisfaction with neighborhood were resolved by both of the groups who moved but not by the group who did not move. Since a greater proportion of non-movers were female, the question arises whether or not women are more rooted to their homes than men.
Harel and Harel (1978)	Cedar Coordinated Services for Seniors provided coordinated services, including social work, nursing, outreach, and home aide, to both the age-integrated and age-segregated sections of a public housing project for low-income residents. The age-integrated section had about 25% elderly tenants.	A goal of the study was to compare the impact of coordinated services upon residential stability, relocation, institutionalization, and survival between the two groups. These variables were monitored yearly from 1972 to 1975. Pre-testing found the two groups to be similar regarding factors such as demographic characteristics, health, social involvement, physical and mental functioning.	Residents in age-segregated buildings tended to utilize nursing, home aide, and social work services more than age-integrated residents. During the four years of the study, the age-segregated residents also had higher degrees of residential stability and survival rates. Age-integrated residents had a lower rate of institutionalization.

TABLE 7-10 Continued

Source	Description of Program or Study	Study Design	Selected Findings
Lawton (1980)	A controlled study of the impact of planned housing and on-site supportive services upon elderly residents. Study goals included the measurement of impacts upon physical, psychological, social functioning and competence in self-maintenance; the differential effects of housing environments; differences between those who applied and did not apply for this housing.	A longitudinal group control method was used with samples of residents from 12 sites interviewed prior to residency and after one year of residence. The sites, studied in the early 1970s, represented low-rent public housing, lower middle-income section 202 housing, and non-subsidized section 312 housing.	Although poorer in functional health than the controls, the rehoused were higher in morale, more satisfied with housing, more involved in social activities, more satisfied with their current situation. Full-service residences appeared to attract tenant groups who were less functionally competent and more vulnerable to passivity. The most efficient way to predict resident well-being after one year of residency is to measure at the time of admission the specific factor that is of interest.
Sherwood et al. (1981)	Highland Heights Apartments, in River Falls, MA, is a low-income, federally sponsored, medically oriented housing project for the physically impaired and elderly. Specialized aspects include hardware and layout specifically designed for the physically impaired, an on-site outpatient clinic, availability of health and other community services as	A quasi-experimental study (1970 to 1976) with matched controls to evaluate the impact of Highland Heights on the health and well-being of its residents. 228 residents were matched with 228 applicants on a number of factors, including ethnic group, closeness of children, characteristics of household and residential mobility, sex, age. Impact up to five years was	A significant positive impact on rate of LTC institutionalization over five years and mortality over four years. Experimentals were more satisfied with their housing, although there was no significant impact upon morale. Experimentals were more likely to be hospitalized but, over three years, there was still a cost-benefit ratio of 2.21. Analysis of a subgroup of deinstitutionalized residents resulted in positive findings regarding service utilization, mortal-

	well as physical and occupational therapy.	studied regarding housing, health, social and emotional variables.	ity, satisfaction with services, and social life.
Home Repair: Ferguson, Holin, and Moss (1983)	An evaluation of seven home maintenance demonstration projects for the elderly (Cincinnati, Cleveland, Boston, Greensboro, Hot Springs, Philadelphia, San Francisco). The demonstrations, begun in 1980, provided minor repairs and maintenance, home inspections, and client referral assistance. They differed in size, structure and auspices, and the home maintenance experience of personnel. Clients were homeowners, met section 8 eligibility criteria, and were 62 or older.	Administrative analysis of operations and costs, surveys of client attitudes and satisfaction, and a survey of other existing programs were used to determine client needs, appropriate delivery systems, costs, and benefits to the target population.	90% of the clients interviewed were satisfied with their repairs; one-third claimed that the program affected their ability to remain in their homes. The demonstration has shown that (1) a program must have the elderly's trust (word of mouth and referrals from other programs attracted clients), (2) it must provide a wide range of repair services, (3) the agency should have experience in the delivery of housing-related services, (4) costs must be low.
Lowy (1984)	The Housing and Living Assistance Program (1980 to 1983) under the aegis of a neighborhood community development and services	An outside agency studied the organizational aspects, services delivered, and outcomes of the project; methods included telephone in-	120–140 contacts were made monthly regarding an average monthly caseload of 15, demonstrating the intensity of effort needed to resolve client issues. Most of the clients

TABLE 7-10 Continued

Source	Description of Program or Study	Study Design	Selected Findings
	agency in Boston (United South End Settlements) provided a range of services, including help with fuel assistance and property tax problems, help with minor home repairs, financial assistance for repairs, in order to help older homeowners maintain their homes and remain in the community.	terviews with 18 program users and non-users.	needed assistance with only one problem. 3 out of 18 homeowners interviewed stated that the program contributed to their ability to stay in their homes.
Shared Housing: Howe, Robins, and Jaffe (1984)	Homeshare, a component of Independent Living Inc., a private, nonprofit service agency for the elderly, arranges intergenerational matches between elderly homeowners and student/younger employed persons in Madison, WI. The program recruits, screens, matches applicants, oversees a contract, and provides follow-up services such as renegotiation and problem solving. The elderly receive services (e.g., personal care, chores) in exchange for room/board.	A qualitative study (1983) based upon interviews with 34 pairs of elders and their roomers, program staff, and community service agency personnel. Findings address the administrative structure and staffing characteristics of the program as well as its impact upon elders and students.	70% of the pairs interviewed described their experience as an "unqualified" or "qualified" success. The 30% failure rate appeared to be often due to live-ins' being pressured for more companionship than they had expected, or elders feeling "expected" services were not met. The programs may defer institutionalization and save costs since the frail elders would probably have not been able to remain at home without a live-in resident.

lar interest are the encouraging findings regarding a small group who entered the housing project from a nursing home. These deinstitutionalized persons did much better than their controls on service utilization, satisfaction with services, social life, and mortality.

Two studies of home repair programs (Ferguson, Holin, and Moss, 1983; Lowy, 1984) presented positive information based on follow-up contacts with users. However, no comparison groups were used. Finally, we identified only one study of shared housing (Howe, Robins, and Jaffe, 1984). This was a qualitative study based on interviewing 34 pairs of elders and their roommates, who had assisted in making these housing arrangements. Seventy percent of the pairs were judged an unqualified success, and the authors speculated that the program deferred admission to institutions and saved costs. Of course, this type of evaluation does not include persons who explored the idea of home-sharing and found it unappealing.

Taking this evidence together, we conclude that there is much we still do not understand about housing choices and their effects, and about systematic programs to improve the ability of the functionally impaired to live independently through manipulating their housing or making services more available where they live. However, the positive findings in the few studies of services in housing, and particularly in the Sherwood study, are too promising to ignore.

MISCELLANEOUS OTHER PROGRAMS

The evaluation of program effectiveness in other areas related to long-term care is spotty and tends to defy categorization. Several such studies are summarized in Table 7-11. Here we found a number of programs, often one-shot demonstration projects or programs under waiver, that were either directly a part of long-term care—emergency alarm and response systems and special transportation efforts for the disabled, for example—or at least indirectly related, such as wellness education demonstrations, or senior center programs.

We were surprised to find no studies on the effectiveness of telephone reassurance programs. In a related area, namely telephone-connected emergency alarm and response systems, however, an ambitious, well-designed study of "lifeline" is available and presented interesting findings (Sherwood and Morris, 1980). The system evaluated was designed to automatically contact and send client-identification information to an emergency service when activated. The investigators used a controlled design to analyze the impact of the system over a 14-month period on three subgroups of frail elderly: those severely disabled as well as socially isolated, those severely disabled but not isolated, and those who were isolated and moderately disabled. The program was found to have the most positive

TABLE 7-11 Miscellaneous Other Programs

Source	Description of Program or Study	Study Design	Selected Findings
Colen and Soto (1979)	A statewide survey of about 200 California social service agencies that attempted to identify programmatic activities and techniques that are successful in attracting, engaging, and serving minority aged participants.	One hundred twenty-five self-administered questionnaires (63% response rate) were analyzed to determine the program characteristics (e.g., outreach, organization, special activities, staff) that correlated with success in serving aged minorities. Programs were defined as successful if their minority population was at least equal to their percentage in the catchment area served.	Variables associated with program success: emphasis upon consumer input that assures confidentiality; location near other vital services; emphasis upon basic needs such as nutrition, employment, health screening; programmatic use of ethnic holidays and events; rapport with minority leaders; minority persons on program staff and boards. These factors varied, depending upon the minority group in question.
Dorosin and Phillips (1979)	"Share A Fare," Kansas City, MO, is a user-subsidized transportation service targeted to those 65+ or certified as non-ambulatory. Program staff (City Hall) enroll participants, dispatch trip requests, pay disbursements. Nonprofit social service carriers as well as taxicab and medicab companies participate. Riders use free coupons, subsidized by a ½¢ city sales tax, in addition to paying about 50¢ a ~~rid~~	A descriptive evaluation of the program's administration, operations, costs, and impacts on a clients for the first 20 months of operation (1977–78).	After 18 months the project had grown to 13,000 enrollees at 10,724 trips per month. Costs per trip were $2.92; total subsidies did not appear to match the transport costs of nonprofit agencies but provided a steady funding source, supplemented by agency funds. Report emphasized that administration by the city provided legal, marketing, planning expertise, and a single coordinating power.

Bass and Rowland (1980)	A study, by the Gerontology Program at the University of Massachusetts/Boston, of the impact of increased fuel costs on Boston elders paying for their own heat.	A non-probablistic stratified sample of 108 elderly, 62+, with incomes under $10,120 annually. In-depth, open-ended interviews were given and the thematic frequencies of the interviews were analyzed.	The problems or concerns mentioned by the highest percentage of elderly persons were the need to take "heat-saving measures" (30%); changes in one's standard of living (21%); the need to seek financial or other assistance (11%); changes in living arrangements such as closing off part of the house (10%); nutrition and health problems (6%).
Sherwood and Morris (1980) Ruchlin and Morris (1981)	"Lifeline" is an emergency alarm system attached to the telephone. It can automatically seize the line, dial the number of an emergency service, and send identifying information by means of digital code. The unit can be remotely activated or can be set to dial automatically if the client is unusually inactive.	Five hundred fifty-one potential users, with a mean age of 75, were randomly assigned to experimental and control groups, and measured at baseline and at 14 months on utilization of health services, costs, indices on quality of life. Three subgroups were studied: Group 1=severely disabled and isolated; Group 2=severely disabled but not isolated; Group 3=isolated and moderately disabled.	Findings were mixed for Groups 1 and 3, but the program had positive impact on those who were severely disabled but not isolated. These Group 2 experimentals used significantly fewer health resources, had fewer days of institutional care, had higher scores on quality of life (reduced anxiety, increased confidence). Net savings were at a cost/benefit ratio of $7.19.

TABLE 7-11 Continued

Source	Description of Program or Study	Study Design	Selected Findings
GAO (1982c)	In 1982, GAO surveyed the special efforts of transit systems to comply with federal rules requiring that federally assisted transit programs make their systems accessible to the elderly and handicapped.	The data were based upon interviews with 10 Regional Urban Mass Transportation Offices and telephone surveys on 18 large, 29 medium, and 37 small transit systems in urban areas. Topics surveyed included accessibility of systems, types of paratransit systems, transit system efforts to work with local representatives of the elderly and handicapped.	Forty-eight percent of the bus systems interviewed and 28% of the rail systems offered regularly scheduled life-equipped buses or cars. Eighty percent of the systems offered some type of paratransit system, usually with shorter hours and less days of service; highest priority was given to medical or work-related travel. Handicapped/elderly representatives thought that coordination and consultation could be improved.
Lalonde and Hooyman (1984)	The Wallingford Wellness Project, begun in 1979, was a 21-week health promotion training program for volunteers aged 54+. Group process, behavioral change methods, and health-related information/skills were essential components in a curriculum that integrated physical fitness, stress management, nutrition, and environmental awareness.	A nonrandom design in which 90 participants and 44 controls (selected from similar residential areas) were compared at baseline, six months, and two years after the program. Self-administered questionnaires measured variables such as health knowledge, risk to heart attack/stroke, number of health problems, health attitudes, health behaviors, and morbidity.	At six months there were significant positive improvements regarding health knowledge, risk of heart attack/stroke, mental health, self-responsibility for health. At the two-year follow-up, life style and health knowledge had been sustained; other variables had returned to pre-test levels. There was no impact upon health status or health services utilization.

Cohen (1983)	The geriatric department of a private, non-profit agency used two approaches to service delivery: a decentralized, team-centered approach in which team members shared cases and had direct control over ancillary services/staff; a hierarchically supervised approach with one-on-one casework in which workers had no direct control over ancillary staff.	All 1,628 clients admitted in a two-year period were assigned "equally" to team or control (hierarchical) groups. A subsample of 250 clients was compared on functioning and client satisfaction variables, using the PGC Multi-Level Assessment Instrument.	No difference between the clients of the two groups in satisfaction with services. The team approach intervened more quickly in crises and was superior in working with complex cases. The control group institutionalized clients at twice the rate of the team group. The team approach appeared to be less costly (no figures given).
Kempler and Gallup (1984)	The Growing Younger Health Promotion Program, Boise, ID, consisted of a core of four two-hour workshops on physical fitness, nutrition, stress management, and medical self-care. Participants were recruited through neighborhood information parties hosted by seniors. The neighborhood groups were encouraged to continue as a focus for support.	Self-administered questionnaire responses were gathered at baseline and six months following the program on changes in nutrition, stress/social factors, fitness, and medical care for 1,658 participants. Pre- and post-biometric measures were also taken on a subsample of over 300. Cost impacts on Parts A and B Medicare were measures.	Significant positive changes in fitness, nutrition, stress/social factors, and medical care behaviors; significant positive changes at six months in systolic blood pressure, weight, body fat, flexibility, serum cholesterol. No reductions in Medicare costs were demonstrated for the 12 months following the program.

TABLE 7-11 Continued

Source	Description of Program or Study	Study Design	Selected Findings
Ralston (1984)	A critical review of the research literature on senior centers, including analyses of research design and findings in the areas of program models, quality of programs, correlates of senior center use.	Available empirical research from the past 20 years was reviewed in terms of population sampled, study design, variables investigated, statistical analysis, major findings. Recommendations were made for the directions of future research.	Little research has been done to evaluate the effectiveness of senior center programs; there is some consistency regarding lack of effectiveness in research on educational goals. Findings are mixed on the correlates of senior center use (race, socio-economic status, social contact), although non-users appear to have poorer health and users tend to be more involved in group activities.
Schneider, Chapman, and Voth (1985)	Two senior centers in Arkansas were studied to determine (1) who used centers and (2) effects of the programs.	A panel of seniors was studied before centers began and two years after implementation. A random community sample (N=149) and a sample of persons screened for the centers (N=251) were used. Frequent participants (i.e., those attending once a week or more) were compared to others in both samples.	Seniors attending centers were active and at low risk of institutional care. Those attending were no different from nonattendees in attitude, behavior, and subsequent rates of entering nursing homes.

impacts, not upon the most severely disabled *and* isolated group, but upon the group that was severely disabled and not socially isolated. The authors speculated that the first group, without even social supports to meet many needs, simply had too many deficiencies for a limited intervention such as "lifeline" to meet. The findings again emphasize the importance of accurate targeting.

Two studies on transportation programs for the disabled described efforts more than they presented findings on effectiveness. The General Accounting Office (1982c) found that, since the issuance of a 1981 interim rule rescinding previous requirements that federally assisted mass transit systems be made accessible to the handicapped, only 30 of 83 bus systems and 6 of 14 rail systems still intended to reach the level of accessibility previously required. A study of "Share-a-Fare," a user-side subsidy transportation program for the elderly and disabled in Kansas City, Missouri, emphasized the effectiveness of using city management to coordinate a variety of systems—medicab companies, taxicabs, and social services carriers—in meeting transportation needs (Dorosin and Phillips, 1979). The program appeared to have minimal impact, however, on taxicab use, and the city subsidy was too low to match the transport costs of nonprofit agencies.

Evaluations on the effectiveness of wellness and health promotion programs have had mixed results. A two-year follow-up study of the Wallingford Wellness Project, a 21-week health promotion program for those aged 54 years or older, found that although some improvements in life style and health knowledge had been sustained, there had been nonsignificant impact upon health status or health services utilization (Lalonde and Hooyman, 1984). In another health promotion program, "Growing Younger" in Boise, Idaho, Kempler and Gallup (1984) found some positive impacts upon health status and behavior at six months but were not able to demonstrate any reductions in Medicare costs for the 12-month period following the program.

In another area, Cohen (1983) studied the impact of a team system of service delivery upon the elderly clients of a family service agency. In comparing an organizational style in which workers shared clients and jointly managed cases in a traditional one-on-one approach, she found that although there was no impact upon client satisfaction, teams were able to respond more quickly in crisis situations and had a lower rate of client institutionalization. Additional results appeared to be lower costs and higher staff morale.

Although not directly related to long-term care, three other studies should be mentioned under this section. Ralston's review of senior center research is helpful in underscoring the need for more research on the effectiveness of senior center programs for the elderly. He found that what few studies there were in the area of program effectiveness focused on educational programs. He suggested the need for more program evaluation, further exploration of senior center models, and more rigorous studies on the correlates of center use (Ralston, 1984). A study of the effects of participating in senior centers in two rural Arkansas counties was conducted in two phases: one to determine who used the center and the other to study program impacts. Programs tended to reach active seniors not at risk of institutional care. Those who attended the centers showed no significant difference from nonattendees two years later on attitude, behavior, use of other services, or institutionalization rates (Schneider, Chapman, and Voth, 1985). In another study, Colen and Soto (1979) surveyed about 200 California social service agencies in order to identify program techniques that were successful in attracting and maintaining elderly minority clients. Key variables included assurances of confidentiality, location near other vital services, programmatic uses of ethnic holidays and events, minority participation on agency boards, and minority staff.

CONCLUDING COMMENT

The programs reviewed in this chapter (and in the previous one on home care and day care) do not stand alone. Ideally, they must be mixed and matched to create a well-organized system of long-term care to meet a community's need. Perhaps an effort to evaluate these programs in isolation is unfair. Their potential effectiveness is highly dependent on the other system components. Moreover, the goals and likely effects of many programs are quite limited, and yet they are often examined singly for wide-ranging results.

Systems can, of course, be designed to emphasize some long-term care components over others. In Chapter 10 we discuss evidence about how to approach an effective system of care. But, the next chapter turns to the nursing home, the form of long-term care that predominates in influence and public expense.

8

Nursing Homes

This chapter considers the effectiveness of long-term care in nursing homes. In the United States, the nursing home dominates long-term care both in influence and in public expense. Statistics on nursing home use have generally been the basis for estimating how much long-term care is needed in the country (Chapter 2), and nursing home care accounts for the lion's share of service financed by public programs (Chapter 3). In fact, community long-term care programs have largely been envisaged and promoted as more humane or cheaper "alternatives" to the nursing home (Chapter 4). Yet, given the complex relationship between the nursing home and other community long-term care programs, a simplistic dichotomy between nursing home care and community care cannot be sustained.

A nursing home can provide a wide range of health and social services to residents and to persons in the community as well. For example, nursing homes can offer home care, day care, home-delivered meals, hospice, geriatric evaluation, emergency alarm systems, specialized housing, and many other long-term care programs discussed in the previous two chapters. Thus, a nursing home may operate a variety of programs at the facility and in detached locations, and its clientele may be residents or may live elsewhere.

For residents, the nursing home is a setting for a package of services, not a single program. Many of the elements we have considered separately as community programs could be, or are, part of care provided within and by a nursing home. For example, organized opportunities for residents to serve as volunteers, supportive programs for family caregivers, mental health programs, geriatric assessment, and hospice could be offered by a nursing home for its residents and evaluated for distinctive effects.

Finally, a nursing home is a housing program, which may well be evaluated for its desirability, convenience, attractiveness, and ability to satisfy its "tenants." For residents, the nursing home is, above all, the place where they live.

Furthermore, residents of nursing homes can derive benefit from programs offered by community long-term care and aging programs, though they seldom have good access to such outside programs. For example, transportation for medical and social purposes, community-based day programs, or community mental health programs offered by organizations other than the nursing home can be used by selected nursing home residents with good effect. Such blending is less common in the United States than in other countries. For example, in some countries, nursing home residents do leave their facilities for specialized day programs or rehabilitative efforts. Or, community workers employed by outside agencies come to the nursing home to give services to residents. In some Canadian provinces, home care agencies even go to nursing homes to provide various therapies, and, therefore, the rolls of public home care programs include clients living in nursing homes (Kane and Kane, 1985). A person for whom a nursing home proves the least restrictive environment for long-term care has a just claim to services that are available to others who receive their long-term care at home (for example, transportation systems for the disabled). At the very least, residents of nursing homes are due the same protective social services to guard their safety, civil rights, and financial resources as people living in the community.

In summary, the nursing home could be viewed as a community itself with a responsibility to provide and arrange all forms of long-term care, or as a hotel-like setting where services can be conveniently delivered, or something between these extremes. But, undisputably, the relationship between care in or by a nursing home and care in or by community-based programs is complex. The body of evidence on effects of nursing homes or the effects of programs within the nursing homes is extensive, but disorganized and hard to apply. In addition, much of the evidence about community long-term care programs could also be applied to improving care in nursing homes.

STUDIES AVAILABLE

Material about nursing homes is voluminous, although well-designed, meaningful studies about outcomes for residents are few. Even after we excluded most descriptions of what nursing home care is and opinion pieces about what it should be, a large body of research remained. We make no claim to comprehensiveness in our selection. Allusion to all the studies we identified would yield a tedious catalog, and attempts to find every last study would have had diminishing returns. Instead we characterized the research on nursing homes according to major themes and trends, and tried to distill consistent messages about the effectiveness of facility care.

We have divided our material about nursing homes into the following categories:

- Studies that examine the effects of particular clinical techniques or programs on the well-being of residents, or that suggest factors associated with well-being of residents. These usually are conducted within a single nursing home.
- Studies of ways to define, maintain, or improve the overall quality of care in nursing homes. Somewhat unfortunately, these studies tend to make the nursing home, rather than the resident, the object of analysis.
- Studies of the effects of staffing patterns and other administrative aspects of organizing nursing home care.
- Studies of how nursing homes are financed or reimbursed that might suggest effective ways to get the most for the money, as well as the incentives introduced by payment policies.

Some studies were beyond the scope of this review. We excluded studies comparing nursing home residents to some hypothetical population "appropriate" for nursing home care according to state policy. We also excluded studies of the effects of specific medical, pharmacological, or other therapeutic procedures on the physical health of nursing home residents. Health care, broadly construed, should benefit nursing home residents equally as well as patients of similar age and health status anywhere else.

Finally, we made no attempt to collect medical care evaluation (MCE) studies, which examine the ability of the nursing home to effect improvements in the care of specific problems where deficiencies have been noted. The MCE study methodology, which was developed first for quality assurance in the hospital, is part research and part intervention. It follows a stylized pattern with the following steps: selection of a topic thought to reflect inadequate care (for example, treatment of skin ulcers, use of antibiotics, use of restraints, or falls), development of criteria for proper treatment of that problem using consensus methods, audit of residents' records to determine the extent of the problem in a facility, introduction of an educational or other systematic intervention to improve care practices, and reaudit to determine whether care has improved. Federal regulations require nursing homes to conduct MCE studies annually, and their results constitute a large body of process-oriented work, which for the most part is unpublished, inaccessible, and without much generalizability (Kane et al., 1979a,b).

GOALS OF FACILITY CARE

Establishing the goals for diffuse programs such as home care or day care is difficult enough—the objectives of care in nursing homes are even harder to articulate. Different circumstances may suggest different goals. Often difficult value choices are implied, but the decisions about goals are better made deliberately than inadvertently. The following general effects have been examined in studies of nursing home care.

Prolongation of life, treatment of disease. Many nursing home residents are nearing the ends of their lives; some are in nursing homes to die. In individual cases, some residents will prefer a quick death without heroic medical interventions to a longer accumulation of days. At the same time, residence in a nursing home should not mean abrogating one's right to receive accurate and prompt diagnosis of physical problems and treatment geared toward improving functioning. We may all too easily accept medical indifference out of a confused striving for policies that permit people to die decently in a machine age. Death rates are, therefore, hard to interpret, but a sudden rise in death rates or a large number of unexpected deaths in a particular nursing home would surely be worrisome.

Maintenance or improvement of physical functioning. This may be a reasonable goal for many residents, but, just as death rates are expected to be high, many residents of nursing homes are expected to decline in functioning over time. Such measures are thus best expressed in terms of reasonable expectation. Functional decline may be slowed rather than re-versed. Moreover, we do not want to establish functional expectations for nursing home residents that would, in turn, encourage staff to withdraw their help under the guise of enhancing the residents' "independence."

Discharge home or to a lesser level of community care. For some propor-tion of nursing home residents (for example, candidates for physical rehabilitation or persons needing time to convalesce after a hospital stay), an expeditious return to the community would be the ultimate test of effectiveness. For others, life in the community might be more constrained and restrictive than it could be in an excellent nursing home. If so, discharge is hardly an appropriate goal for that group of residents.

Reduced use of acute hospitals and emergency rooms. This goal may make sense from a cost-savings perspective, but will only be desirable from the residents' perspective if they can get the medical and nursing care they need as well or better in the facility.

Emotional well-being. It seems a reasonable goal that nursing homes minimize residents' anxiety and depression. But the heterogeneous popula-tion in nursing homes makes further specification difficult. Some people are in nursing homes because of a chronic mental condition; one expects competent treatment for those diseases. Others may become depressed, anxious, and demoralized because of the environment; one expects that routines, programs, and opportunities be established to diminish that result. Still others may be depressed because of the physical and social circum-stances that necessitated the move to a nursing home; facility personnel should try to alleviate psychic pain as much as possible, but they cannot rewrite life's harsh scripts. The facility is challenged to sort out appropriate candidates for various psychological therapies, as well as to recognize when residents are emotionally hurt by unnecessarily restrictive facility policies, and to develop appropriate responses.

Social well-being/involvement. Life goes on after admission to a nursing home. People should be able to maintain their interests and social relationships to the best of their ability. Unfortunately, this irreproachable platitude translates poorly into measurable goals for nursing home residents. The individual's capacity for social interaction and intellectual life tends to be decided by professional judgment, and indeed such judgments can also become self-fulfilling prophecies. If people are treated as though they no longer have intellectual interests, friendships, plans, and purposes, they deteriorate rapidly and those very capacities diminish.

Improved cognitive functioning/lessened "behavioral" problems. Substantial numbers of nursing home residents are cognitively impaired, but how effectively specific programs can minimize or improve cognitive functioning is unclear. Wonders can be worked for the relatively small group whose dementia-like symptoms are due to reversible causes such as drug toxicity, untreated organic disease, or depression. The goals for others may be physical comfort and apparent contentment (perhaps measured by absence of distressed reactions and visible signs of pleasure) rather than improved cognitive abilities. The success of nursing home care can be reflected in the frequency of disruptive behavior such as violent outbursts or wandering. It is hard, however, to distinguish between outcomes that are important for the demented resident (such as less agitation, tearfulness, and overt distress) and outcomes that may be important for the comfort of other residents, the peace of mind of relatives, or the convenience of staff.

Satisfaction. For the cognitively intact who can describe their reactions, satisfaction with the care and the environment may be the best "gold standard" of the effectiveness of the facility. Even here, however, qualifications must be made. Residents usually lack the technical knowledge to evaluate the quality of health care or to know what has been left undone or done too vigorously. In that sense, satisfaction may be a necessary but not sufficient indicator of quality. Furthermore, people adjust their expectations to deprived circumstances; it is possible that the facility where complaints abound is doing a better job in maintaining a sense of purpose in the residents than one where satisfaction is uniformly expressed. In that sense, the facility that is responsive solicits expressions of dissatisfaction. Finally, satisfaction is difficult to measure accurately given that many residents are vulnerable and deeply dependent on caregiving staff. This term may be too impersonal to indicate the importance of providing services in a way that allows the recipient to retain his dignity and to feel like a person rather than an object. It means that the food served should taste good and be attractively presented. The facility should allow privacy. Patients should feel that help will come promptly when they call.

Therapeutic or programmatic efforts in nursing homes can be directed at one or more of these goals. Logically each effort should be targeted at those within the facility who are likely to benefit, and the intervention should correspond to the goals sought and the outcomes measured. Nursing home residents are, above all, a heterogeneous group. They vary in their physical health, functional abilities, and prognoses. They vary by age, education, interests, values, and preferences. They also differ in their cognitive abilities and capacity for decision-making. And certainly the type and availability of social resources outside the nursing home range widely. It is unreasonable to suppose that a particular intervention is useful for all residents. It is equally unreasonable to expect all outcomes—including some that are mutually incompatible—to flow from a single intervention.

EFFECTS OF INTERVENTIONS AND PROGRAMS ON INDIVIDUAL RESIDENTS

Studies of Interventions

The first area for review gets to the heart of the matter—how treatments, techniques, and programs in nursing homes affect the individual residents. Much has been written on this subject, but relatively little has been studied. Table 8-1 summarizes studies that described an innovative intervention and made at least some attempt to evaluate its effects. Taken as a whole, this literature has several limitations.

- Studies tended to be confined to single nursing homes. We found almost no instance where an intervention was studied in more than one facility.
- Sample sizes tended to be small.
- Sample members were often selected by staff as "people capable of participating," or they were self-selected. In other studies, criteria for selection were simply unspecified.
- Attrition tended to be high. Typically, those who died before the study was over were dropped from the analysis.
- Interventions were rarely replicated. Table 8-1 reads like a catalog of innovative ideas that have been tried somewhere—once.

Despite these criticisms, the cumulative information in Table 8-1 is quite revealing. The interventions illustrated in the table fall into four rather imprecise categories: (1) clinical programs with a therapeutic intent offered to selected residents or family members (for example, reality orientation therapy, reminiscence groups, or behavioral therapies); (2) changes to make the environment more pleasant, interesting, or responsive to human need (for example, a resident's welcoming committee, a resident-published magazine, juice and coffee for residents in the hour before breakfast); (3) interventions designed to increase interaction between the nursing home and the outer world (such as programs to bring nursing home residents to senior centers or to involve them with children); and (4) efforts designed to give nursing home residents more choices and sense of control over their lives. These are by no means mutually exclusive categories. Some interventions may employ several mechanisms. For example, a program may be designed to increase a resident's sense of control and simultaneously use strategies that allow residents choice in and control over contact with outside visitors. (See, for example, Schulz, 1976.)

The least effective interventions studied in nursing homes may well be the formal therapeutic efforts. Six studies in Table 8-1 are typical. Two dealt with reality orientation therapy, a popular intervention to orient cognitively impaired persons to the world around them. Gubrium and Ksander (1975) argued that the intervention's lack of effect on the residents was predictable given that highly contrived and structured efforts to emphasize time and reality during therapeutic sessions were negated by staff attitudes the rest of the time. In a randomized experiment comparing a "sheltered workshop" where residents made gifts to a reality orientation group, MacDonald and Settin (1978) found that the residents in the workshop made significant gains, whereas those in the reality orientation group did no better than an untreated control.

Following only two subjects, Baltes and Zerbe (1976) studied the effects of operant conditioning on self-care of dependent residents. This study is illustrative of many studies with single subject design, where positive effects have been produced in a handful of selected residents (in this, transforming nonfeeders into self-feeders). Berger and Rose (1977) also did a behaviorally oriented study among a much larger group of residents. Although their experiment with efforts to make residents more socially assertive and effective showed an immediate increase in skill, the effect was limited to the learned situations. It neither transferred to other situations nor sustained its effect over time. In a small study comparing 15 depressed residents who were equally randomized to psychotherapy, pet-assisted psychotherapy, and no treatment, both treatment groups improved depression scores significantly more than the untreated control (Brickel, 1984). During 15 minutes left alone with the animal, members of the pet-assisted group interacted socially more than when they were without the pet. This was measured by the subject's being within three meters of another person and listening or speaking to that person. In our view, however, this is a trivial result, the expected outcome of a contrived situation, and, therefore, hardly merits being defined as social interaction. On a more optimistic note, Berghorn and

TABLE 8-1 Effects of Innovative Interventions on Individual Nursing Home Residents

Source and Intervention	Subjects	Design	Findings
Effects of Therapeutic Efforts:			
Gubrium and Ksander (1975) Daily brief reality orientation (R.O.) sessions with small groups plus "24-hour R.O." reinforcement by staff.	Demented residents in two large nursing homes. Selection criteria unclear.	Observations of R.O. groups and life on ward. No systematic description.	No findings quantified. Authors question that any positive effects were likely. Residents were sometimes bribed to attend sessions; format required them to give "correct" answers corresponding to R.O. board rather than true reality, and time-oriented behavior was devalued in wards though stressed in R.O. sessions.
Baltes and Zerbe (1976) Operant conditioning program to get persons to feed themselves.	Two residents. A stroke patient aged 79 and a woman aged 67 who was not a self-feeder.	Single subject reversal design.	Positive effects in eating behavior were achieved.
Berger and Rose (1977) Skill assessment training sessions in which groups of residents were taught how to solve daily situations through modeling, coaching, and rehearsal.	From 160 residents 90 were deemed cognitively and physically able to participate and a sample of 27 was drawn from 40 of these who volunteered.	Twenty-seven residents were randomly assigned to training or one of two control groups (a discussion group control and a nontreated control). Three hour-long training sessions were conducted using eight selected situations. Assessment occurred at baseline, at end of experiment, and eight weeks later.	Experimental group was better than controls in behavior role play test after training but not in eight weeks. There was no carryover to the way the subjects would handle other situations not modeled in training.

MacDonald and Settin (1978) Reality orientation (R.O.)—group of five met for 15 50-minute sessions over five weeks for reminiscence and repetitive R.O. activities. Sheltered workshop—participants made gifts for children in group of five.	Thirty residents selected by staff from volunteers meeting minimal functional criteria (mobility of at least one arm, adequate visual, vocal, and auditory functioning).	Ten persons randomized to each of R.O., sheltered workshop, or control group that received assessment only.	Analysis of covariance found that sheltered workshop group had significant gains in life satisfaction scores and staff-perceived "social interest." No differences for R.O. group and nonsignificant *drop* in life satisfaction scores. No differences in observer-rated ward behavior (NOSIE scale).
Brickel (1984) "Pet-assisted" therapy for depression—i.e., therapist brought dog to sessions and resident could pet it.	Fifteen male residents of a single VA facility who tested as depressed on Zung Scale (from 50 selected for testing).	The 15 subjects were randomly assigned to regular psychotherapy, pet-assisted psychotherapy, and an untreated control.	Both psychotherapy groups improved significantly on Zung Scale compared to untreated group. Behavioral observation showed more social interactions when with the pet than without.
Berghorn and Schafer (1986) Discussion groups for reminiscence.	Ninety-nine residents in 30 facilities.	Randomized experiment. Drop-out was high.	Significant change in self-reported health, perceived friendliness of other residents, and life satisfaction, but no data given.
Effects of Improving Milieu: Friedman (1975) Resident welcoming committee.	Self-selected small committee of alert residents.	Anecdotal only.	Residents found satisfaction in serving as welcomers. They resented welcoming cognitively impaired residents and resented changed resident mix.

TABLE 8-1 Continued

Source and Intervention	Subjects	Design	Findings
Blackman, Howe and Pinkston (1976)	Thirty female residents, most very impaired and two-thirds said to be "confused."	Single group reversal design to examine attendance in solarium and pro-social, interactive behavior when activity took place and when it was withdrawn.	Residents were more likely to congregate in solarium and engage in proactive social behavior in presence of refreshments.
Offering coffee and juice in the solarium in the hour before normal breakfast time of 7:30 A.M.			
Koger (1980)	One hundred and four of 210 residents deemed capable of participating. Eighty-four agreed and 50 were randomly selected.	Randomized trial.	Life Satisfaction Index increased for experimental group. Participation in activities did not.
An eight-week writing workshop and production of a resident-written semiannual 26-page magazine.			
Effects of Community Contact:			
Hirsch (1977)	Fifty-five facilities in Baltimore were eligible to send residents.	Data collected on homes that inquired, homes that chose to participate, and residents who actually participated. No outcome measures or control group.	Forty-four of 55 homes made initial inquiry, 34 sent a staff member to center, and 22 arranged a visit of at least one group of residents; 144 residents made 4,370 visits in a 30-month period; 17% of the 144 visits 56 times or more and 28% visits 5 or fewer times; 11 residents were discharged to community and 6 of these continued at center.
A senior center activity program was made available to nursing home residents.			

Solon et al. (1977) Interaction promoted between nursing home residents and institutionalized mentally retarded through a series of alternating visits.	Five selected residents in the state hospital for the retarded and self-selected residents of a nursing home.	Impressionistic and informal observations of project staff.	Authors asserted that program benefited the core group in both institutions who made visits and stimulated residents on the periphery. In fact, few people in either institution were involved and elderly were unenthusiastic about foster grandparent role. Program petered out.
Wallach, Kelley, and Abrahams (1979) High school students visited residents of a Veterans Administration nursing home care unit with one-to-one contacts and group discussions.	Project started with ten students from one school and 10 residents and expanded by the fourth year to include 80 residents and 80 students from three schools.	Evaluation in year three was a before-and-after study of 10 patients new to the program that semester. Sickness Impact Profile (SIP) was given by program staff before and after semester.	Significant differences in three scales from SIP: daytime sleeping, mobility/confinement, and social interaction. Increased patient self-sufficiency was *not* noted.
Newman, Lyons and Onawola (1985) Ten selected psychology students at community college received training on aging and visited two nursing home residents each for three hours a week through semester. During visits students did activities with their residents.	Staff selected 40 from 185 residents and based on profiles, the students picked residents to visit. Twenty residents selected.	Uncontrolled study. Resident outcomes evaluated by a semi-structured interview on satisfaction and a clinical assessment procedure (record review, discussion with nurse).	Subjective reactions of residents were positive and clinically 83% maintained or improved their health status at the end of the program. ADL functioning also improved.

TABLE 8-1 Continued

Source and Intervention	Subjects	Design	Findings
Effects of Choice and Control:			
Langer and Rodin (1976)	Forty-seven cognitively intact residents in a Connecticut nursing home.	Quasi-experiment with 44 residents on a comparable floor used as control subjects.	Experimental subjects were rated more highly by nurses on alertness, active participation and sense of well-being as well as behavioral measures of the same variables.
Residents were given choice to care for a plant. They also received independence-inducing message and a choice of times for movies.			
Schulz (1976)	Five nursing home residents randomly assigned to each visiting condition.	Groups receiving visits under the condition of predictability or of control were compared to each other and a control group that received random visits, and a group receiving no visits.	The subjects with the control and the predictability did better than the group with random or no visits on health status indicators (e.g., rated health, use of medication), "future commitments scale," perceived happiness, and hopefulness.
Residents received student visitors under two conditions: (1) they could predict time of visit because they were told in advance; (2) they could choose and control time of visit.			
Grey (1978)	137 residents.	No control, but mortality in unit was compared for one year before and after the move.	Mortality rate 14% in year after move compared to 30% in previous year. Functional status also improved.
Residents being moved to a new building received elaborate preparation including group discussions, involvement in room selection, family involvement in packing.			

Study	Sample	Method	Results
Mercer and Kane (1979) A five week system-wide intervention. Administration delivered an independence-evoking message to residents as a group, reinforced a week later by a visit in residents' room; choice of a plant, opportunity to repot the plant, and invitation to a newly organized residents' council.	All residents over age 60, ambulatory and able to communicate in one Arkansas nursing home (N=40).	Quasi-experiment in which the 40 eligible residents from experimental home were compared to the 35 eligible residents from a matched control facility.	Analysis of covariance found that compared to the control, experimental group had significant reduction in Beck Hopelessness Scale score, an increase in activities, and improved staff ratings of behavior.
Banzinger and Roush (1983) Residents given a choice to manage a bird feeder and received an independence-evoking message.	Forty residents aged 57–96 in one Ohio nursing home.	Fourteen persons randomized to receive independence-evoking message and choice to feed birds; 13 persons received dependence message and no bird feeding choice, and 13 persons were in control group; measures were taken two weeks before and three weeks after the start of the intervention.	Analysis of covariance found that the responsibility/bird feeder group compared to the two controls had greater improvements in self-reported control, happiness, and activity on nurse ratings of similar variables.

Schafer (1986) reported positive effects on self-reported health, perceived friendliness of other residents, and life satisfaction for those who participated in reminiscence groups in a randomized experiment involving almost 100 residents of nine homes; however, dropout of subjects was high and no specific data were given about the extent or duration of the effects.

Efforts to improve the milieu of nursing home residents by adding pleasant routines or thoughtful opportunities for interesting activities are likely to pay off in increased well-being. Three such examples are shown in Table 8-1. In an admittedly subjective study, Friedman (1975) reported that the addition of a resident welcoming committee had positive effects both on the newly arrived persons being welcomed and the small, selected group of welcomers. (However, the welcomers resented greeting cognitively impaired arrivals and even resented their admission to the community.) The other two studies in this category had rather rigorous designs. Koger (1980) found that participation in writing and producing a residents' magazine increased the life satisfaction of the experimental group. It had no effect on their participation in activities, perhaps because the other activities had not interested them in the first place. Finally, Blackman, Howe, and Pinkston (1976) used a single group reversal design to see if juice and coffee before breakfast would entice more residents to congregate and socialize appropriately in the solarium where the refreshments were served. Elaborate measures of "proactive socialization," as well as simple counts of persons in the solarium, both proved the value of the intervention. Unfortunately, the nursing home chose to discontinue this sensible, inexpensive intervention once the study was over. Furthermore, the study raises a question of fundamental values. Is it necessary to prove the benefit of every single intervention in a nursing home setting? Can we not assume some services are worthwhile simply as decent, humane things to do? Moreover, must we evaluate each service in terms of improved physical, mental, or social functioning? Would expressions of satisfaction be sufficient justification for the juice and coffee?

The next four studies, none of them controlled, illustrated efforts to break down boundaries that scholars suggest (e.g., Dobrof, 1984) divide the nursing home and the community at large. One study arranged for high school students to visit nursing home residents (Wallach, Kelley, and Abrahams, 1979), and another (Newman, Lyons, and Onawala, 1985) used psychology students for the same purpose. Before-and-after measures showed significant effects on health status and psychological or social well-being. Hirsch (1977) reported on a program that allowed residents to become members of a nearby seniors center program and Solon and colleagues (1977) described efforts to promote interactions between residents of a nursing home and children in a facility for the retarded through alternating visits. Not surprisingly the latter effort generated minimal enthusiasm in the nursing home. Although the authors would likely disagree, we view this strategy as conceptually flawed because it accentuates differences between nursing home residents and those on the outside. It links nursing home residents to a stigmatized group rather than regularizing their opportunities for a full life. The program with senior centers, which is intuitively more appealing, was made available to 55 nursing homes in Baltimore. Most facilities failed to follow through with making the arrangements, and, although some residents participated to good effect, nursing homes tended not to sustain the program.

Perhaps these studies point out that it is easier for facilities to encourage outsiders to come into the nursing home than to facilitate residents leaving it. (Liability issues and staffing requirements both inhibit the latter.) Unfortunately, getting out of the facility would open a more varied array of opportunities for those capable of using them. But, if facilities seem unenthusiastic, there is equally little evidence that community agencies and other organizations, including clubs or churches, make vigorous efforts to reach out to nursing home residents, particularly to bring the residents away from the facilities. Tydeman (1981) polled all Area Agencies on Aging (AAAs) to examine any programs concerning nursing homes. About half the AAAs responded, and, of these, only 148 had any programs in nursing homes at all. The bulk of the efforts described were ombudsman and friendly visiting programs, information and referral, public education, and guides to nursing home selection. Efforts to integrate residents into other AAA programs or the community, or to enlist nursing home residents as volunteers, were less frequent although isolated interesting examples were found.

By now, impressive theoretical and empirical literature supports the premise that if nursing home residents perceive that they have choices and control over their life, they will experience better outcomes. Taken together, such studies confirm the existence of "learned helplessness"—a phenomenon of depression, abrogation of decision-making, and inability to perceive a relationship between one's own actions and outcomes. Learned helplessness arises when persons feel out of control and is associated with morbidity and even mortality.

Thus the main focus of the last set of studies from Table 8-1 was not the intervention itself but the *choice* offered to residents. For example, Langer and Rodin (1976) offered not just a plant, but the opportunity to accept or reject it. They also provided the residents on the experimental floor with a message in a speech from the administrator (later reinforced by one-to-one repetition) that asserted that they were expected to make decisions, combined with a choice of evenings to watch movies, if desired. This study showed positive effect on a wide range of subjective and objective measures. Most ingenious among the latter was an unobtrusive measure of activity levels; tape was affixed the bottom of wheelchairs and the more wear on the tape, the greater the level of activity was judged to be. Mercer and Kane

(1979) used a similar administrator's speech to induce independence in an experimental group, combined with the opportunity to choose to care for a plant and a later opportunity to participate in a residents' council. A later study used an independence-inducing message, combined with an opportunity to choose to tend a bird-feeder (Banziger and Roush, 1983). All three studies gave the comparison group similar attention, but used a dependency-inducing message reinforcing that the nursing home would care for their needs.

In a different variation on the learned helplessness theme, Schulz (1976) found that residents realized positive effects from having control over other human beings. In his study, college students visited specific nursing home residents under various conditions. The best results occurred when residents could control the timing of the visits, though merely being informed about the timing of the visits in advance also had a desirable effect. Randomly timed visits with no prior notice had no more effect than no visits at all. Along the same lines but without an elegant study, Grey (1978) showed that the mortality rate and functional ability of a group of residents who were moved to another facility as a result of renovation actually improved. She attributed this to the careful preparation of the residents and their active involvement in making choices for the new setting.

Taking such studies together, they show that slight interventions in a nursing home can have a measurable effect on the well-being, functioning, and even mortality of nursing home residents. Morning coffee before breakfast, a chance to feed the birds or to take care of a plant, contact with animals, or work on a magazine have all been the independent variable in randomized studies where the experimental group has done significantly better than the control group on the outcomes examined. The theory of learned helplessness and the benefits of increased perception of choice and control offer an explanation for some effects. But even interventions with less impeccable theoretical underpinning seem to have beneficial effects, suggesting that in the relative deprivation of a nursing home, almost any beneficial attention may make a difference. (The exception seems to be various forms of stylized reality orientation therapy, perhaps because the target group is the cognitively impaired and the goals are inappropriately keyed to improved condition.) In general, almost any intervention seems able to produce a measurable benefit, regardless of how small or inexpensive the effort.

Despite the propensity of interventions to show effects, programmatic change has proceeded slowly and uncertainly. Bennett (1983) surveyed more than 1,000 facilities to determine the extent and range of innovative programs and the factors associated with ever having or retaining such programs. Only 274 facilities responded, describing 488 programs. Religious programs and arts and crafts predominated; community outreach was least often arranged, and active rehabilitation programs were also sparse. Program attrition was relatively high. Many of the programs cited were no longer in existence. Particularly vulnerable were outreach efforts, programs of self-governance, and programs to enhance social adjustment.

Studies of Factors Associated With Residents' Well-Being

In addition to studies of interventions, some studies (summarized in Table 8-2) described factors associated with the well-being of residents in nursing homes and, thus, point the way to interventions that might be helpful. Dudley and Hillery (1977) documented the problem provocatively by pointing out that nursing home residents, in comparison to residents of other "total institutions" like dormitories, monasteries, and communes, experienced very high deprivation of freedom and sense of alienation. (Perhaps nursing home residents have less choice about entering the community and less freedom to leave it than members of the comparison communities.) Similarly, Stein, Linn, and Stein (1985) documented that persons entering nursing homes expected a high level of stress. Harel and Noelker (1982) showed that the best predictors of well-being for nursing home residents included the perception of choice in entering the facility and receiving visits from preferred visitors rather than a general count of visitors.

It has commonly been assumed that residents of nursing homes experience detrimental "transfer trauma" when they move to another facility. But according to a secondary analysis of relocation studies (Schulz and Brenner, 1977), conflicting findings about the effects of such moves on the institutionalized elderly could be reconciled. When the residents wanted to move, when they perceived the move as an improvement, and when they could predict the routines at the new facility relocation they tended to have considerable good and few bad results. These studies thus provide further data supporting the important of choice and control in the nursing home.

The debate on the existence, nature, extent, and causes of transfer trauma is far from over. A series of studies in Utah (Borup, Gallego, and Heffernan, 1979, 1980; Borup and Gallego, 1981) suggested that transfers *improve* mortality rates. These data have in turn been criticized methodologically (Horowitz and Schulz, 1983; Schulz and Horowitz, 1983), particularly because of likely bias in the sample against including those most vulnerable to negative effects of transfer. The topic has significance beyond the niceties of research design. On the one hand, concern over the dangers of relocation can become a convenient excuse to leave people in substandard facilities. On the other hand, if, as it seems likely, control and choice and other factors associated with relocation make a difference in results, the Utah studies should not be used as justification for casual relocations between (or even within) nursing homes.

Miller and Barry (1976) showed a correlation between physical abilities and the likelihood that a resident would have an outing away from the

TABLE 8-2 Selected Studies of Factors Associated with the Well-Being of Nursing Home Residents

Source	Purpose	Study Design	Findings
Miller and Barry (1976)	Determine the frequency and duration of off-premise activites, the reason for the visit, and the relationship of the accompanying person.	In two White Plains nursing homes, the trips of those who elected to leave the facilities for any reason other than hospitalization were studied through log for six-month period.	35% of the census in the two homes left the facility once during the period ($N=65$) and 645 outings. Physical abilities associated with more frequent outings, and cognitive impairment with less frequent outings.
Dudley and Hillery (1977)	Study the relationship between deprivation of freedom and alienation in various institutional settings.	Monastaries, military colleges, dormitories, sororities, cooperative housing, boarding schools, communes and homes for the aged were compared in freedom deprivation (measured by questions about former freedom compared to present) and alienation.	Homes for the aged residents had highest scores on alienation and second highest on freedom deprivation of any group.
Schulz and Brenner (1977)	Reconcile conflicting findings in studies in trauma associated with the relocation of frail elderly.	The authors identified and reviewed previous studies of relocations from home to institution, and home to other community residence.	Authors identified factors associated with absence of relocation trauma: older person chose to relocate, older person viewed the move as an improvement, and the previous environment had similarities to former environment.

Snyder et al., (1980)	Determine what distinguishes wanderers from nonwanderers in facilities, and what prompts wandering, and which forms it takes.	Eight residents of a SNF were randomly selected from a group of identified wanderers and matched with nonwanderers by sex, nursing floor, level of care, mode of ambulation, mental status, vision, and hearing. Subjects were observed at intervals.	Wanderers had more behavior problems, lower MSQ, and more psychological problems. No difference in age, diagnosis of heart disease or stroke, sex or marital status. Wandering patterns classified as goal directed/searching; industrious; non-goal directed.
Barton, Baltes, and Orzech (1980)	Study of the relationship between independence-supportive and dependence-supportive behavior of nursing home staff and independent or dependent behavior of residents.	Seventeen staff members and 36 residents were observed and rated during morning care for 23 days.	Independent behavior of residents was *not* reinforced but dependent behavior is followed by supportive reactions from staff.
Greene and Monahan (1982)	Determine factors associated with receiving visitors in nursing homes.	Two hundred ninety-four residents in Arizona facilities were studied to model predictors of receiving visits. A variety of functional, psychological, and behavioral items about residents were collected from staff.	Level of ADL was positively related to visiting. Length of stay was negatively related. Psychological indicators were irrelevant. Proximity to relatives made a difference—a 16-mile increase in distance was associated with decline of .5 visits per week.

TABLE 8-2 Continued

Source	Purpose	Study Design	Findings
Harel and Noelker (1982)	Study how social integration of residents was related to their well-being in nursing homes.	Fourteen for-profit and non-profit facilities in Cleveland were studied through 10 randomly selected residents on "self-care" floors of each.	Best predictors of well-being (measured by PGC morale scale, self-reported satisfaction with care and self-reported life satisfaction) were self-rated health, choice to live in a facility, positive feelings about admission, and receiving visits from *preferred* family and friends (not total number of visits).
Hendy (1984)	Examine the effects of different pet presentations (no pets, stuffed pets, video-taped pets, and live pets) on sociability and health activities of nursing home residents.	Thirteen ambulatory subjects in county nursing home in Pennsylvania were selected from those regularly using day room before lunch. Observations made four days per week in 45 minutes before lunch for eight weeks with random determination of which animal presentation was used. Observations of behavior were made directly.	Live pets produced significantly more of the following effects: proximity to others, talking, smiling, ambulatory, alertness to surroundings, and eating a variety of foods offered at lunch. Women were more influenced than men. Moreover, the number of people in the day room also had an effect on all the outcomes.

Study	Purpose	Methods	Findings
Retsinas and Garrity (1985)	Examining factors associated with friendship between nursing home residents; who forms friendships and what predicts loners?	Friendships measured by staff observations and rating of friendship score. All 145 nursing home residents in single home were studied.	Thirty-five percent of residents were loners with no friends. Mobility was positively correlated with number of friends and negatively with being loners. Tenure was negatively associated with friendship. Friendship dyads were more likely to be formed by people located near each other (87% of 110 dyads) and relatively close in age (70%).
Stein, Linn and Stein (1985)	Determine extent to which nursing home residents expect stress on admission.	Two hundred twenty-three patients in 10 nursing homes received questionnaire about expected stress in the facility within a few days of admission. Five factor-produced scores were correlated with demographic, functional, and other measures.	Most were ambivalent or neutral about admission and anticipated difficulty in adjusting. Though no residents were expected to go home, 68% held this expectation. Residents who were depressed, had low self-esteem, or pain scored high on all factors of anticipated stress. The better educated had more concern about kindness of care; married persons more likely to score high on "severance anxiety" factor.

facility. However, they leaped to the conclusion that, therefore, activities should focus on the less able residents. Barton, Baltes, and Orzech (1980) carefully studied the interactions of staff and residents during morning care routines, noting that the staff encouraged dependent behavior and discouraged independent behavior by rewarding those who asked for help by providing that assistance. This study led the authors down the slippery slope of ill-advised interpretations. Though they seemed to judge assistance to residents as "dependency-inducing," much of the behavior so labeled might have been helpful assistance from staff, which should be encouraged. Given that residents are often physically dependent, their ability to exercise the choice and control that has been deemed so helpful might actually be contingent on staff members' willingness to accede to residents' requests on residents' timetables.

Greene and Monahan (1982) showed that visitors to nursing home residents strikingly decreased with length of the residents' stay and also with the distance between the nursing home and the home of the visitor. The first factor may be associated with increasing disability of long-stay residents and inertia of visitors, though it also may be a reaction to the way the setting responds to visitors. The second factor, however, emphasizes the importance of helping people find a nursing home located close to their friends rather than shunting them to the first available bed. On a more positive note, Retsinas and Garrity (1985) documented that nursing home residents can and do form friendships despite the odds against it. Friendship pairs tended to fall in a similar age range and live in the same vicinity in the facility.

Hendy (1984) manipulated a variety of pet-associated stimuli for a small group of residents in the day room before lunch. Compared to no pet stimulus, stuffed animals, and videotaped animals, live animals were associated with smiling, talking, alertness, ambulation, proximity to others, and eating well at lunch. The author noted that the number of people in the day room also was associated with these results, suggesting that people may be even more important than pets. (In passing, the authors explained that women and men had separate day rooms, so the intervention was done separately at each location; we were struck by the possibility that changing these segregated conditions might have helped more than the pet presentations!)

Implications

The implications of the material we have reviewed seem inescapable. The preponderance of the evidence is that in a nursing home little things mean a lot, and that the choices and control that are so important to Americans throughout their lifespan actually sustain health and well-being in long-term care facilities. The niceties that a caring staff member might think of to improve the environment will make a difference if one bothers to study them. Indeed, such niceties might be even better if tailored to individual preferences and requests. At this point, we recommend fewer studies and fewer interventions organized as "therapy." In contrast we prefer deliberate efforts to create a climate for choice and for normal life, at least for cognitively intact residents. At present, it is easier to receive pet therapy in a nursing home than to have a pet, to receive music therapy than to listen undisturbed to music, to receive reminiscence therapy than to have the opportunity for quiet, pleasurable conversation and reminiscence. Now that the point has been made that nursing home residents, like other people, prosper when their dignity is respected, when they can do what they prefer and like, and when they can continue interests within and outside the facility as they individually desire, the time is ripe for an overhaul of routines, expectations, and programs to allow these changes to come about.

QUALITY, REGULATION, AND STAFFING

So far, this discussion has explored evidence about how particular programs in nursing homes might affect particular groups of residents. But a nursing home is much more than an intervention or technique. It is a dwelling place, a source of intimate care and assistance, and, for persons with limited functional abilities, almost a complete way of life. It is the sum of all its routines, rules, programs, and activities, its opportunities and its restrictions, its physical setting, and its people—both the other residents and the staff. Considerable effort has been devoted to studying what constitutes a good or, at least, an adequate facility, and what factors are associated with an acceptable quality of care or quality of life. A much smaller body of studies examines the effects of regulatory efforts to ensure quality. This section discusses evidence about quality itself and about efforts to assure quality. Also, because the caliber and circumstances of nursing home staff are intimately related to quality of care, we review the spotty evidence about the effects of various staffing or administrative patterns.

Table 8-3 presents a highly selected, but illustrative, group of studies that examined what affects the quality of nursing homes, the effects of various regulatory efforts, and the advantages and disadvantages of particular administrative or staffing patterns. Almost none of the studies were experiments—an accurate reflection of the state of the art.

Quality

As Chapter 4 described, quality of care and quality of life can be judged on the basis of achieving the outcomes sought and implementing approved processes of care in response to particular conditions, or maintaining

TABLE 8-3 Selected Studies of Quality of Care, Administration and Staffing Patterns, and Regulation in Nursing Homes

Source	Description/Purpose	Study Design	Selected Findings
Quality of Care: Linn, Gurel, and Linn (1977)	A study comparing the relationship between nursing home characteristics and differential outcomes of patients placed in several homes. One thousand male patients were transferred from a VA Hospital in Miami to 40 nursing homes during a nine-year period. At transfer, physicians rated the patients as to expectations of outcomes within six months.	Patients were measured at baseline and six months following on physical functioning using the Rapid Disability Rating Scale; they were also classified at follow-up as improved, the same, deteriorated, or dead. Data were also collected on the patients' location at follow-up as well as on 15 variables measuring nursing home inputs.	Patient survival was related to the nursing home characteristics of more RN hours per patient and high meal ratings; improved RDRS scores were related to RN hours, higher cost, better physical plant, higher meal ratings, and better appearance of patients in the homes. In contrast to patients still in the home or rehospitalized at six months, discharged patients were associated with facilities having better medical records, higher professional staff-patient ratios, and more RN hours per patient.
Hay (1977)	A study examining the characteristics of "superior" facilities.	One hundred facilities (three-fifths proprietary) in 42 states were identified as "superior." Data derived from interviews with administrators. No comparison group except for comparison with national staffing norms.	Administrators of superior homes were focused on rehabilitation. Superior homes did not have a higher ratio of nursing staff, PTs, OTs, or dieticians compared to the average, but they had a higher ratio of social work and activities staff.

Florida Department of Health and Rehabilitative Services (1981)	A descriptive and evaluative study of clients and nursing homes served by Florida's Medicaid program. The study addressed (1) the efficiency of nursing home monitoring activities, (2) client characteristics, (3) factors influencing admissions, (4) characteristics and quality of nursing homes.	In 1978 data were collected on 268 Florida nursing homes certified for Title XIX funds. Study methods included the surveying of state monitoring and services field staff, and of nursing home administrators; reviewing samples of client Medicaid report forms; reviewing licensure deficiency reports and ombudsman complaints.	State field workers tended to rate the nursing homes highly in the areas of cleanliness, accessibility to visitors, safety, and nurses' attitudes toward patients; low ratings were in areas such as stability of staff, prevention of theft, provision of rehab therapy and social services, recreational services, handling of trust funds for patients. Higher quality of care ratings appeared to be associated with factors such as smaller size of home, higher aide-to-patient and nurse-to-patient ratios, smaller proportion of Medicaid patients.
Fottler, Smith, and James (1981)	A study of the relationship between profits per patient day and four measures of quality of patient care (nursing hours per patient day, non-nursing hours per patient day, total hours per patient day, staffing ratio) in a sample of proprietary nursing homes in California.	Through interviews and survey questionnaires, data were collected on 43 of 46 nursing homes located in the same geographical area; annual state financial and facility census reports were also used. Profitability was defined as total annual revenues minus costs divided by total annual patient days. Multiple regression was used, controlling for the variables of size, occupancy rate, percent of Medicaid patients, administrator experience, and the administrators' monitoring of nursing home trends.	Profit per day was significantly related to the three quality measures of nursing hours, total hours, and staffing ratio. Percentage of Medicaid patients was significantly related to all four quality measures. None of the other independent variables were related to more than one "quality" variable.

TABLE 8-3 Continued

Source	Description/Purpose	Study Design	Selected Findings
Epstein (1981)	A comparison of the quality of care in VA-owned nursing homes and community nursing homes.	Three benchmark community homes were selected to represent adequate, minimal, and inferior homes. Raters compared a random stratified sample of VA homes and the three benchmark community homes on quality of services, staffing patterns, quality of environment, and patient needs.	The VA compared favorably to all three community homes on all four indicators. The overall care was adequate in 50% of the VA homes and at least minimal in all but one.
Greene and Monahan (1981)	Study of factors associated with quality of care in chain and non-chain nursing homes in several Arizona counties.	Quality of care was defined by proxy of direct resources available for patient care. Using sample of homes in Phoenix, Arizona, authors did regression analysis to determine factors associated with quality.	For-profits had poorer quality than nonprofits. Chains managed by an office in distant communities had poorer quality (nursing/patient ratio) than chains managed locally.

Elwell (1984)	A study of the relationship between ownership type and quality of care offered in old age institutions (OAIs) in northeastern New York State. Proprietary, voluntary, and government ownership were compared according to nursing staff distributions and expenditures in the areas of administration, rehabilitative services, social services, nutrition, and housekeeping.	A health system agency's information system provided 1976 data from the annual reports of 493 non-federal SNFs in New York State. Analysis of covariance was used to isolate the effects of ownership while controlling for per diem cost, proportion of patients functionally impaired according to the DMS-1, proportion of Medicaid patients, size of the institution.	Contrary to the literature, no negative correlations were found between Medicaid and any of the quality measures—a finding that may be specific to New York. Government and voluntary SNFs allocated more money per patient day than proprietary facilities in each patient service area measured. Government SNFs offered significantly more nursing and other professional hours than voluntary or proprietary facilities; voluntary facilities offered more staff physician hours and had a lower proportion of patients in multiple-bed rooms.
Spalding (1985)	A study to determine what residents perceive as important elements of quality of care and life in nursing homes, and their views of a regulatory system.	More than 400 cognitively intact, selected residents in 10 areas of the country participated in an iterative process of three "focus group" discussions on quality. Content analysis of the sessions was done.	Residents emphasized the importance of well-trained, responsive, and kind staff, food, privacy, and opportunity for choice.

TABLE 8-3 Continued

Source	Description/Purpose	Study Design	Selected Findings
Regulation: Gardiner and Maloc (1984)	A descriptive and evaluative study on current policy issues in nursing home regulatory enforcement.	The descriptive and evaluative findings were based on reviews of the literature and government hearings, as well as interviews with enforcement officials. Federal, state, and agency-level roles were reviewed and recommendations for policy change were made.	States, initially having only drastic measures such as revocation of licenses to enforce compliance, are now adopting intermediary sanctions such as fines, suspension of admissions, reclassification, public ratings. Major problems include delays in implementation, lack of staff, the potentially adverse impact of fines on quality of care in the sanctioned home, problems of interagency cooperation, ambivalence in the perception of consultation vs. policing roles.

| Jost (1984) | A presentation of descriptive and evaluative information on the enforcement of quality nursing home care in the legal system. Problems, state responses, and proposed federal initiatives were presented in areas such as the investigation and initiation of action, the use of counsel in hearings, case preparation and presentation, impact of judicial system on enforcement. | A review of the literature as well as presentations of data gathered from interviews with licensure/certification agency staff, legal counsel, consumer advocates, nursing home ombudsmen, and attorneys representing providers. | Problems associated with the effectiveness of enforcement include surveyors' confusion over the role of consultant vs. investigator, lack of coordination between state offices, inadequate documentation, lack of training and experience on the part of state lawyers, inadequate preparation of witnesses, difficulties in obtaining testimonies from physicians, delays in the processing of administrative and juridical appeals. Although states are taking some steps to address these and other problems, financial support, training, and dissemination of data on successful efforts is needed. |

TABLE 8-3 Continued

Source	Description/Purpose	Study Design	Selected Findings
Zimmerman et al. (1984)	An evaluation of three state demonstrations in nursing home quality assurance processes (New York, Massachusetts, Wisconsin). The demonstrations, implemented in the early 1980s and designed to test a "screening" approach as an option to traditional survey methods, are analyzed in terms of their impact upon quality of care and resource utilization.	The evaluation consisted of three case studies that differed in design. Old and new systems were compared in terms of the detection of deficiencies, their correction, their reappearance in a subsequent survey. The new systems were also compared to independent measures of care, including the Quality Assessment Index developed especially for the Wisconsin demonstration. Analysis included the use of regression such as size of home, SNF beds, private-paying patients.	The new systems were found to reduce the time spent by surveyors in activities, although a reallocation of time from higher-quality to poor-quality facilities was not supported by the findings. When compared to alternative measures of quality of care, they performed reasonably consistently over the three states. It was concluded that the demonstration findings gave moderate support for the federal government to design a survey and inspection of care processes based on screening and sampling principles—either as a replacement or supplement to the current system.
Johnson (1985)	An evaluation of the use of intermediate sanctions by the states, including civil fines, receivership, enforcement of residents' personal rights, public disclosure, and other sanctions. Recommendations were made for	An analysis of common experiences shared by several states, based upon interviews with professionals, Institute of Medicine case studies, hearings, and a review of the literature.	*Civil fines* are most effective when they can be imposed swiftly (e.g., without court order) and have a range sensitive to the severity of the violation. Statutory obstacles limiting *litigation* in some states (fear of multiple suits) should be removed in the light of patients' lack of access to

	the role of the federal government.		attorneys and fear of retaliation. Effectiveness of *consumerism* depends upon access to information and assumes that there are free market forces to influence nursing home proprietors. Public disclosure has produced mixed results and is most effective when supported and used by advocacy groups. Recommendations for the federal role include a federal private right of action, federal mandates on the use of certain sanctions, development of a uniform management system making data available to consumer advocates.
Institute of Medicine (1986)	A study of how nursing homes should be regulated to effect quality.	Data base for study included existing literature, a survey of all state regulatory units, intensive case studies in selected states, transcripts of public meetings conducted around the country, commissioned papers and conferences, and expert opinion.	Recommendations included: a strong federal presence in nursing home regulation, outcome-based standards, increased emphasis on quality of life and civil rights, a case-mix-adjusted survey process, better training for surveyors, data collected from direct interview or observation of patients, and stronger enforcement (including intermediate sanctions).

TABLE 8-3 Continued

Source	Description/Purpose	Study Design	Selected Findings
Staffing/Administration: Gehrke and Wattenberg (1981)	A study identifying the social work tasks and assessing the activities of social service consultants and designers in the nursing homes located in two central Illinois counties.	A pre-tested questionnaire listing 48 social service tasks was distributed to 13 designees and 7 consultants from 16 proprietary or non-profit facilities. Respondents ranked the importance and rated the frequency of the tasks, in addition to responding to open-ended questions.	Both designees and consultants gave similar ranking to the social service tasks: those relating to planning residents' care were seen as most important and most frequently performed. Six of the first 10 tasks ranked by both groups were maintaining care plans maintaining plans in residents' records, keeping statistics, deciding who needed services, helping residents adjust, and helping staff to understand residents' problems. Designees were often active in counseling residents but only occasionally active in work with families. Consultants seldom participated in the development of nursing home policies and tended to provide their services to particular residents rather than the total population.

| Mercer and Garner (1981) | A study of the role and responsibilities of social work consultants in long-term care facilities in Arkansas. | By means of a mailed questionnaire (1979), data were collected on a random sample of 49 untrained social work designees representing Arkansas' 232 nursing homes (89% response rate); data were also collected on 28 of 42 MSWs providing consultation in the state. In addition to demographic data, information was collected on functions performed by the consultants, satisfaction with the consultative process, and the extent and manner in which designees were evaluated by consultants. | The consultants appeared to see themselves as both working for the designee rather than for the facility and as supervisors more than as consultants. Their role perception appeared limited to direct practice areas, neglecting administrative and programmatic aspects such as assisting with problems of morale, acting as a channel of communication to the administration, teaching the administrative aspects of the designee's job. |

TABLE 8-3 Continued

Source	Description/Purpose	Study Design	Selected Findings
Stryker (1982)	An investigation of the impact of 17 internal management interventions upon personnel turnover in nursing homes.	19 nursing homes located near Minneapolis-St. Paul, with annual turnover rates in personnel of 70% or higher, participated in a two-year study in which they reported detailed turnover data quarterly and agreed to engage in at least five managerial actions. The Fisher Exact test was used to correlate managerial interventions with turnover rates. The facilities were similar in size, ownership, number of employees, number of unionized employees.	The homes that were successful in reducing turnover were those that had intervened with more than twice as many managerial actions than the unsuccessful homes and had four times as many significant interventions. Significant interventions were increased supervision of new employees, supervisor training, revised personnel policies, increased recruitment efforts, avoidance of use of personnel pools.

Halbur (1983)	A study of the relationship between the job turnover rate of nursing home staff and three structural factors: opportunity structure (e.g., supply-demand ratio for nursing home staff), organizational structure (e.g., ownership, size), and control structure (e.g., wages, promotion opportunities).	The source of the data was a 1978 study of nursing personnel in 122 North Carolina nursing homes. Multivariate analysis was used to regress the job turnover rates of RNs, LPNs, and NAs on the independent variables of unemployment rate, supply/demand for nursing jobs, ownership, size, wages, fringes, and ratings on facilities' opportunities for promotion, decentralization in decision making, communication among staff.	All three structural factors had a significant impact upon turnover. General measures of the state of the economy and supply of nursing personnel were closely related to turnover. Larger facilities had more turnover, although for LPNs and RNs this was mediated by the provision of life insurance and pensions. In general, fringe benefits impacted turnover more than wages. Personal leaves negatively affected the turnover of RNs and were perhaps used by them for professional advancement.
Waxman, Carner, and Berkenstock (1984)	A study of the factors associated with job turnover and satisfaction among nursing home aides in seven proprietary facilities.	Two hundred thirty-four aides from seven randomly chosen SNFs in the Greater Philadelphia area were interviewed and administered scales on job satisfaction and perception of institutional milieu. Data were gathered on turnover rates, and independent sources were used to rank the facilities in overall quality. Kendal's Rank Order Correlation and analysis of variance were used to determine between-home comparisons.	The turnover rate was not explained by the "quality" ranking of the facilities, nor by wages and benefits. The two factors that appeared to at least partially explain job turnover were related to amount of supervision and administrative control: where turnover was lower, the home was perceived as being administratively more loosely organized and less rigidly controlled. The authors speculated that job turnover had more to do with management style than wages and benefits.

TABLE 8-3 Continued

Source	Description/Purpose	Study Design	Selected Findings
Barney (1981)	A study to demonstrate the feasibility and effectiveness of nursing home community councils as a vehicle for community involvement with nursing homes.	Under an AOA grant, the University of Michigan established "community councils" that included nursing home residents and friends as well as interested public. Two models were tested: an advocacy model and a service model. Evaluation was qualitative.	The advocacy model had no staying power. It also proved impractical to meet outside the facility. Authors recommended a service model and that staff be excluded from membership but permitted to observe.
Kahana and Kiyak (1984)	An examination of the relationship between the attitudes of nursing home staff	Eighty-six of 243 employees of four nursing homes were observed randomly in a	The more positive the stereotypes about aging the subjects held, the less likely they were to be positively

	and their behavior toward residents.	three-month period. Their demonstrated affect was measured on a scale that included positive, neutral, and negative, and specific behaviors with clients were observed. Findings were correlated with previously measured attitudes.	supportive in behaviors toward the elderly.
Aiken et al. (1985) Williams (1985)	A study to examine the effects of establishing relationships between nursing homes and schools of nursing in a national demonstration project.	These articles presented theoretical hypotheses about likely effects of the interventions on both residents and nursing students. Independent evaluation is pending.	Not applicable. In theory positive effects on quality of care and cost (through less hospital and medical use) were expected. Some cautions were raised about the possibility of increased exposure to heroic interventions and "medicalizing" nursing homes under the model.

acceptable structural characteristics of facility, program, and staff. For example, the proportion of residents with new bedsores is an outcome criterion, regular turning of bed-bound residents is a process criterion for preventing bedsores, and the requirement that all nurses' aides have received formal training in the care of bedsores is a structural criterion. Research in quality, in part, attempts to establish links between structure and processes, on the one hand, and outcomes on the other.

Despite the attention given to examining the factors associated with improved quality in nursing homes, the work unfortunately often has a circular nature. Because desirable outcomes have been elusive to define, an input measure, such as the ratio of nursing service staff to residents, is often used as a sign of quality. Then, all other indicators are examined for their relationship to the likelihood of a high ratio of nursing service staff to patients.

Support for this strategy was derived from a study that examined the outcomes of residents transferred from the Miami Veterans Administration Hospital to 40 nursing homes over a nine-year period. Patients survived longer in nursing homes that had more RN hours per patient and higher ratings of meals. Improved scores on a Rapid Disability Rating Scale and discharge home were also related to RN hours, meal ratings, and some other structural indicators (Linn, Gurel, and Linn, 1977). Subsequent studies have used staffing measures themselves as indicators of quality and have attempted to find correlates of a high nurse to patient ratio. For example, Epstein (1981) used this approach, in part, to assert that nursing home care units in Veteran's Administration Hospitals are of higher quality than other nursing homes outside the VA. This simplistic approach has limitations. Using four slightly different staffing measures as signs of quality, Fottler, Smith, and James (1981) found that most nursing home characteristics did not correlate with most measures; only the percentage of Medicaid patients was significantly (and negatively) related to all four.

The Florida Department of Health (1981) used similar circular logic in comparing the ratings made by nursing home inspectors with objective descriptors of the homes. Highly rated facilities tended to have higher nurse-to-patient ratios and aide-to-patient ratios, and fewer Medicaid residents. They also tended to be smaller. Generally, inspectors rated homes highly in areas like cleanliness, safety, and accessibility to visitors, but poorly in relation to provision of rehabilitation, social services, activities, recreation, providing trust funds, or even preventing theft.

Given that 80% of nursing homes are operated for a profit, considerable effort has been devoted to determining the relationship between ownership and quality. Here again the reasoning is more often based on resources than results. Two such studies are described in the table. Elwell (1984) suggested a relationship between nonprofit status and resource driven measures of quality. Greene and Monahan (1981) suggested that nursing home chains in

Arizona were of higher quality when administered locally rather than by distant management. Here the measure of quality was a nursing staff to patient ratio. Despite a widespread conviction that nonprofit facilities are of higher quality on the average, no conclusive case has been made. The proprietary industry points out, with justification, that voluntary nursing homes tend to have higher reimbursement rates as well as other sources of outside funds and claim that better quality is related to money rather than ownership. (This argument is blunted as an argument in favor of the proprietary sector because a proprietary nursing home is highly unlikely to attract the philanthropic support that enables the improved care.)

Hay (1977) took an intuitive approach to delineating elements of quality. He polled administrators of 100 facilities in 42 homes that were identified as "superior." Almost all the administrators expressed an orientation toward rehabilitation. Interestingly, superior homes did not have a particularly high ratio of nursing staff to patients (though they did have a slightly higher than average representation of RNs), nor did they have an advantage in dietitians, occupational or physical therapists; but they did have more social work and activities staff. Although three-fifths of the sample were proprietary homes, few were members of chains.

Unfortunately, most existing studies of quality fail to get at the heart of the matter. They tend to use easily measured indicators of quality that are structural in nature.

One exception was a study organized by the Coalition for Nursing Home Reform (Spalding, 1985) that systematically determined the opinions of a large number of articulate nursing home residents on what constituted a high quality of care and of life. Residents pointed to matters such as the courtesy and competence of nurses' aides, privacy and opportunity for choice, private rooms, quantity and quality of food, and a wide range of specific items that are rarely used by professionals. There has been virtually no effort to determine what factors are associated with the kind of quality indicators mentioned by the residents. Furthermore the residents' nominations for indicators of quality are much more elusive, subjective, and difficult to measure than simple staffing ratios.

Regulation

The next group of studies in Table 8-3 deals with the effects of regulatory efforts themselves. Only one such study had a quasi-experimental design. The rest attempted to describe factors associated with effective regulation.

Gardiner and Maloc (1984) pointed out the weaknesses in the legal remedies available to enforce existing nursing home standards. Similarly, Jost (1984) identified factors associated with ineffective enforcement, including the difficulty of getting adequate documentation, the difficulty in getting testimony from physicians, poor preparation of witnesses, and generally inadequate training of everyone involved (inspectors, lawyers, and so on). Johnson (1985) analyzed the effectiveness of various intermediate sanctions available (that is, sanctions less drastic than closing a facility). A system of civil fines was regarded as particularly promising.

On a different level, Zimmerman et al. (1984) evaluated quasi-experiments in three states (Wisconsin, Massachusetts, and New York) to streamline the processes of inspecting nursing homes. These changes were designed to give regulatory relief to homes with good prior records, while allowing more resources to be spent inspecting and trying to improve or sanction homes giving poor care. The study did not examine whether homes exempted from thorough review under the new systems maintained their records when the incentives of inspections were removed. Moreover, the time saved in inspecting facilities deemed better or in doing more stream-lined procedures was *not* reallocated to increased inspection of the poorer facilities.

Using all these and other data, the Institute of Medicine (1986) conducted a two-year study of how nursing homes should be regulated. The study committee recognized that the supply of beds (which allows for or constrains consumer choice) and the reimbursement rates will affect quality. However, it concluded that regulation can have an independent positive effect on quality and that a strong federal presence is needed. It, therefore, set forth an agenda of sweeping reform that would have, among other things, weighted standards more toward quality of life and residents' rights, inspected quality by examining the actual outcomes of the care instead of the procedures undertaken, collected information rather than relying on medical records and discussion with staff, introduced surprise inspections, allowed graduated levels of inspection based on screening of outcomes, and rendered enforcement swifter, more appropriate, and more stringent. At this writing, it is unclear which, if any, of these and other recommendations will be implemented.

Staffing/Administration

Inevitably the quantity, makeup, and quality of nursing home staff influence the care and lives of nursing home residents for better or worse. Diagnosis and treatment of health problems depend on the acumen of nursing staff, medical directors, and attending physicians. Activities and programs will be no more varied and stimulating than the imagination of the staff entrusted to organize them. Furthermore, the administrator in charge and the director of nurses set the tone for care and establish the internal quality controls. It is commonly acknowledged that life and care in a nursing home can plummet or dramatically improve with changes in management.

At the bottom of the staffing pyramid are the nurses' aides, who tend to be paid minimum wages, receive perfunctory training, and find themselves catapulted then into difficult roles that combine heavy labor with portentous responsibility. It is nurses' aides who spend the most time with the residents, who attend to their intimate needs, who make the difference as to whether the residents can establish a sense of control despite functional dependence. It is also the nurses' aides who must make decisions about when a physical symptom should be brought to the attention of a nurse or other professional. The common designation, "nurses' aide" or "nursing assistant," is, in fact, a misnomer for the role. In the sense that the paraprofessional employees in the nursing home fulfill all the plans of the professional staff and consultants, including the physical therapists, the social workers, and others, they might better be called "care aides" or "care assistants." To the extent that they are the front line helpers of the residents, they might better be called "resident assistants," and indeed this is the term suggested by the nursing home residents who participated in a landmark session on *their* view of quality in nursing homes (Spalding, 1985).

Pessimists see little opportunity to improve staffing in nursing homes. They point to the extremely low levels of professional staff and nonprofessional support required by the regulations and note that a minimum expectation quickly becomes a maximum in a profit-maximizing environment where reimbursement levels are fixed. Innovation in creating new personnel configurations is discouraged when administrators must also meet prescribed expectations for certain staff and consultants, and are vulnerable to criticism from rule-bound regulators. Pessimists also note the absence of a career ladder for the aides and point out the inevitability that the positions will be used either as stepping-stones for talented people (often immigrants, members of disadvantaged minority groups, or students and housewives temporarily unable to participate in the labor market) or as hiding places for the untalented and unambitious.

Against this bleak scenario, however, are the examples of how staff can be assisted to generate a higher quality of care and life. Despite the disincentives in the reimbursement system and the disadvantage of low wages, administrators report that it is possible to reorganize the work force to produce a more motivated, skilled, and, therefore, effective group. Among the strategies reported anecdotally are the following: assigning each aide as primary care coordinator for a small group of residents, with the responsibility to be alert to those residents' needs and wishes; teaching aides in a systematic way the observations that they should make, the routines they should perform, and, most important, the *reasons* why, developing a supervisory structure that is supportive to the problems encountered by aides and a training program that is truly relevant to their practical dilemmas. Typically, structural changes are needed to undergird such change; for example, a record system might need adjustment so that it can be properly used by semi-literate staff, it may be necessary to readjust staffing levels for more evening and weekend coverage, it may be that new professional roles and positions—such as nurse practitioner, or attending pharmacist—should be organized.

Research in this general area is extraordinarily underdeveloped. The evidence is thus largely indirect. Hints can be gleaned from management research, which has long asserted that people who understand the reasons and the importance of their work and who experience appreciation and rewards for jobs well done will respond by finding the work more interesting and engaging. These axioms are then strengthened by case reports that describe heightened morale and lower turnover among nursing home staffs when the work is more thoughtfully organized. Geriatric specialists also regularly return from Europe with the wistful conviction that it is possible to develop a capable, socially oriented cadre of attendants who are not so highly educated that they are unaffordable, but who are dedicated to the well-being of residents and can foresee a pleasant career in caring. It seems to happen in England, Western Europe, and other countries.

Because long-term care is essentially a question of personal services, there are a number of issues that could address better ways to deliver care, but they have not been the subject of contemporary research. A fundamental goal in establishing a program of long-term care is to provide a setting where residents can receive humane and compassionate care. How do we motivate minimally paid staff to care about the people they serve, especially when many of these residents may be incapable of normal communication? What is the basis for satisfaction from such work? One test of nursing home care may be whether an aide comes quickly and cheerfully in response to a request for assistance, but this is not the stuff of research.

There are a number of important researchable questions that have not been well asked. We have not systemically explored the use of better information and feed-back systems to motivate aide performance. We often hear great debates about the need for more and better professional training for nursing home staffs, but there is scant evidence that such training makes a sustained difference. Anecdotal data suggest that much of the high turnover rate among newly hired aides could be dramatically reduced if more effort were directed toward initial orientation and training, but no well documented proof is yet available to support such an investment strategy. The nursing literature is replete with debates over the value of primary care nursing, but nothing of that kind has been carefully tested in the nursing home setting. Would care really be better if it were more professionally delivered? If one were prepared to invest the money required into nursing home care, would it be better to buy more trained staff or more better-motivated paraprofessional staff?

The possibilities for meaningful research into how to improve the way staff work in nursing homes are legion. It is all the more dismaying that the subject has barely been studied given that the nursing home constitutes a natural laboratory to try new arrangements on an experimental basis. It would be entirely feasible to use control groups and to determine whether, *from a resident's perspective*, new ways of selecting, training, and deploying staff made a difference in their functioning and quality of life. Armed with information based on observing and interviewing residents, those who wish to change the incentives that operate in nursing homes would have a much better case for regulatory and legislative reform.

Having stressed the importance of staffing and administrative patterns, the evidence presented in the last section of Table 8-3 is somewhat anti-climactic. It is descriptive, not experimental; it fails to probe outcomes from a resident perspective in any depth; and no studies systematically studied the effects of changes at the aide level. Nevertheless, the material provides glimmers that new ways of staffing nursing homes may provide better results. (In Chapter 9, we present evidence about effective ways to deliver medical care in nursing homes. Effective uses of nurse practitioners, pharmacists, and medical directors, as presented in that chapter, also depended to some extent in developing changed expectations for the large paraprofessional work force.)

Social work in nursing homes could conceivably provide a focal point for emphasizing the elusive quality-of-life issues so important to residents. Two descriptive studies dealing with the practice of social work in nursing homes (Gehrke and Wattenberg, 1981; Mercer and Garner, 1981) pointed to the inadequacies of social work programs, which in most facilities in most states are staffed by a designated nursing home employee (the social service designee) with minimal consultation from a professionally trained consultant. Both studies showed the professional consultants took an inappropriately narrow, nonprogrammatic approach to their roles, spending their time consulting about or assessing particular patients and negating their influence on the well-being of a larger group of residents, the competence of the designee, or the quality of the social work program.

In some facilities, the staff changes 200% or more in the course of a year. Turnover of staff, including nonprofessional nursing staff, is widely believed to account for problems in quality and unnecessary costs of nursing home care. Staff turnover is thus used as a proxy for poor quality. Stryker (1982) found that turnover was significantly reduced in homes with strong managerial practices including orientation and supervision of new employees, training of supervisors, and systematic recruitment efforts. Halbur (1983) identified structural factors associated with lower turnover, pinpointing not only labor-force characteristics (that is, the supply of other low-income jobs) but also fringe benefits. The latter had a greater impact on turnover than wages. A more recent study reinforces earlier findings. Waxman, Carner, and Berkenstock (1984) showed that high turnover is associated with loose administrative control and minimal supervision, rather than lower wages and benefits or poorer rankings of the quality of facilities. These findings have face validity. Work in nursing homes tends to be poorly paid and difficult, but administrative practices that equip nursing assistants with skills and a sense of purpose for what they do and provide them with supervision, support, and feedback on their performance are more likely to engender commitment and job satisfaction. Another study of nursing home staff provided counterintuitive results. Those staff observed to be supportive and friendly toward residents as opposed to those observed as impatient and angry held more negative stereotypes and fewer positive stereotypes about aging. Furthermore, those with positive stereotypes that the elderly merit care and attention were less likely to engage in supportive behaviors that fostered the residents' individuality. Perhaps paternalism is associated with conventionally positive attitudes (Kahana and Kiyak, 1984).

The last entries refer to organizational features in nursing homes. Barney (1981) conducted a demonstration to organize "community councils" in nursing homes. These were to be organizations of residents, friends, and interested members of the general public. Two models were attempted—one that emphasized advocacy and one emphasizing service. The former met outside the nursing home in a neutral place. The evaluation—actually a case study of implementation—suggested that the advocacy model was unworkable, but the service models could become viable. The author recommended that staff members not be accepted as members of a community council, but that they be permitted to attend as observers to defuse staff anxiety. Finally, we note the formation of "teaching nursing homes," in this case nursing homes affiliated with schools of nursing. Aiken and her colleagues (1985) and Williams (1985) described the model theoretically and the likely effects of such an affiliation in upgrading the quality of care. A national evaluation of this program is currently underway.

EFFECTS OF REIMBURSEMENT POLICIES

Ideally, nursing home reimbursement should promote desirable outcomes across the triptych of long-term care; that is, the way nursing homes are paid should encourage a high quality of care, promote equitable access, and control excessive costs. In reality, long-term care reimbursement policy for the past 10 years has emphasized the objective of controlling costs to the exclusion of other objectives. The 1980 Omnibus Reconciliation Act changed the Medicaid law to allow states greater flexibility in setting rates and establishing rules for reimbursing nursing homes (General Accounting Office, 1983). Many states that in 1978 had reimbursed nursing homes on the basis of their reasonable costs had by 1982 moved to a fiscally tighter perspective type of reimbursement system (Harrington and Swan, 1985).

Nursing home reimbursement systems can be broadly categorized as retrospective, prospective, or flat-rate systems. Retrospective systems set the rate for the nursing home after the actual costs (or charges) are known.

Prospective systems pay according to rates set in advance, regardless of specific costs incurred. Usually base-year costs, adjusted for inflation, are used to set such rates. In flat-rate systems, homes are paid a fixed-rate per diem for each resident, whatever their cost experience (Holahan and Cohen, 1984). Rather than use a flat rate for all residents in all facilities, states can set class-specific or facility-specific rates, or combinations of both. Reimbursement systems also vary widely according to factors such as the cost components allowed in the rate, ceilings established, allowances for capital costs, incentives and disincentives used to influence occupancy rates, quality of care, and the kinds of persons admitted to the facilities (Harrington and Swan, 1985).

Studies of Effects of Reimbursement

Although money is surely a powerful persuader in an industry dominated by investor-owned corporations and small profit-making businesses, surprisingly little information is available about how the manner and amount of payment actually affect the product. Table 8-4 draws together five studies that made some comment on the effects of reimbursement policies. Three dealt with state Medicaid programs, one evaluated the consistency of fiscal intermediaries who administer nursing home claims for Medicare, and one tested how the industry might respond to incentives deliberately built into reimbursement policy. Only the latter used an experimental design, whereas the others were based on surveys or secondary analysis of data.

Harrington and Swan (1985) analyzed changes in Medicaid rates for skilled and intermediate facilities and in expenditures per recipient from 1979 to 1981. Comparing retrospective payment systems to three types of alternative prospective systems, they found that the states with the alternative systems had lowered skilled rates about 8.6% more than the states with retrospective rates, but no differences were noted for intermediate care rates. The investigators had no data on the average Medicaid expenditures per recipient per day of nursing home care, but they did predict total expenditures per recipient by reimbursement type. Hardly surprising, the lower rates of the alternative systems translated into lower expenditures per person.

Using data from the 1977 National Nursing Home Survey, Holahan, Cohen, and Scanlon (1983) compared nursing home costs per day, controlling for such variables as scale, ownership, type of residents, proportion of Medicaid residents, and wage levels. They judged that changing to a prospective or flat-rate system would have saved states using retrospective systems about five dollars a day or an average of 20% of per diem costs at that time. They also found that the characteristics of the residents— popularly dubbed "case mix"—were important in explaining the cost per day. Given the limitations of the data, they measured case mix rather

TABLE 8-4 Effects of Reimbursement System

Source	Description of Program or Study	Study Design	Selected Findings
Smits, Feder, and Scanlon (1982)	A study to determine the extent and nature of differences between claims reviewers from fiscal intermediaries and professional standards review organizations (PSROs) in granting or denying the claims of Medicare beneficiaries.	Nine hypothetical cases were presented on the telephone to a nonrandom sample of claims reviewers from 18 intermediaries and PSROs; the organizations represented different geographical locations varying in the use of Medicare skilled nursing facilities. Reviewers were asked to make a claim determination and to state the factors used in their decision.	In only two cases did the 18 reviewers approach consensus: Three reviewers decided to cover very few cases; almost half decided to cover most of the cases. When the reviewers agreed or decided on coverage, they tended to measure and assess coverage criteria—stability, restoration potential, need for institutional care—in different ways.
Holahan, Cohen, and Scanlon (1983)	A discussion and analysis of the relationship between nursing home costs and type of reimbursement system, as well as other variables, including type of ownership, wage rates, Medicaid participation, patient mix, occupancy rates, capacity. Reimbursement systems were categorized as retrospective, prospective, and flat rate.	Using data on nine states from the 1977 National Nursing Home Survey, average total cost per day as well as disaggregated costs per day (health, operating, and fixed costs) were regressed against traditional cost study variables. The variables were used to control for effects of scale, including ownership, case mix, reliance on Medicaid and other facility characteristics.	States with prospective and flat-rate reimbursement systems have per diem costs that are about 20% lower than states with retrospective systems. Other factors such as wages, capital costs, proportion of Medicaid patients in the home, case mix had significant impact upon nursing home costs. Controlling for case mix, proprietary homes were found to be less expensive than non-profit or government homes.

| Harrington and Swan (1985) | An analysis of the impact of four different Medicaid nursing home reimbursement systems upon SNF and ICF reimbursement systems, SNF and ICF reimbursement rates, and expenditures per recipient. Retrospective reimbursement was compared to three alternatives: prospective facility-specific, prospective class, and combination. | Secondary source data on state Medicaid nursing home reimbursement methods and rates from 1978–82 were compiled and analyzed; rates and expenditures were regressed on dummy variable representing systems that are alternatives to retrospective reimbursement. | States with each of the alternative systems have average daily SNF and ICF rates for each year (1978–82) that are at least $10 lower than those for states retaining retrospective systems; also, alternative systems in general and prospective facility-specific systems in particular, have SNF changes in rates across the four years that are lower than those of the traditional system. The lower-rate effects appeared to translate into lower expenditures per recipient. |
| Holahan and Cohen (1984) | A summary of interim findings from the case studies of eight states' Medicaid nursing home reimbursement systems. Systems were examined in terms of the strengths of their cost containment incentives as well as their impacts upon quality of care and access. | Cost report data were taken from eight states (New York, California, Massachusetts, Illinois, West Virginia, Minnesota, Georgia, Connecticut) for the years 1978 to 1980; states were chosen because of their large share of the industry and because they represented different reimbursement systems. States were compared on the bases of operating costs, Medicaid capital costs, Medicaid days, expenditures for patient-related and non-patient-related items. Further analysis, using multivariate methods, is in progress. | States with "weak incentives" for control of operating costs had up to 5.75 higher cost growth rates and higher cost increases in Medicaid vs. private patient homes. Reimbursement systems had stronger effects on high cost than on low cost homes. In states with strong cost controls, facilities appeared to curtail cost growth by limiting patient-related costs (nursing, social/leisure, and dietary services). Facilities appeared to expand Medicaid access in response to rate controls, but this was most likely a short-term response. |

TABLE 8-4 Continued

Source	Description of Program or Study	Study Design	Selected Findings
Meiners et al. (1984) Jones and Meiners (1984) Thorburn and Meiners (1984) Weissert et al. (1983)	A nursing home reimbursement system, sponsored as a demonstration by the National Center for Health Statistics, was designed to provide payment incentives for (1) admitting highly dependent Medicaid residents who otherwise might remain inappropriately hospitalized, (2) meeting outcome goals of some patients, (3) discharging and maintaining some patients in the community. Admission and outcome incentive rates were tied to patient characteristics and their corresponding costs of care; discharge incentive rates reflected vacant bed costs and staff efforts to effect the discharge.	Thirty-six proprietary, Medi-Cal-certified nursing homes, grouped according to size and location, were randomly assigned to a treatment (incentive system) or control group. During the 30-month demonstration (1980–83), extensive assessments of patient ADLs and special conditions were made at baseline, throughout treatment, and following discharge. Patients were graded in increasing dependency levels from A to E, with C level as the breakeven point, requiring no additional reimbursement.	The experimental nursing homes did experience a significant decrease in some low dependency patients and a significant increase in patients with the highest level of dependency (E), but not enough for the reduced length of hospital stay to offset program costs. There were no significant differences between experimentals and controls in attainment of outcome goals. Experimentals discharged more patients to lower levels of care than controls, once discharge plans were made, but the incentives did not appear to encourage facilities to identify candidates for discharge. Discharge usually involved a lower level of institutional care rather than deinstitutionalization.

crudely by the percentage of residents needing assistance in toileting and eating and the percentage of residents receiving skilled care. Reaffirming earlier research (e.g., Bishop, 1980), they also noted that proprietary homes were less expensive than nonprofit or government homes even after case mix was considered. This study was limited by its inability to suggest cause and effect; the data were cross-sectional and permitted only associations to be made.

A case study of eight states analyzed the effect of various cost containment incentives (such as percentile ceilings, inflation allowances, administrative salary controls, and efficiency bonuses) on operating and capital costs (Holahan and Cohen, 1984; Holahan, 1985). The authors found that such incentives work as intended, and especially affect higher-cost rather than lower-cost homes. The annual percentage change in costs per day between 1977 and 1980 differed as much as 5.75%, ranging from an average reduction of 68 cents in the state with the strongest incentives (Illinois) to an average increase of $5.05 for the state with the weakest incentives (Minnesota). Although strong controls on capital transactions also lowered rates of growth in costs, they had adverse effects upon new investment in capital stock. The study also compared the effects of rates related to resident characteristics on the likelihood that residents would be admitted. The results were offsetting. Illinois, which based its payment rates on the level of patient impairment regardless of actual expenditures, encouraged access of those needing heavy care but did not increase nursing home expenditures for nursing care. In contrast, the West Virginia system, which increased ceilings on nursing costs as actual costs rose according to increased levels of resident impairment, encouraged expenditures on nursing but had no effect on access for the highly impaired.

The authors also looked at the general impact of cost containment incentives upon quality of care and access. Measuring quality of care circuitously, in terms of changes in expenditure patterns for costs directly related to patients (that is, routine nursing, social and leisure services, and dietary services), they found that in states with weak incentives the costs related to patient care generally grew faster than the other costs. This was also true for facilities serving predominantly private patients. But in high-Medicaid, high-cost homes under moderate or strong cost containment incentives, non-patient costs grew faster than costs directly related to patient care. The authors recommended that reimbursement systems be divided into three components. To safeguard quality, reimbursement for patient care services (nursing, social work, activity personnel, food) should be based on the facility's own costs—either prospectively or retrospectively—with minimal cost containment incentives. Non-care operating costs should be based on a flat rate or a facility-specific prospective rate. Capital cost reimbursement should be based on the principle of a fair rental, recognizing the appreciation of facilities over time and thereby encouraging good maintenance and long-term ownership.

Smits, Feder, and Scanlon (1982) examined the administration of nursing home claims under Medicare. Presenting hypothetical cases to claims reviewers at 18 different, geographically dispersed offices of fiscal intermediaries and review organizations, they found a remarkable lack of consensus among the reviewers. They tended to differ in how they applied criteria on key points such as the ability of the client to use outpatient services, the instability of the patient (and concomitant need for skilled nursing), and the type of documentation required. The authors recommended more centralized review with oversight by Medicare's central office rather than its ten regional offices, as well as more training for claims reviewers.

Finally, one experimentally controlled demonstration examined whether incentives tied to payment could alter the behavior of facilities (Weissert et al., 1983; Meiners et al., 1984). Incentive payments were tied both to resident characteristics and to outcomes to encourage facilities to admit heavy care patients and to discharge them to the community or to lower levels of institutional care. Thirty-six Medicaid-certified skilled facilities in San Diego were assigned to either the experimental group with incentives or the control group without incentives. Extensive data were collected about residents upon their admission, and a rate structure was implemented based upon previously determined amounts of nursing service time required for five types of residents. The data also formed the basis for determining whether certain outcome goals—for example, elimination of tube feeding and improvement in number of ADL dependencies—had been achieved for certain residents. Finally, discharge incentive payments, based upon the cost of vacant beds and of discharge-planning efforts, were established and certain patients were nominated for efforts to effect a discharge.

The demonstration was unable to show that such an incentive system was cost-effective in terms of reducing the need for hospital care. The experimental nursing homes did admit more heavy-care residents, eliminating some of the more expensive days waiting in hospitals that those patients would have used. But the savings were less than the program costs. No significant differences were noted in attaining outcome goals for residents, and although the experimental homes did discharge somewhat more patients to a lower level of institutional care or to the community, the homes were reluctant to initiate aggressive discharge planning despite the incentives. The researchers commented that the disappointing results may have been due to long delays in starting the program and, particularly, to misunderstandings of the incentive structure by staff at the participating facilities. Thus incentives and training for line staff might have been needed as well as the general payment incentives (Meiners et al., 1984; Thorburn and Meiners, 1984; Jones and Meiners, 1984).

Current Concepts of Reimbursement

Two forms of prospective payment are now vying for attention in discussions of nursing home reimbursement. Based on some of the work already discussed, case mix approaches have been implemented in a number of states. The approach, a variant of the prospective payment system now in place for Medicare reimbursement of hospitals, is attractive to facilities because it pays them proportionately to their efforts. The alternative approach shifts the emphasis from the processes of care to its outcomes, thereby linking quality and cost more directly. Although case-mix reimbursement is being adopted enthusiastically, neither payment method has been well evaluated, and outcome-based reimbursement has not actually been attempted.

Case-Mix Reimbursement. Earlier discharges from acute hospitals under the pressure of prospective Medicare payments for hospital stays, combined with the increased availability of community care for the less impaired subset of the dependent elderly, has been perceived as creating a sicker clientele for contemporary nursing homes. Indeed, the nursing home population has become gradually more impaired in a trend that predates those two shifts. The National Nursing Homes Surveys of 1973 and 1977 show that the resident population has become more functionally disabled over the four-year period (General Accounting Office, 1983).

The resultant pressure for a reimbursement system that recognizes the differences in cost of caring for various types of residents has led states to introduce some form of case-mix reimbursement. The systems developed in nursing homes, such as the RUGs (resource utilization groups) in New York State, differ from DRGs (diagnosis related groups) in hospitals in one major respect. In hospitals, the institution is paid for an entire admission on the basis of the patient's status on admission. The measure of hospital resource intensity is basically the length of stay. The measure of resource intensity in the nursing home is derived from staffing hours per day. The resident is periodically reevaluated, and the rate is adjusted according to the resident's current status.

The advantage of a case-mix approach is that it removes disincentives for accepting heavy care cases and avoids excessive payments for light cases. The systems are predicated on the assumption that there are substantial differences in the costs of caring for residents with different characteristics and that such differences are primarily attributable to personnel costs. Most case-mix systems calculate the costs of care by putting a price on the additional time to provide services that are associated with various markers of disability—for example, tube-feeding, incontinence, inability to dress or transfer, or aggressive behavior. Each service is costed on the basis of the average time taken to provide it. Alternatively, cost has been related inductively to case mix by examining the total amount of care given to each patient and estimating the proportion attributable to each problem. For management purposes, these analyses are usually compiled into a series of case profiles, not altogether different from the old levels of care except for their greater detail and presumed basis in empirical data (Grimaldi, 1985; Fries and Cooney, 1985; Cameron, 1985).

Case-mix reimbursement provides negative as well as positive incentives. The most obvious criticism pertains also to most cost-based health care financing: the more disabled and dependent the patient becomes, the more the facility is paid. Yet a rational system should provide incentives in the opposite direction. But the case-mix approach has subtler problems. The basis for calculating component costs is a set of time and motion studies of personnel in traditional nursing homes. Unfortunately, as already discussed, the relationships between inputs and outputs of nursing home care have not been strongly demonstrated. Further, the care modeled to determine costs is generally custodial (though a rehabilitative approach is surely more desirable) and tends to be heedless of social and psychological aspects of care. Many of the standards embodied in the time and motion studies are directly tied to professional orthodoxies about the need for care delivered by certain kind of personnel working for certain increments of time. Little is substantiated by empirical evidence that shows such care is efficacious.

Most time and motion studies are flawed by an assumption that only one task is done at a time. Little provision is made for joint production despite anecdotal evidence that efficiencies can be achieved by creative ways of grouping tasks. In that sense, the time values might be too great. In another sense, however, *more* time may be needed than generally allowed. Certainly encouraging a person's independence is more time consuming than simply providing services. Another subtle bias lies in the kinds of items measured. Work sampling depends on observable behaviors. For some time, payment schedules for physicians have been criticized because they greatly favor performing technical tasks that can be counted and billed. Time spent solving a problem or even speaking to the patient draws a lower payment rate. It is unfortunate to create the same biases in nursing home payment that have been decried in payment systems for hospitals and physicians.

In summary, although appealing to many policy-makers, case-mix reimbursement systems are worrisome because they are possibly based on inaccurate assessment of real time needed for important tasks and because, even if the assessments of time spent according to type of patient were accurate, these values merely codify a status quo that is not particularly a desirable model for humane care producing good outcomes. Finally, the case mix method definitely discourages a facility from trying to render the residents more independent. Such an effort costs more money than is generally allowed for in the studies and results in a lower payment once the task is accomplished. Although case-mix methods are in place in Illinois, Ohio, West Virginia, Maryland, Washington, and, more recently, Minnesota and New York, the studies of those programs concentrate on creating the systems rather than examining their effects.

Outcome-Based Reimbursement. Case-mix methods do offer a solution to one very real problem—the disincentive that fixed payment systems impose on admission of residents with need for heavy care. What kind of alternatives are available that would prevent discrimination against very time-consuming residents, while producing incentives that promote the well-being, improvement, and independence of the residents? In several of the long-term care interventions described earlier in the chapter, we noted rather dramatic evidence of major improvements in residents' functioning as a result of rather subtle interventions. It, therefore, seems appropriate to create a climate that provides incentives for good outcomes and leaves the field as open as possible to creative approaches. If outcomes were monitored and achieved, we might be prepared to be more flexible about processes and shun orthodoxies. We might also be able to note that some methods for achieving desirable outcomes require less intensive manpower than others. Casual observation already suggests that within cost-constrained systems of care, great variations in quality and outcome are seen. Some institutions have demonstrated an ability to achieve substantial improvements in the resident's functioning at no greater expenditure than those institutions performing largely custodial tasks.

A system of rewards must not be based on outcomes alone. Any educator knows that the performance of a school's graduates is related to the quality of the students admitted in the first place. Similarly, any effort to reward outcomes of nursing home residents must take into account the characteristics of those residents when they were admitted (in the language now prevalent, the case mix of the facility). Thus, proposals to reward outcomes do not rely on rewards simply for better or worse results, but rather use an approach that compares the observed outcomes against expected outcomes, deriving the latter from empirical data about the usual course of similar residents. Such calculations are well within the capabilities of modern sophisticated techniques for multivariate analysis. The outcomes could be compared with professionally established norms or expectations, or against a statistically derived set of standards. The latter appears more free of bias, but the former might be used until sufficient experience has been accumulated to make a transition to the more empirical approach. In either case, appropriate statistical adjustments would be made for the characteristics of the individual residents.

An alternative approach might be to use the outcomes of groups of patients, where the patients have been grouped according to similar characteristics. Researchers at the Hebrew Rehabilitation Center for Aging in Boston have done preliminary work using data collected on a large population of residents to test the feasibility of such an approach (Morris, Sherwood, and Bernstein, 1984).

The most elaborate modeling of outcome-based reimbursement has been done at The Rand Corporation (Kane et al., 1983b). For each of eight major outcome areas (medical status, ability to perform daily activities, pain and discomfort, cognitive abilities, affect [especially depression or anxiety], participation in social activities, significant social interactions, and satisfaction with care and the living environment), measures were developed and tested for reliability across raters and over time (Kane et al., 1983a). Virtually all the data came from interviewing and observing the residents, and the functional abilities were, whenever possible, demonstrated rather than reported. The assessment system was then applied to all residents in four facilities in Los Angeles at the time of the resident's admission to the facility or the study and at six-month intervals for five cycles thereafter. In general, the results of the research suggested that the future status of residents on the eight outcome areas could be reliably predicted. Major changes in status at the time of discharge (that is, discharge to the community, discharge to hospital, death) were less accurately predicted but sufficiently so to allow the development of appropriate reward systems.

Under such a system, patients need not improve; they just have to do better than similar patients receiving good care. Nursing homes would be rewarded when residents did better than expected, penalized if they did worse, and be unaffected if the resident continued along the expected course. The reward was expressed as a prognostic adjustment factor (PAF), a number greater than one if the resident did better than expected, less than one if the resident did worse, and one if the outcomes were as expected. One could use a number proportional to the extent to which the observed result deviated for better or worse than expected, or simply reward or penalize any better or worse outcome. The PAF is then multiplied against a base cost rate, which again could represent all costs of caring for that resident or only the variable costs. The nursing homes' payment for operations would be the sum of the cost times the PAF for all residents in the home. Thus although a nursing home would be rewarded if the majority of its residents did well, not all residents need do better than expected.

Such a system permits redistribution of resources among nursing homes, because the norms for expected performance would be shaped by overall performance of the industry. Homes that consistently did well would be rewarded financially and be encouraged to expand. Those doing poorly would receive less than costs and would be appropriately targeted for further investigation. Economic pressures might encourage such facilities to withdraw from the market.

At a time when the nursing home industry is asking for clearer market signals, an outcome-based reimbursement system is one way of defining more precisely just what is wanted from the industry. Of course, such a system requires decisions about how to weight achievements of one kind of outcome compared to another. This calls for value judgments expressed as social policy. We have explored this issue by measuring the preferences of various constituencies concerned with nursing homes (providers, residents, family members, regulators, even state legislators). Using simple methods, we established the relative importance different constituencies place on the different outcomes (Kane, Bell, and Riegler, 1986). The very act of measuring preferences elicits useful dialogue about what is really being sought in nursing home care.

One concern about an outcome-oriented approach is the cost of administration. In the initial study, observers spent an average of a little over an hour with each resident. However, a less expensive and intrusive approach might well be feasible. Subsequent work has suggested that much useful information could be gained from records if the facility were required to keep records appropriately. (Such an approach would have the secondary advantage of potentially improving care). Using even extant record systems, we were able to achieve about the same level of prediction for gross outcomes on discharge as with the more intensive data collection efforts (Lewis et al., 1985). One would still have to do spot validity checks with appropriate penalties for falsification of records. Moreover, the system would be difficult to manipulate because data at one point in time are used to predict subsequent outcomes and the outcome data for the previous period becomes the baseline data for the next time period. This system has the added advantage of being self-correcting. As the data base grows the accuracy of the prediction increases.

Is reimbursement based on outcomes consistent with reimbursement based on case mix? The answer is affirmative only at the time of initial admission to a facility. Later case-mix systems carry an incentive that increases payment as the resident's status deteriorates, while outcome-based reimbursement does just the opposite, increasing payment when the resident does better than expected on the outcomes of interest. Thus a system using both approaches produces a set of off-setting incentives that would be confusing and dysfunctional. But case mix could be recognized at the time of admission, using the patient's baseline status as a basis for greater initial payment. The experiment of Meiners and his colleagues discussed in the previous section suggests that such an incentive system can encourage greater access to sicker persons.

CONCLUSION

This chapter has presented some tantalizing indications of what is possible in the nursing home, although little has been definitively established. The large array of information about the effectiveness and effects of care in nursing homes leads to an inescapable conclusion: More is known about how to improve nursing home care than society currently has the will or organizational channels to bring about. In many instances, the efforts at regulation have had the side effect of constraining innovation. Too many of our standards are based on discipline-derived definitions of professional needs unsupported by evidence of increased effectiveness.

Some changes will surely cost money, and others imply no extra cost except an upheaval in standard practices of staffing and routines. Some ideas that are promising for improving care and the quality of life have not been systematically studied. Prominent among them would be separate units (or even facilities) for persons with severe cognitive impairment. This controversial idea is currently being tested for its marketability in the private sector; it seems logical that the needs of both the cognitively intact and the cognitively impaired could be better met if the groups could live separately, because ideal programming differs enormously for the two groups. In our opinion, a compromise position is likely to benefit neither group, leading to overprotection and infantalization, as well as diminishing the environment of the lucid while unnecessarily restricting the demented.

The nursing home is best conceptualized as one location, among others, where long-term care occurs; it should not be sharply contrasted to community care. It is a form of care very much in transition. In all likelihood the future will see many new species of such care with varying emphases placed on different components. In such a context attention is better directed to assuring that the goals of care are met, leaving more flexibility for the ways by which they are reached. We do not want to lose sight of the twin missions implied by the term "nursing home": care and a place to live. By either measure we still have a long way to go.

9

The Relationship Between Long-Term Care and Acute Care

By its very name, long-term care implies a relationship to acute health care. But it is a mistake to think of that relationship as merely sequential, with long-term care following when acute care is finished. The interaction is much more dynamic. Certainly many long-term care "careers" begin with an acute illness and a hospital stay. Just as often, however, an episode of long-term care begins with care at home but includes one or more admissions to the hospital. Most importantly, long-term care and acute care must often be provided simultaneously. As this book has emphasized, just as the artificial distinction between the medical and social models of care is dysfunctional, so too is the artificial separation of acute and long-term care. The need for acute care does not disappear when a person begins receiving long-term care. In fact, the opposite occurs. On the average, long-term care clients use about twice as much acute care as do their age-matched peers (Leutz et al., 1985).

Persons with functional impairments requiring home care or nursing home care surely need competent primary medical care, appropriate medical and surgical treatment of acute conditions, and palliative medical care during the end-stages of terminal illnesses. (We have already seen that geriatric assessment units and hospices fall into a no-man's land between acute and long-term care.) Provision of adequate health care is essential for effective long-term care, but some orchestration between acute and long-term care programs is required for efficient long-term care. Coordination and systematic efforts are even more necessary because many physicians spend shorter times at each encounter (that is, in an office visit, a hospital visit, or a nursing home visit) with a person over 65 than with a younger person whose problem is likely to be less complex (Kane et al., 1981). Furthermore, older people often fail to disclose symptoms to professionals (Brody and Kleban, 1981).

Effective care of the frail elderly requires a long-range perspective. Rather than being construed as single events of hospitalization or other discrete interventions, care of the functionally dependent elderly is more appropriately viewed as an extended episode composed of transitions from one functional state to another. The general slope for the population, and eventually each individual, will be downward, though some individuals will make marked improvements along the way or experience interspersed "highs" and "lows." For many, the episode of long-term care will continue (at varying intensity) until death, but some will recover enough functions so that the episode ends with self-care. Each intervention should serve to improve functioning when possible and, at least, minimize deterioration and improve the quality of life.

Activities undertaken as part of acute care (either primary care or hospital care) have particular potential for long-range effects on future functional status, use of services, and costs. Those grappling with how best to organize and provide acute care for long-term care recipients are hampered by lack of *longitudinal* information about the effects associated with various patterns of combining acute and long-term care for the frail elderly. Such information is even more elusive because of artificial programmatic separations between acute and long-term care, codified in regulations for Medicare and Medicaid.

This chapter considers a relatively small body of research on movement between long-term care and acute medical care. We review studies on three general topics:

- movement of persons from acute hospital care to long-term care;
- movement of persons receiving formal long-term care to acute hospital;
- medical attention for persons in nursing homes.

The next chapter deals with the effectiveness of various efforts to improve long-term care systems by changing the balance between nursing home care and community care, targeting long-term care services more accurately and efficiently, or changing financial coverage and incentives. Frequently, such improvements in long-term care programs have been expected to result in less use of acute hospital care and physician services, with associated economies. But, as this chapter shows, the relationship between acute care and long-term care is so intimate that demonstrations intervening on the long-term care side alone may be doomed to less than optimal results. In fact, some of the change may need to occur in what is now considered the acute care sector.

MOVEMENTS FROM HOSPITAL TO LONG-TERM CARE

Despite the often repeated statistic that about half the nursing home admissions in the United States originate from acute hospitals, the information on patients' movements from hospitals to nursing homes is surprisingly slim. We cannot confidently estimate the proportion of elderly hospital patients who enter the hospital from the community and are discharged directly to nursing homes. Very few investigators have asked the question that way, and, because of the fragmentation between acute and long-term care, such statistics have had little practical value to hospitals and are not collected routinely.

A few investigators have tried to trace what has happened to persons discharged from hospitals and identify characteristics associated with admission to nursing homes. Four such studies are summarized in Table 9-1. Each was severely limited by its reliance only on information available in the hospital records or in abstracted versions of such data. The first two used data abstracted by professional standards review organizations (PSROs), and the other two were based on audits of hospital records.

An early study used data from the PSRO in west Los Angeles to examine discharges from the community hospitals and one teaching hospital in the region (Kane, Matthias, and Sampson, 1983). About 9% of persons over 65 discharged from those hospitals were admitted to nursing homes. Overall, women were more likely to go to nursing homes than men, and the age distribution of those going to nursing homes closely paralleled the age distribution in nursing homes themselves. But for persons who had been in a nursing home prior to the hospitalization, the effects of sex and age were much less evident. Persons in that subgroup almost inevitably returned to a nursing home on discharge unless they died in the hospital.

This earlier effort was replicated on a larger scale using PSRO data from four areas; namely, rural California, west Los Angeles, Utah, and South Carolina (Kane and Matthias, 1984). The regression model developed to fit the initial results remained constant over two separate years in west Los Angeles but did not fit the data for other parts of the country, suggesting that nursing home use varies from region to region. Individual explanatory models varied in their components, with age the only consistently strong predictor in all the geographic areas studied. The interaction of multiple diagnosis with age also emerged as a significant predictor in three of the four areas studied. The rate of discharge from hospital to nursing home in the four locations averaged at about 9%, but also varied considerably from region to region.

Because both these studies used extant information abstracted by the PSROs, pertinent information on functional status was unavailable. In contrast, the following two studies reviewed hospital records to identify

TABLE 9-1 Studies of Movement from Hospital to Nursing Home

Source	Description	Study Design	Selected Findings
Kane, Matthias, and Sampson (1983)	A pilot study of 10 non-teaching hospitals and one large area teaching hospital in West Los Angeles, CA; records of nursing home patients admitted directly from acute hospitals are studied to better identify those at nursing home risk.	Two data sets (taken from professional standards review organization case records) of patients aged 65+ and discharged in 1979–80 were analyzed; variables included age, sex, race, admission source, disposition, length of stay, diagnoses, surgical procedures.	Of the 9% discharged to nursing homes, those aged 85+ were ten times more likely to be institutionalized than those aged 65; females were twice as likely as males; those diagnosed with mental illness were more likely than those with physical illness. Adjusting for differences in patient source, characteristics, and type of treatment, the teaching hospital was less likely than the nonteaching hospitals to discharge patients to nursing homes.
Kane and Matthias (1984)	A statistical model was developed to predict which patients admitted to a hospital from home would be discharged to a nursing home.	A logistic regression model was applied to a 1979 sample of cases from hospitals reviewed by professional standards review organizations in Riverside, CA; Utah; South Carolina; and West Los Angeles, CA.	Age was the only consistently strong predictor across all four geographical areas. Multiple diagnoses interacting with age was a strong predictor in three areas. Other variables—sex, mental diagnoses, orthopedic surgery—varied in their relative importance among areas.

| Lamont et al. (1983) | Data on elderly persons admitted to a 290-bed county community hospital in California were studied to determine what demographic, medical, and sociologic characteristics recorded at admission predicted change in functional status and discharge to a nursing home. | The medical records of 205 patients, aged 75+, discharged in 1981, were analyzed; information collected included demographic variables, admission source, discharge location, diagnosis, procedures, complications, social support. Clinical judgments were made on how the hospitalization fit into the patients' general course of recovery or deterioration. | The most important predictors of functional deterioration were older age, especially 85+, and abnormal mental status. When discharge location was compared to admission source, 47% of the patients remained at the same level of care following discharge; the rest required a higher level. Elderly surgical patients were three times likelier to return to baseline functioning. |
| Davis, Shapiro, and Kane (1984) | A study on the extent to which persons aged 75+, admitted to a university teaching hospital, received supportive care or nursing home placement at discharge. | The medical records of 233 consecutive patients admitted to the medical service of the hospital in 1979 were reviewed. Demographic information was collected from admission data; charts were reviewed for evidence of hospital-associated complications and discharge diagnoses. | Few medical patients (6%) were newly placed in nursing homes; 65% returned to the same level of care as on admission; 10% returned home at an increased level of care; 18% died or were discharged to another acute care facility. Of the variables studied (age, female sex, being unmarried, and abnormal mental status during hospitalization), only abnormal mental status significantly correlated with nursing home placement. |

factors associated with discharge to nursing homes. Both were confined to persons over 75, who have a greater risk of nursing home use.

Lamont and his colleagues (1983) reviewed the medical records of over 200 patients over age 75 who were discharged from a community hospital in Los Angeles in 1981 to determine what information at admission predicted functional status and destination at discharge. Of the 209 patients studied, 145 had been admitted to the hospital directly from the community. Of these, 19% were discharged to nursing homes. As expected, those admitted from facilities either died or returned to a nursing home. The only factors in this study that distinguished those discharged to nursing homes from the others were abnormal mental status and increasing age. To the extent they were adequately represented in the hospital record, factors such as sex, marital status, insurance status, race, social support, primary service in which the patient had been treated, and complications in the hospital failed to differentiate those who ended up in nursing homes.

In a parallel effort, Davis, Shapiro, and Kane (1984) reviewed the records of 233 patients over age 75 discharged consecutively from the medical service of a teaching hospital. Only 8% of the sample had been admitted from a nursing home and only 6% were discharged to a nursing home. Characteristics associated with discharge to a more dependent level of care (which included board and care, sheltered housing, or more intensive home care) were Medicaid coverage, female sex, and impaired mental status, but only the latter was associated with discharge to a nursing home. Unlike in other studies reported here, age was not associated with probability of discharge to a nursing home.

As the foregoing studies suggest, little systematic information is available about discharge from a hospital to long-term care, and none of it pertains to discharge to community-based long-term care. Unfortunately, relevant studies are difficult to mount because hospitals do not routinely record functional status on admission and discharge or information about other potential risk factors such as social support. Although half the nursing home patients are admitted from a hospital, a much smaller proportion of hospital patients are discharged to nursing homes (somewhere between 6% and 9% of those over 65 and 19% of those over 75 in the four studies discussed).

With the new pressures of prospective payment, hospitals are increasingly interested in facilitating discharge and Medicare is increasingly interested in controlling potential misuse of nursing homes and home care. Under these conditions, the stage is set to pay closer attention to the characteristics of hospitalized patients that may make them likely candidates for long-term care, or at least post-acute care. We anticipate that medicine regulations will soon mandate at least rudimentary information on functional status and social support elements in each hospital chart. Such an expectation would enable more meaningful study of the effects of hospital practices and payment systems on the quality of aftercare for the elderly.

If hospital discharge planners want to prevent nursing home admission, they will need to target patients more precisely than simply by age 75 and above. Factors intuitively thought to be important, such as marital status and general social support, are imperfect predictors of nursing home use. Moreover, they may be inappropriate bases for policies directed toward eligibility. Poor mental status may be the best indicator that a hospital patient is likely to enter a nursing home, though not necessarily a good marker for nursing home admissions that could or should be prevented. In fact, none of these data indicate the appropriateness of the nursing home admission, the effectiveness of the hospital stay in minimizing the need for subsequent long-term care, or the adequacy of the decision-making process that led to a nursing home admission or an alternative long-term care plan. The data on geriatric assessment units presented in Chapter 7 strongly suggest that specialized physical and social assessment combined with short-term treatment can alter the trajectories of persons bound for a nursing home.

MOVEMENT FROM LONG-TERM CARE TO ACUTE HOSPITAL

We know little about transitions from hospitals to nursing homes and other forms of long-term care, and we know even less about transitions from long-term care programs into acute hospitals. Such information can be gained by following the paths of people who are discharged from long-term care facilities or home care programs, following them beyond the first destination. Indeed, without such studies, some data on length of stay in nursing homes can erroneously lead to a belief that many residents leave the nursing home after a short stay and never return. In fact, many of those who go to hospitals simply pass through a revolving door back to the same or another nursing home.

Statistics generated by state Medicaid programs and others tend to count each nursing home admission as if a new person were involved. Only a few studies have diligently followed persons from nursing home to hospital and back again. But a picture can be pasted together from a series of snapshots and a small amount of continuous footage from these longitudinal studies. Table 9-2 summarizes several studies pertaining to this theme.

The study by Lewis and her colleagues (Lewis, Cretin, and Kane, 1985; Lewis et al., 1985) provides the best data on the fate of persons discharged from a sample of nursing homes. This study began with a population of persons discharged from nursing homes and followed them for two years. The usual course was circular travel. Of those discharged from the nursing home, about a quarter went home, a third died, and most of the rest went to a hospital. Almost all who survived the hospitalization returned to a nursing

TABLE 9-2 Studies of Movement from Nursing Home and/or Community Long Term Care to Hospital

Source	Description	Study Design	Selected Findings
Lewis, Cretin, and Kane (1985)	The authors examined the natural history of care and use of health services following discharge from a sample of nursing homes until death or two years after discharge. Subgroups of patients are identified on the basis of survival and use of services.	A random sample of 24 nursing homes, stratified according to bed size, was identified from 47 facilities in the San Bernadino area of California. Data from the medical records of 197 persons who were admitted to a nursing home for the first time were collected on characteristics at admission, length of stay, discharge status; four patient classification groups were developed, and length of life from admission until death at the end of the study was examined using a life table analysis.	Of 123 persons who survived the initial nursing home discharge, 39% were transferred between nursing home and hospital two or more times and 21% were transferred four or more times. There were four subsets of patients: single admission patients who died quickly; single admission patients with good functional status who returned home; multiple admission patients, either alive or dead, who tended to be incontinent, and confused with poor functional status.
Lewis et al. (1985)	A study of the relationship between patient characteristics on admission to a nursing home and subsequent outcomes at discharge and two years after, including discharge to home, transfers to SNFs, transfers to hospitals, death.	A random sample of 529 patients from 24 nursing homes (San Bernadino, California) was followed from discharge in 1980 through 1982. The relationship of patient characteristics, nursing care needs, and social supports to outcomes was analyzed by both univariate and logistic regression techniques.	Upon discharge, 28% of the sample went home or to community facilities; 36% went to a general hospital, where 11% died; and 25% returned to nursing homes. Of 529 discharges, only 38 were alive and at home at the end of two years; 401 were dead. Mental orientation, urinary continence, functional status, hip fracture, and dementia were predictors of immediate and follow-up outcomes.

Gordon, Kane, and Rothenberg (1985)	A study of acute hospitalization coming out of a 229-bed home for the aged; the symptoms and signs leading to hospitalization, the diagnosis established, and the various outcomes were explored.	Data on a stable population of 239 persons hospitalized 503 times in a four year period (1977–81) were analyzed; subjects were traced for one additional year. Variables included demographics; level of care before admission, at discharge, after one year; symptoms on admission; diagnoses; treatment; length of stay. Logistic regression was used to determine predictors of mortality at six months.	Four variables were significantly associated with death at six months after first hospitalization: age, hospital complication, surgical procedure, diagnosis of acute myocardial infarction. Of those surviving their first hospitalization, 23% returned to a higher level of care; at one year, 36% had died and 17% of the survivors were at a higher level of care.
Stark, Gutman, and McCashin (1982)	A study examining transitions between acute and long-term care, including (1) the number of admissions to LTC directly from acute care settings versus the community; (2) the number of LTC persons hospitalized at least once in the 12 months after admission to LTC; (3) the outcomes of these hospitalizations.	Descriptive data were presented on 3,518 clients admitted in 1978 to home care or nursing home services at any one of five levels of care in two health unit areas—one urban and one semi-rural—of the British Columbia Long-Term Care Program.	About 20% of new admissions to the LTC program were from an acute care hospital. Only 36.8% of the admissions were to nursing home care, mainly at the urban study area. About 75% of the clients had no acute care admissions in the first year, and about 50% of those with such admissions returned to the facility and care level from which they had come.

TABLE 9-2 Continued

Source	Description	Study Design	Selected Findings
Stark et al. (1984)	A preliminary analysis of home and facility, level-of-care changes, and program attrition for the three years following initial admission to British Columbia's Long-Term Care Program. The program provides pre-admission assessment, client placement, and periodic review for clients at five levels of home care or facility care.	Data were presented on 1,241 home and 409 facility clients newly admitted to the LTC program in two study areas in 1978, and follow-up data at one, two and three years. Particular attention was given to contrasting home and facility clients at both the lowest and highest levels of care.	54% of clients admitted to the lowest level of home care were still in the program after three years, about 50% at the same place and level of care. A higher proportion of home care clients under 75 than facility clients remained unchanged at year 1. 25% of those admitted to the highest level of care at home and 14% admitted to the highest level at facilities remained in the program for three years. Moves to a lower level of care from the highest level were infrequent.
Stark and Gutman (1986)	A 5-year follow-up of 1,653 persons newly admitted to British Columbia Long-Term Care Program in 1978 (1,241 to home care and 412 to nursing homes). All persons in the LTC program were assigned a level of care from 1 to 5, connoting need for service.	One urban and one rural area were selected for the study, and LTC clients were followed through existing records.	Of the home care group, 34% were still in the LTC program (14% receiving home care at an unchanged level, 7% receiving home care at higher level, and 12% in facility), 39% had died and 27% were discharged. Of the facility group, 29% were still in the program (13% at an unchanged level of care and 2% in home care), 39% had died, and 32% were discharged from the program.

home (but not necessarily the same one). Of those who went back to the community, about a third remained there two years later. Looking at the data another way, virtually all of those in the community two years later had been discharged to the community initially from the nursing home.

The factors associated with discharge from a nursing home were primarily functional. Neither age, sex, nor marital status were related to the discharge destination; but patients with greater ADL independence, continence, and mental orientation were more likely to go home. Those who died in the nursing home were more likely to have had reduced functional status, to have been incontinent, or to have been disoriented. Diagnoses were indicators of outcome in only a few cases. Patients with cancer and dementia were more likely to die, either in the nursing home, in the hospital, or in a second nursing home, whereas patients with hip fracture were more likely to go home (Lewis et al., 1985).

Gordon, Kane, and Rothenberg (1985) followed all those who were hospitalized in a sectarian home for the aged for a two-year period. The outcomes of the hospitalizations differed according to the reason for hospital admission. Overall, of those admitted to a hospital for the first time, 9% died and 19% of the survivors went to a more dependent level of care in the same or another facility. (Three levels of care were measured in the study—residential, intermediate, and skilled.) One year later, almost 40% had died and 17% were at a more dependent level of care than at the outset of the study.

Stark and her colleagues (Stark, Gutman, and McCashin, 1982) examined the rate at which a group of elderly persons receiving long-term care in both community and nursing homes were hospitalized. A little over 20% of the patients from long-term care facilities were hospitalized in the first year. Being hospitalized was unrelated to the level of care prior to the hospital admission or after it, even when the patient had multiple admissions. (The province of British Columbia, where the study was done, recognizes five levels of long-term care.)

In a subsequent study, the same investigators (Stark et al., 1984) traced the course of clients admitted to community and institutional long-term care programs over three years. About half remained in the same type and level of care at the end of the first year, but only 20% were unchanged after three years. Among both facility and community clients, the rate of change was greatest for those at the more dependent levels of care. In facilities, for example, those at the least dependent level had a mortality rate of 19% after three years compared to 48% among those at the most dependent care level. For home care clients, the comparable rates were 25% and 42%. The rates for discharge from long-term care during the same three year period were 28% for the least dependent and 38% for the most dependent in facilities, and 21% for the least dependent and 33% for the most dependent in home care. Among facility clients, the discharge rates seemed to level out by the second year, whereas they remained fairly continuous over the three years for those receiving care in the community.

A five-year follow-up of the same group of long-term care clients in British Columbia (Stark and Gutman, 1986) accentuates our point that long-term care should be seen as an extended episode. Of a group enrolled in home care in 1978, 34% were still in care five years later, 39% had died, and 27% had been discharged and were still living at the five-year follow-up. Of the 34% still in care, 14% remained at the same level of care at home, 7% were in a higher home care level, and 12% had moved to a facility. Of those in a facility in 1984, 29% were still in the program (2% of these had moved to home care, 39% had died, and 32% were discharged and still living five years later). Unfortunately, the discharge rates are ambiguous; those discharged home without care and those discharged to an extended hospital classification were both included in this count. Even so, Stark and Gutman's study suggests that many long-term care users remain stable in their needs for many years and that some improve in functioning, though more decline.

Two other data sets, which have already been discussed in this book—one from Manitoba and one from Massachusetts—offer useful longitudinal information relevant to transitions. These are summarized in Table 9-3. Shapiro, Roos, and their colleagues have linked a survey of elderly people in Manitoba to the records for that province's Health Services Commission, which administers the universally insured hospital care, physician care, and personal care home benefits. This unique data set (which included sub-samples of persons in senior housing projects, senior hostels, and nursing homes) provides interesting insights into the asymmetric ways services are used. Roos and Shapiro (1981) noted that about one-tenth of the elderly population accounted for about a third of the ambulatory care visits and three-quarters of the hospital days. Similarly, Mossey and Shapiro (1985) noted that elderly Manitobans established highly consistent patterns for using physician care. In an eight-year study, 60% of the sample maintained an identical pattern of physician use for at least six of those years. Again the overall use was skewed, with 15% making seven or more visits per year. Interestingly, increased age was related to increased physician use only for males.

When the utilization data were analyzed according to the older person's place of residence, an interesting pattern emerged. Residents of nursing homes used many more physician services than any other group (an average of 9.7 visits per year compared to 7.4 visits to people in senior housing and 5.3 to elders in the general community). But those in nursing homes used the *fewest* hospital days of any group (an average of 4.2 hospital days for nursing homes compared to 4.9 for the general community and 6.3 for those in senior housing). Given that the nursing home group was likely to be frailest, it seems that some of the needed care must have been given in the

TABLE 9-3 Longitudinal Studies

Source	Description	Study Design	Selected Findings
Roos and Shapiro (1981)	A study of institutionalized and noninstitutionalized elders in the province of Manitoba, examining the distribution of health services utilization among the elderly, the consistency of physician visits over a two-year period, and the relationship between usage and such variables as place of residence, health status, and income level.	Two parallel, random, stratified samples were drawn and matched according to area, sex, and institutional or noninstitutional residence ($N=4805$); respondents interviewed in 1971 on 517 separate measures were linked to all physician and hospital contacts made during the 12 months before and 12 months after the interviews. Utilization data were taken from government files.	8.8% of those interviewed made 35% of all ambulatory visits; 3% used 47% of all the hospital days in the year before the interview, and 10% used 78% of all hospital days in year 2. The mean number of hospital days increased with age. Males used more hospital days and females had more ambulatory visits. Service utilization was also related to residence, self-reported health status, and number of self-reported health problems.
Shapiro (1983)	A study of the hospital utilization patterns of elderly decedents as compared to elderly survivors; the relationship of age, sex, and impending death was examined in relationship to volume of hospital use.	Data were collected on a subsample of 3,169 elders, taken from the six-year Manitoba Longitudinal Study on Aging (1970–77). Survivors and decedents from the original cohort were measured after three years on admission rates, average number of hospital days, and percent of each group using 1–17 or 18+ days in the hospital. Utilization was measured on a yearly basis.	Decedents (5% of the population) used 20% of the total hospital days. Impending death raised the odds of hospitalization 6-fold for those aged 68–74; 7-fold for those 75–84; 5-fold for those 85+. Once admitted to the hospital, decedents are 5½ times more likely than survivors to use 18+ hospital days. Advancing age lowered the relative odds of high use among decedents, but sex had almost no effect.

TABLE 9-3 Continued

Source	Description	Study Design	Selected Findings
Shapiro and Webster (1984)	A study describing the admissions, discharges, and changing health status of eight admission cohorts to nursing homes in Manitoba (a system of universally insured nursing home and home care services). Data were compared to the findings in U.S. studies.	Data on all persons admitted to nursing homes for the first time between 1974 and 1981 were obtained from agency records; the information included numbers of long-term care beds, occupancy rates, costs, and characteristics of users. Changes in the level of care and reasons for discharge were extracted for each cohort at the end of every year.	About 15% of each first admission cohort died by the end of year 1; about 33% died by the end of year 2; about 50% were dead by year 4. Data suggested, however, that about 20% would survive over an 8-year period. About 40% of Level I admissions (lowest level of care) and 30% of Level II survived over six years, and almost half of each remained at their respective levels. Less than 20% of Levels III and IV survived six years, and about 80% of them retained the same classification level.
Mossey and Shapiro (1985)	A longitudinal study of ambulatory use of physicians by older persons, aged 65+, over an eight-year period in the province of Manitoba.	A random sample of 2,029 elders in the community from 1970–77 was obtained from the provincial government's universal health insurance program. Claims filed by physicians for the payment of ambulatory physician visits by these elders were used as the source of data.	60% of the subjects visited physicians with similar frequency per year for six or more years; 22% regularly made two or less visits a year; 14% made 7+ visits per year. Age was unrelated to level of use among females but males 75–79 and 80+ were more likely to be medium or high users. The weak association between age and level of use and a yearly increase in the percentage of high users suggested that cohort effects were a primary determinant of use.

Branch et al. (1984)	A six-year prospective study estimating the functional status of white elders living in the community according to age, gender, and previous functional status.	A Massachusetts statewide stratified area probability sample consisting of 1,625 elderly respondents was interviewed in 1974, with follow-ups in 1976 and 1980. A six-item index (Branch) and a four-item index (Katz) were used to measure the ADLs of bathing, dressing, transference, eating, personal grooming, and walking.	About 50% of the sample remained independent in ADLs for the 6-year period; those aged 85+ had 3 times the probability of being dead or dependent, and 7–9 times the probability of being in a nursing home. Of those dependent at baseline, one-quarter to one-third regained independence at the end of 15 months; one-fifth at the end of five years.
Branch (1985)	A study of the relationship between personal health practices (physical activity, sleep, smoking, alcohol use, meals) and point-incidence physical limitations for initially physically robust elders living in the community.	391 elderly respondents from the second wave (1976) of the Massachusetts Health Care Panel Study reported no physical limitations on the Rosow-Breslaw Functional Health Scale; variables on this sample were used to predict incidence of disability at the third wave of the study (1980).	After controlling for age, health status, income, and the influence of other health practices, only "slowed down physical activities" (for women) and a history of smoking cigarettes (for men) were found to be associated with the subsequent development of physical limitations.

facility itself, and perhaps the increased physician visits enabled such a policy (Roos and Shapiro, 1981).

One of the factors closely associated with increased use of health care services is impending death. Although those who died represented only 5% of the elderly sample, they accounted for 20% of the hospital days. Looking at it another way, the odds of someone who died being hospitalized was five to eight times greater than those of a survivor (Shapiro, 1983). Ironically enough, the Manitoba studies suggested that one of the best predictors of impending death is the individual's own perceived health status. This self-reported evaluation was a better predictor than either physician judgment or previous use of health care (Mossey and Shapiro, 1982).

Shapiro and Webster (1984) traced the course of cohorts admitted to Manitoba's personal care homes. The general pattern over eight years showed a discharge rate (essentially a mortality rate) that averaged about 10% annually, with a more rapid rate during the first two years and the steadiest state during the last four years. The mortality rates were highest for those at the more dependent levels of care (Manitoba recognizes four levels). At the same time, the study showed evidence of improving function as well. About 15% to 20% of surviving persons who had been admitted to more dependent levels of care moved to lower levels over the study period.

The Massachusetts longitudinal study of community-dwelling elderly has focused most on the risks of nursing home admission (which were discussed in Chapter 2) than on movement from long-term to acute care. Nevertheless, a few observations are pertinent here. Branch and his colleagues (1984) have shown that the health course of older persons is more dynamic than might be expected. Although the rate of dependency increases with age as one would predict, movement in the opposite direction is also shown. About half of the subjects lost at least one ADL function over the six-year period of the study, but a fifth of those who were initially dependent regained the lost function in the same period.

In related studies (Branch, 1985; Branch and Jette, 1984; Branch and Nemeth, 1985) attempts were made to associate the onset of disability with the health practices of the elderly. This effort is instructive in pointing out several pitfalls associated with such work even in longitudinal studies. None of the factors proved statistically significant in discriminating the dependency rate, but two statistically significant associations remained after other factors had been controlled for. Among the men, the significant factor was a history of cigarette smoking; among the women, it was a reported slowing down in physical activities. This latter measure illustrates confusion of a risk factor with an indicator of a condition already underway. Reminiscent of the Manitoba data on the predictive power of self-reported health, it suggested that older persons have a sense of impending change in their health status.

Like the information about movement form hospital to long-term care, the data on movement in the opposite direction (or, more broadly, the overall experience of those receiving long-term care) is inconclusive and based on scant evidence. The data do suggest variation in use of services from one older person to another, and from region to region, with no clear predictors of heavy use or of deterioration. The data on use of health care services are obviously sensitive to public policy about the appropriate use of acute care services for those in institutions. Once again, we have virtually no information about the appropriateness of use of acute services—whether it was too much, too little, or the wrong thing—nor could we locate studies of special programs designed to make the acute episode more effective for persons already receiving long-term care.

MEDICAL ATTENTION IN NURSING HOMES

As Chapter 8 suggested, medical care in nursing homes receives mixed to poor reviews both on availability and quality. However, only a few studies have looked specifically at the way primary care is given in nursing homes, and fewer have intervened to change that delivery systematically. Table 9-4 summarizes five studies of patterns of care and five intervention studies. All the latter used a strategy of adding personnel (nurse practitioners and/or pharmacists) rather than changing the structure of physician practice alone.

Some of the earliest studies suggested medical neglect. Solon and Greenawalt (1974) showed those patterns in the Pittsburgh area; and a few years later, a Utah study (Kane, Hammer, and Byrnes, 1977) showed the same phenomenon. Although nursing home residents were seen by physicians in a relatively timely manner, the care was superficial. About two-thirds of the patients had been seen by a physician in the previous month, but there were few instances when there was even the most elemental record that the patient had been directly observed, such as any physical examination findings suggestive that the patient had been literally examined or any changes in drug regimens. In the same spirit, Willemain and Mark (1980) showed that the frequency of physician visits to nursing homes was determined almost entirely by the mandated rate of visits necessary for the resident to be recertified as eligible for the care. A small scale study of the prescribing patterns of physicians in one California nursing home showed numerous drug errors, many of them potentially dangerous (Segal, Thompson, and Floyd, 1979).

Using Medicare Part B claims data, Mitchell and Hewes (1982) studied the behavior of physicians in Michigan apropos of their work in nursing homes. Less than half of the general practitioners, internists, and cardiologists had made even one nursing home visit in the previous month, with

TABLE 9-4 Studies on Medical Care for the Long-Term Care Elderly Population

Source	Description	Study Design	Selected Findings
Descriptive Studies: Solon and Greenawalt (1974)	A study of the extent of physicians' participation in nursing homes.	38 nursing homes (84% response rate) in Allegheny County, PA, responded to a mailed, one-page questionnaire, including questions on the number of physicians participating, the frequency and length of their visits, and their jurisdiction over medical affairs.	14% of active physicians in Allegheny County (includes Pittsburgh) participated in nursing homes: 74% were involved in only one home; 20% in two homes; 6% in three or more. The average monthly, per-patient time for lowest level of care facilities was 17 minutes; for highest level of care facilities, 68 minutes. 53% of for-profit homes and 81% of nonprofit homes claimed they had a physician serving as medical director.
Kane, Hammer, and Byrnes (1977)	A study of the ways in which nursing home patients receive medical care in Salt Lake County, UT. Utah facilities are classified according to three ascending levels of care/service offered: personal care, intermediate, comprehensive. Medical attention is required annually, quarterly, or monthly for the three levels, respectively.	For six separate, randomly chosen weeks (1974), records for 2,071 patients in 60 of 69 nursing homes were abstracted. Sources of data were nursing home staff and companies holding Medicare-Medicaid contracts for providing transportation for patients. Data on each patient trip listed point of origin (nursing home), point of delivery (source of care), type of payment.	About 65% of the patients had been seen by a physician within a month, but there were fewer new observations (45%), records of exams (25%), or prescription changes (40%). A substantial amount of medical care was found to be delivered outside the nursing home: an estimated 3.6 patient trips per bed per year were made. 55% of the care was at the university hospital; 27% of the trips were to the offices of various specialists. Less than 5% of the trips led to hospitalization.

| Segal, Thompson, and Floyd (1979) | A study of the patterns of drug prescribing and utilization in a skilled nursing facility in California, and their relationship to potentially adverse drug reactions. | A sample of 50 patients attended by seven physicians was randomly drawn from 250 patients at a SNF facility. Their health care records were analyzed according to such criteria as drug interactions, indications for the use of the drug, adverse drug reactions. | The average number of drugs per patient was 7.06 with a total of 353 drug orders for the 50 patients. Of the 353 prescriptions, 40% were given without a corresponding diagnosis indicated in the record, 31% were given at inappropriate intervals, 22% were at potentially toxic dosages, 20% had possibly caused clinically significant adverse reactions, and 9% had probably caused clinically significant drug reactions. |
| Willemain and Mark (1980) | A study of the distribution of intervals between physician visits in nursing homes and their impact upon quality and cost of care. Suggestions were made for using a system of "stochastic" regulation of physician services to allow for greater freedom in responding to patients' needs. | Data were taken from a 1976 Boston City Hospital "Nursing Home Telemedicine Project" in which patients at 10 nursing homes received physician visits on the basis of need and without the restraints of current reimbursement regulations or frequency of visits. The distribution of visit intervals was compared with the conventional system of physician coverage in eight matched "control" nursing homes. | The distribution for ICF and SNF experimental patients, with visits made in response to randomly occurring episodes of acute illness, was geometric, whereas the distribution for the controls was dominated by a mode around the minimum reimbursable level of 30 days. The medium interval for experimentals was 10 days; for controls, 22 days. |

TABLE 9-4 Continued

Source	Description	Study Design	Selected Findings
Mitchell and Hewes (1982)	An econometric study of physician behavior in Michigan nursing homes, presenting data on the frequency and type of physician visits, the relationship between reimbursement rates and visits, characteristics of physicians who do not make visits, and reasons for physicians' reluctance to visit nursing home patients.	1980 Part B Medicare claims (including such data as diagnosis, location of service, type of visit, physician specialty, reasonable charge as determined by Medicare), a survey of a final sample of 978 physicians, and Census Bureau data on county market characteristics were merged into a single file for descriptive and econometric analysis.	Only 41.4% of general practitioners, internists, and cardiologists had made any nursing home visit in the previous month. Cardiologists were least likely to visit. 66% of all visits were provided by 5% of the physicians. Major reasons for not visiting were reimbursement-related reasons (32%), dislike of nursing homes (14%), too much time (20%), few nursing home patients in practice (20%). Econometric analysis concluded that physicians were not more likely to visit if fees were higher, given the travel time.

Interventive Study:			
Kane et al. (1976)	The Nursing Home Demonstration Project (1973–74) was developed to test the effectiveness of a combined care program of direct services, staff education, and community coordination provided by teams of nurse practitioner and social worker. The teams used a specially designed problem-oriented record.	13 intermediate-level nursing homes in Salt Lake City were randomly allocated to one of 3 study groups: care given by a nurse practitioner supported by a physician and pharmacist (medical group); care given by the above plus a social worker (combined group); no changes in care other than the addition of a social worker (social group). Functional and behavioral changes were measured at 2-week intervals; detailed cost records were kept.	The "combined" team identified and resolved more patient problems, especially social problems, than the other approaches; it also was more effective in decreasing the number and dosage of patient medications. Positive functional status change was greater for the "combined" group, whereas positive behavioral change was greater for the "social group." Average annual patient medical costs were about $300 less for the "combined" group than for the "social" group, more than offsetting project costs.
Master et al. (1980)	A nonprofit group practice of five physicians, three nurse practitioners and physician assistants was established in Boston in 1977 to provide a continuum of care for ambulatory, homebound, and nursing home patients in inner city neighborhoods. The practice was linked to four neighborhood health clinics, three home care programs, and a teaching hospital.	Between July 1977 and April 1979, the project collected data on such variables as demographic characteristics, first-listed diagnosis, hospital admissions and days, and level of care for nursing home residents; cost and revenue data for health center, nursing home, home care, and hospital components were also collected. Data on hospital admissions and days were compared with data from studies on "comparable" and aggregate populations.	The hospitalization rate for the nursing home patients was 3995 days/1000 patients per year, in contrast with a rate of 7198/1000, found in a 1975 Boston study of nursing home patients. The ambulatory patients' rate of 559/1000 contrasted favorably with an expected rate of 1300/1000 for a population with a mean age of 50.

TABLE 9-4 Continued

Source	Description	Study Design	Selected Findings
Gryfe and Proctor (1984)	At Jewish Home for the Aged in Toronto, Ontario, a 370-bed facility, medical care was provided by a closed group of 6–7 physicians, each committed to visit weekly their assigned unit of 43–51 patients. At least one physician was scheduled for a routine visit each weekday morning and would see acutely ill persons on other units as well as attend their own. In 1979, medical attendance was increased to twice weekly for each physician and a family practice resident also began rotating through the facility.	The effects of doubling the frequency of medical attention and adding the residency program were studied by a time series comparing hospitalization rates and mortality rates for all residents during the four years before the change and three years after. Facility budgets and hours of nursing care were also collected.	The increasing rate of hospitalization in the three years before the intervention was abruptly reversed without any difference in average annual death rates for the two time periods. This lower hospitalization rate occurred despite increasing morbidity measured by needed nursing hours. The costs of the increased medical and nursing services delivered in the home were less than the cost of avoided hospitalizations. Authors calculated an annual average savings to the provincial government of over $300,000.

Thompson et al. (1984)	As one of two pilot projects authorized by the California Assembly, clinical pharmacists, under the general supervision of a family practitioner physician, assumed responsibility for drug management of geriatric patients in a Los Angeles skilled nursing facility (1982–82).	A nonrandom pre-test, post-test design in which an experimental group of 67 (under the management of two clinical pharmacists) were compared to 72 controls who received traditional patient care. Measurements were taken for a year previous to and a year following the program's beginning on such variables as demographics, mix of diagnoses, number of drugs, discharge, hospitalization, and mortality. In the study year, subjects had an average of 1.4 less drugs per patient than the controls. Subjects also had significantly more discharges to lower levels of care, less hospitalizations, and a lower mortality rate.
Weiland et al. (1986)	Initiated in 1984, the Academic Nursing Home (ANH) Program in the Nursing Home Care Unit of Sepulveda VA Medical Center utilizes geriatric nurse practitioners, backed by geriatric physician faculty and internal medicine residents to provide a program of improved care, interdisciplinary training, and research.	A staggered implementation of the program allowed for comparisons on outcomes between clients of the new ANH program and those from wards in which the program was not yet implemented. After a four month period, patients were compared on morale, care satisfaction, mental and functional status. In addition, pre and post comparisons were made on mortality and discharge for a year before and after the program's implementation. The experiments had significantly lower rates of transfer to acute care hospitals (17% vs. 32%), greater improvement in functioning (23% vs. 6%), in morale (49% vs. 32%), and in maintenance or improvement of satisfaction (76% vs. 38%). The rate of community discharge significantly increased for the long-stay patients (20% vs. 7%).

cardiologists least likely to visit. About two-thirds of the visits were made by 5% of the physicians. A special survey of almost 1,000 responding physicians indicated that the major reasons for not visiting was low reimbursement combined with a high commitment of time needed to make such visits. However, almost 20% acknowledged a dislike of nursing homes as the reason. This was borne out by an econometric analysis that showed no correlation between the "reasonable" charges reimbursable in an area and the frequency of physicians' visits.

A time-honored approach to the failure of primary medical care in nursing homes is the direct attempt to educate, persuade, or coerce physicians into changing their behavior. Indeed such attempts have been made as part of the efforts to improve overall care in nursing homes, such as those done by PSROs in the mid-1970s (Kane et al., 1979a, 1979b). Regulatory requirements for medical directors together with efforts to strengthen their role may have also had a modest effect, but such programs have had little evaluation and quality problems remain. Making primary care a team approach and relegating much day-to-day monitoring to less expensive and more enthusiastic personnel than physicians seems a more promising approach for a nursing home population.

A decade ago, Kane and his colleagues (1976) reported an innovative effort to use geriatric nurse practitioners as sources of primary care for nursing home residents. This care proved cost-effective. Not only was improvement in functional status and resident satisfaction documented, but the savings due to fewer hospitalizations and other associated costs more than offset the cost directly attributable to the new service. Moreover, the program introduced a new system of problem-oriented records in the participating homes and an inservice program for nursing home staff; both focused on improving the abilities of semi-literate attendants. The record-keeping system encouraged the nurses aides to understand better why information was requested and provided alternative actions for reporting deviations observed from patterns of current levels of residents' functioning. Thus as early as the 1970s, an argument was made that Medicaid programs could simultaneously do good and save money by turning the medical care over to a freestanding group in which the geriatric nurse practitioner played a predominant role.

Master and his colleagues (1980) introduced geriatric nurse practitioners as primary care deliverers in an organized program of health care for inner-city older people. These practitioners provided services to older people in their own homes as well as in nursing homes. The report suggested that this program led to a reduction in the expected use of hospital services, thus supporting the concept that improved primary care through nurse practitioners could lead to important savings.

Both the studies mentioned so far used nurse practitioners who were employed independently of the nursing home. More recently, an innovative program in a Veterans Administration Hospital introduced a system of delivering health services for nursing home patients that relied on geriatric nurse practitioners as primary resources in the hospital's associated nursing home unit (Weiland et al., 1986). Preliminary data suggest that the new program had a number of beneficial results including reduction in mortality, fewer transfers to acute care, and improvements in residents' self-care, morale, and satisfaction.

The Veterans Administration program constituted a test in a single setting and, at that, an academically oriented one atypical of most nursing homes. The most ambitious deployment of nurse practitioners as employees of nursing homes was done as a demonstration project in ten western states (Kepferle, 1983). In this program, coordinated by the Mountain States Health Corporation in Boise, Idaho, participating nursing homes designated a registered nurse to receive training as a nurse practitioner in one of four university schools of nursing and arranged a further preceptorship from a local physician once the trainee returned to the facility. The nursing homes committed themselves to using the employee in a direct clinical capacity after the training. Currently the University of Minnesota and The Rand Corporation are conducting a detailed study of the effects on residents and the cost-effectiveness of the program, by comparing 30 homes in the demonstration with matched counterparts without nurse practitioners. Study results are unavailable as yet, but preliminary qualitative findings show that it can be difficult to sustain the clinical role of nurse practitioners as nursing home employees without conscious efforts by the practitioners themselves, the administrators, and the directors of nurses. Once again, the financing mechanism interferes with efficient practice. According to current policies, most of the cost savings effected by the practitioners (for example, in reduced hospitalizations, physician visits, emergency room use, or drugs) will likely accrue to the Medicare program, while in most states the facilities, paid under Medicaid, receive no direct reimbursement for the nurse practitioner's salary.

In the context of a large, sectarian nursing home in Toronto, Gryfe and Proctor (1984) reported the effect of doubling the amount of physician attention and adding a residency program, both of which occurred in 1979. Using time series data from 1975 to 1983, the investigators showed a dramatic reversal of the previous trend to increased use of hospitals for the nursing home population, a finding that occurred despite evidence that the population became more frail and needed more nursing attention as the eight-year study period progressed. The change in physician behavior was deemed extraordinarily cost-effective. Assuming that hospitalization would have increased for the last four years at the rate of increase for the first five (admittedly a large assumption!), they calculated that the government saved about $319,500 a year when the cost of additional medical and nursing attention was subtracted from the imputed additional hospital costs. This estimate may be inflated—obviously other measures might have reduced hospital use independently and no control nursing homes were used—but it seems likely some cost savings were effected. This study challenges the conventional view that a physician's time is the most expensive and should be minimized.

Reacting to the problems of overuse and misuse of medications in nursing homes, another proposed strategy involves a more direct role for a clinical pharmacist. The early study by Kane and his colleagues, already cited, included a pharmacist as an important part of the backup team for the geriatric nurse practitioner. In California, Thompson and his colleagues (1984) directly tested the potential of the clinical pharmacist. He showed that when a clinical pharmacist took direct responsibility for primary care decisions on drug use, the rate of potential drug complications decreased and the quality of care generally improved. In 1985, the Hartford Foundation announced an initiative to improve the patterns of prescribing medications for the frail elderly. Each of the studies funded under that program will have an intervention component and an evaluation.

CONCLUDING COMMENT

Unlike the other chapters in this section, this chapter has largely presented descriptive information about the relationship between acute and long-term care and the movement of persons from one sector to the other. The only interventive studies presented were the few on the use of innovative personnel to provide primary care in nursing homes. Furthermore, we have been unable to derive prescriptive formulas about the ideal way that frail elderly persons should move between acute and long-term care. The studies of such movements for the most part contain insufficient information about the decision processes and how various strategies affect the outcomes for the older person. It would be possible, and indeed desirable, to test the relative effectiveness of alternative strategies for locus of care (e.g., treatment of certain conditions in nursing homes or home care versus admission to hospital), always assuming safeguards for the health of the participants in the study.

One point stands out. The type and quality of acute care received by frail elderly persons before, after, or during the time they receive long-term care has enormous potential to influence functioning for better or worse. And functional status is what long-term care is all about! Drugs, surgery, and other aspects of acute care treatment are powerful tools. Common sense suggests that the way they are used will powerfully shape long-term care. Furthermore, arbitrary changes of location are often said to cause debilitating and even fatal "transfer trauma" in the frail elderly (see Chapter 8), suggesting that moves to hospital and subsequent discharges to yet another facility should be carefully considered and planned.

It is also clear that many frail elderly people move back and forth between acute and long-term care, and that the quality of their primary health care is by no means assured. The designation of what is the sphere of the acute hospital and what falls into the realm of "aftercare" is also arbitrary, the result of professional convention reinforced by financing.

The message from this review is the need to consider the total picture when planning long-term care services. Plans should anticipate change in status and the need to mobilize different services during the course of an episode of long-term care. Special attention needs to be paid to the points of transition from one locus of care to another. In some instances the change can be avoided entirely; in others it may prove a useful opportunity to review the patient's total status and management.

The fragmentation in funding has tended to reinforce a fragmentation in care. Opportunities for timely intervention may be foregone because the potential savings accrue to a different program. Certainly consideration of maximizing efficiency must be interpreted differently depending on the funding context. The pressures on the hospital are beginning to produce repercussions in the long-term care arena. On the one hand, hospitals are vigorously marketing outpatient and aftercare options to the elderly (Brody and Persily, 1984; Evashwick, Rundall, and Goldiamond, 1985). On the other hand, complaints, as yet unsubstantiated, of more disabled persons being discharged prematurely are the harbingers of the need to pay closer attention to the often overlooked interdependency of acute and long-term care. In the opposite direction, improved primary medical care has the potential to reduce the burden on the acute care hospital.

The final chapter in this section turns to a review of evidence about efforts to change the system of long-term care in communities. As we turn to that chapter, we should keep in mind that aspects of the acute care system may also need changing before older people can get the most value from their long-term care.

10

Systems of Long-Term Care

Thus far, we have dealt with long-term care programs one type at a time, a somewhat artificial and limited approach. No single form of long-term care program is essential, and no single form of program suffices to provide strong support for independence among the functionally impaired elderly. Some exchange among services is always possible, and some combinations are expected.

In this chapter, we turn to evidence about efforts to make the system of care work better for the functionally impaired elderly, to identify their problems correctly, and to make available a wider range of community service than would be possible under most current state law. About a score of demonstration projects done over the last 15 years—some with extensive publicity—address the costs and benefits of comprehensive long-term care reform.

In actuality, the research is more modest than the title of the chapter suggests. Although our terminology is conventional, "long-term care system" is a misnomer to describe either the current situation or the changes brought about by the demonstrations. The various demonstration projects in community long-term care were systematic in some ways. They drew on multifaceted services that involved more than one type of organization or provider in the community. They modified eligibility for funded care, provided ways of getting access to that care, and sought to influence the relationships among key actors and organizations in the community. But they fell far short of changing many relevant aspects of care, nor could they be said to have created a coherent system of long-term care. Typically the interventions bypassed physicians, hospital personnel, and others at the boundaries of long-term care.

ORGANIZATION OF THE CHAPTER

The chapter deals with five topics, each representing an increasingly stronger influence on a system of care.

1. *Preadmission screening.* Preadmission screening is an assessment of whether applicants to nursing homes are eligible for admission on the basis of their functional abilities. It should also suggest the best plan to meet the person's needs and preferences. If all nursing home applicants in a community were to receive preadmission assessments, followed by assistance with other plans when indicated, this procedure could be a force for rationalizing a system of care. Because many applications for long-term care occur while the applicant is in an acute hospital and most occur on advice of physicians, a preadmission screening program has potential for narrowing the gap between acute and long-term care. The preadmission screening programs that we discuss below are much more limited.

2. *Community long-term care demonstrations.* The central section of the chapter draws inferences from demonstration projects that broadened eligibility for community long-term care services under Medicare and/or Medicaid and increased the range of covered service. Typically, these projects contained a case management component—that is, a coordinator of care who assessed the need for care, developed a care plan, arranged or purchased service, and monitored the adequacy of service under the plan and the client's well-being. The most recent, ambitious, rigorously designed, and, therefore, influential of these demonstrations was the multisite National Long-Term Care Channeling Demonstration (Kemper et al., 1986).

3. *Case management.* Case management, as already suggested, is a process for coordinating the long-term care an individual receives and/or for allocating that care in a community. Depending on how the case management is conceptualized and organized, it may influence the type of services a person receives and the configurations of providers that flourish in the community. As an integral part of most long-term care demonstrations, case management is somewhat difficult to examine by itself.

4. *Capitation.* The social health maintenance organizations, currently being demonstrated nationally, test the effects of expanding the concept of health maintenance organizations to include some long-term care and socially oriented services in the package of entitlements for enrollees. To date, only preliminary information is available about the implementation of the model (Leutz et al., 1985).

5. *Selected operational programs.* Finally, to the extent possible, we move from demonstration projects to examine available evidence about mechanisms that have been developed as operational programs. Such operational programs include local and state initiatives and programs developed in other countries analogous to the United States. Typically, firm

evaluative data are absent. Whereas demonstration projects present problems for those who would generalize to the likely effects of implementing the program, operational programs—especially those developed statewide—present problems in proving what would have happened in the absence of the program.

PREADMISSION SCREENING

Most information on preadmission screening is descriptive only. Table 10-1 summarizes studies with at least some evaluative components. As mentioned in Chapter 4, most preadmission screening programs in the United States are limited to persons eligible for Medicaid or likely to exhaust their funds and become eligible within a specified, relatively short time (for example, 90 days, 120 days, 180 days) of admission. The Minnesota program (Moscovice, 1985) was limited to Medicaid eligibles and "180-day spend downs" during the time the sample for evaluation was enrolled, but in the fall of 1985 the screening became required of all applicants regardless of their income, assets, or expected source of payment.

Of the five studies in Table 10-1, two were overviews of the practices then occurring. State Medicaid staff provided the information, much of which was impressionistic. Knowlton, Clauser, and Fatula (1982) reported on the status of preadmission screening as of a 1981 survey. At that time, two states—Virginia and Massachusetts—supplied information about program impact. Virginia reported that 20% of those screened over a three-year period had not been approved for admission. The denials varied considerably (from a rate of 10% to a rate of 30%) within health districts, and this variation was attributed to the uneven availability of community care. Similarly, Massachusetts reported on the basis of eighteen months of operation that it had denied admission to about 8% of the applicants, but that 28% of the others who were approved could have been maintained in the community had adequate services been available. Almost all respondents in Iverson's survey (1986) believed that preadmission screening helped decrease the overall cost of long-term care. The state officials who responded perceived a myriad of problems that weakened the effort, including insufficient resources for preadmission screening itself, lack of support from physicians, hospitals, and nursing homes, and insufficient services in the community.

The Virginia program was subjected to a more thorough analysis using a quasi-experimental design (Harkins and Bowlenz, 1982). Comparisons were made among four groups: screened persons who were approved, screened persons who were denied, a sample of frail elderly in the community, and a sample of nursing home residents. At baseline the approved group resembled the nursing home residents in their functioning and the denied

TABLE 10-1 Studies on Preadmission Screening Programs

Source	Program Description	Study Design	Selected Findings
Harkins and Bowlenz (1982)	The Virginia Nursing Home Pre-Admission Screening Program, established in 1977 by the State Department of Health, has as its goals the delaying/avoidance of unwanted or inappropriate nursing home admissions and the control of Medicaid costs. Applicants who are not already in a hospital or nursing home are screened by a three-person team if they are or will become Medicaid eligible in 90 days.	A quasi-experimental design in which two stratified experimental groups (screened NH applicants approved for admission, screened applicants not approved) were compared with two control groups (NH admissions not screened, community elderly at risk) at baseline and two times over six months. The 400 subjects were measured on functional status, use of services, costs of formal services. Committee members were also surveyed on operational procedures.	BASELINE: Those screened and not approved for nursing home admission reported fewer illnesses, fewer days in bed, and a level of dependency less than half of those who were screened and approved. Several approvals did not differ from the nursing home controls on health and well-being measures. Community controls were similar to screened denials. SIX MONTH OUTCOMES: There were no changes across time within or among groups in functional status. Screened denials cost significantly less in total Medicaid expenditures than screened approvals ($1959 vs. $3923); the community controls had fewer expenditures than the screened denials ($122 vs. $1959).

TABLE 10-1 Continued

Source	Program Description	Study Design	Selected Findings
Knowlton, Clauser, and Fatula (1982)	A 1981 Health Care Financing Administration study of state preadmission screening programs, including information on the scope of programs, composition of teams, and the client assessment instruments. Two states also provided information on program impact.	In 1981, Medicaid staff in 49 states and the District of Columbia were telephoned and surveyed on the nature of their PAS programs, if extant. Virginia and Massachusetts supplied data on program impact.	IMPACT: In Virginia, 20% of those screened for nursing home admission had not been approved (1977 to 80). Denials varied from 10% to 30% among health districts, due mainly to lack of alternatives in some communities. In Massachusetts, after 18 months of operation, 8.4% of cases received were denied. 28% of the cases approved could have been maintained in the community if adequate services had been available.
Cairl, Pfeiffer, and Keller (1984)	Comprehensive Assessment and Review for Long-Term Care (CARES) is a pre-nursing home assessment demonstration project initiated in 1981 in Florida (Jacksonville, St. Petersberg, Miami). Goals include the prevention of unnecessary nursing home admissions and control of Medicaid expenditures.	An initial (1982–83) and a second more comprehensive evaluation study (1983–84) were made based upon records from the demonstration projects. CARES I examined the diversion experience for persons referred from nursing homes, hospitals, and community. CARES II examined diversions for only hospital and community referrals.	CARES I: Of those referred to CARES from the nursing home, 23% were determined to be capable of being placed in the community. CARES II: The overall diversion rate was about 20%; at a 120-day follow-up, 55% of those originally diverted remained in the community. Functional measures showed that the diverted clients had scores significantly higher than nursing home patients and similar to elderly community residents.

Moscovice (1985)	Statewide mandatory PAS by a RN/social worker team for all Medicaid eligibles and those who would be eligible within 180 days of admission to a nursing home. (Later the program expanded to include *all* nursing home applicants.) Each county PAS team can deploy special funds to provide home care for financially eligible screeners who stay in the community.	All persons screened in two urban counties (comprising Minneapolis-St. Paul) and two rural counties were followed at intervals for a year to determine placement and changes in functional outcomes, use and cost of services, and type and amount of informal services from family and friends.	Study is in progress; data are still being analyzed.
Iverson (1986)	A study presenting state-by-state and aggregate data on the status of 31 state-administered preadmission screening programs. The study included descriptive data on program characteristics as well as the perceived impact of PAS on the community and the major problems reported with PAS.	State Medicaid and/or PAS officials were contacted by phone to determine if there was a program; subsequent mailed questionnaires, using both closed- and open-ended questions, contained eight sections on factors such as administration, screening process, funding, other services provided, placement recommendations, purpose, and impact of PAS.	Regarding impact and major problems: 43% indicated that PAS helped decrease the overall cost of LTC; 66% felt it increased the supply and use of community services; 64% thought it had little effect on the supply of nursing home care; 30% felt it decreased the use of nursing home care. Major problems were inadequate funding, lack of support from physicians, hospitals, and nursing homes, lack of a coordinated system, insufficient services.

group resembled the community elderly. At follow-up six months later, the functional status of all four groups remained consistent. In the six months, those screened and approved generated average Medicaid costs of almost $4,000, about twice the costs generated by those denied admission. Assuming that the screening really did change the plans of persons not approved (that is, that they really would have entered a nursing home), these findings support the state's contention that the program really did save Medicaid money. On the other hand, the study design relied on incomparable groups to begin with, and, moreover, the total costs incurred for those denied nursing admission were not calculated.

In 1981, a preadmission screening program was initiated in three Florida cities to control Medicaid nursing home costs. In this case, preadmission referred to entrance to the Medicaid program for nursing home coverage. Because many clients were already in nursing homes when they applied for Medicaid, evaluators examined the experience in two ways. First, they looked at all Medicaid nursing home applicants referred for screening regardless of whether they were in a hospital, at home, or in a nursing home at the time. In a subsequent analysis, they eliminated those currently living in nursing homes from the analysis (Cairl, Pfeiffer, and Keller, 1984). Unfortunately for the program, most of the persons screened were in nursing homes already, and discharge proved impractical despite the judgment that 23% of those nursing home residents screened at the time they applied for Medicaid would have been capable of living in the community. In the second analysis, which excluded the nursing home residents, 20% of those screened were diverted, and four months later half of those still remained in the community.

Early experience with preadmission screening programs clearly shows that the screening must work in tandem with reasonably priced community programs to which the nursing home applicants can be referred. Once such community programs are in place, however, the potential cost of the diversion becomes substantial. This is especially true if the costs of community care are borne, in part, at public expense, and if persons financially ineligible for Medicaid receive community care. Operational programs in several states, most notably Minnesota and Pennsylvania, should shed light on the experience of linking preadmission screening to services. In Minnesota, teams of nurses and social workers perform the assessment and also act as case managers for the use of Alternative Care Grant funds that the state allocates to each county on a formula basis. Moscovice (1985) followed the entire population of persons screened in four counties during the first six months that the program was mandated statewide. He is currently examining the nature and costs of their total health and social services in the community and the precise way that family assistance was affected by any alternative care community services added. A similar preadmission screening program linked to services was introduced on a demonstration basis at multiple locations in Pennsylvania. The state is currently commissioning an evaluation of the program's effects.

Preadmission screening seems so rational a concept that it is almost unobjectionable. The caveats, however, are that resources are needed to assist in diverting admissions and that such resources must be targeted well if saving money is the major objective. In Minnesota, the counties initially varied considerably in whom they screened and whom they deemed eligible for services. Later, strapped for funds in their block grant allocations for alternative services, counties tended to limit the assessment screening to those who actually had made application to nursing homes, rather than assessing those seeking long-term care at home. Of course, once application to a nursing home becomes known as a procedural requirement for eligibility for community services, some proportion of people who apply will have no intention of entering a facility.

Finally, the logistical problems in doing prompt preadmission screening, including screening of persons in hospitals, are formidable. Programs must resist the pressure to become perfunctory and routine. Preadmission screening has the potential to force all parties to the decision (prospective residents, family, doctors, case managers, and other health and social service personnel) to take a careful look at the decision to enter a nursing home before it becomes a fait accompli. For this to happen, participants must seriously consider the issues one more time. In the province of Manitoba, where long-term care in nursing homes and in the community is a universal, non-means-tested benefit, all persons entering a nursing home are presented to a multidisciplinary panel that examines the adequacy of medical diagnosis and social planning up to that point (Kane and Kane, 1985). The panel then affirms the decision or (less often) questions it, usually in the form of a request for more evaluative workups. Such a system has enormous potential as a failsafe in the system, but in practice it struggles against large caseloads, insufficient involvement of the primary care physicians, and a certain momentum that resists specialized attention to single cases.

COMMUNITY LONG-TERM CARE DEMONSTRATIONS

Background

As we discussed in Chapter 4, the central issue in developing a long-term care system is frequently construed as developing a cost-effective (or at least an effective, cost-controllable) set of alternatives to nursing home care. By 1972, amendments were added to the Social Security Act that permitted waivers of ordinary Medicare or Medicaid eligibility and service coverage to study the effects of offering different packages of care to a differently defined clientele. In Chapter 6, we discussed the homemaking and day care experiments that used Medicare waivers to test whether the addition of homemaking, day care, or both for persons already eligible for Medicare services (on the basis of being rehabilitatable and needing skilled care for the episode of illness) would benefit by the addition of these more socially oriented services (Weissert et al., 1980a, 1980b). As we saw, the additional benefits were costly, yet failed to reach those in need efficiently. The advantages to the clientele, compared to those without the additional Medicare benefit, proved slight.

Other studies, relying on Medicaid waivers or, less often, Medicare waivers, or, occasionally, a combination of both, have sought to study the effectiveness of benefits for socially oriented long-term care services plus a case management component to make those services more responsive and appropriate to the needs of the persons receiving care. As the demonstration projects evolved (and some have had long lives, moving through distinct phases of program development), the advocacy aspect of case management became blunted, and case management was directed at least equally toward rationalizing access to the new benefits and controlling the overall cost of services.

Also, as the demonstration projects evolved, they boasted increasingly sophisticated study designs. Early case reports on the benefits of adding home services gave way to studies with at least some comparison group (perhaps a neighboring community, or a sample of the general population of elderly in the same community), followed by projects that assessed clientele for eligibility and then randomized them to receive or not receive the benefit.

Studies of the Studies

Twenty years of field studies of coordinated community long-term care have yielded an enormous volume of final reports and journals articles, as well as a small shelf of monographs. Considerable effort has also been made to organize and compare the studies to extract general messages. But analysts preparing summary treatments tend to define the universe of relevant studies somewhat differently and therefore do not produce identical lists.

Table 10-2 lists 15 major studies of coordinated long-term care that figure in many summary treatments. In Table 10-3, we present our own summary material on 13 of that group. (We omitted the Oregon FIG Waiver Project, which was never fully evaluated before the state moved on to operational programs, and the Texas ICF Project, a deinstitutionalization effort; for these two projects, we could not locate sufficient material for analysis). Table 10-2 also shows how eight other summarizers identified and grouped studies for cross-project comparisons.

Greenberg, Doth, and Austin (1981) did one of the earliest comparative studies. They included nine early projects, mingling studies of more narrow interventions, such as the Highland Heights housing study (Sherwood et al.,

1981) and the Medicare-waivered studies of home care and day care (Weissert et al., 1980a, 1980b), with studies of case-managed coordinated long-term care efforts. They were among the first to point out that many of the demonstrations suffered problems of ambiguous goals, poor or uneven implementation, and contamination between experimental and comparison groups. In another early review, Stassen and Holahan (1981) selected five projects (four of which are among the 15 listed in Table 10-2) to represent interventions in coordinated care, reserving studies of day care and home care for separate classifications. Zawadski (1983), who is associated with the On Lok project in San Francisco, edited a monograph that compared 8 of the 15 projects. Aptly titling her discussion "Apples and Oranges," Hughes (1985) distinguished three kinds of studies of home-based long-term care: traditional medically oriented home care (such as Medicare covers); expanded, more socially oriented home care for chronic conditions; and "channeling-like" studies with a case management component. She included 4 of the 15 studies as examples of the latter. In a monograph about case management within the coordinated projects, Austin and colleagues (1985) discussed all but 1 of the 15, and added an additional entry, the Washington Community Based Care Project.

To supplement our own review, we relied mostly on three particularly stringent summary treatments. First, under a HCFA contract to perform "a cross-cutting evaluation" of previous demonstrations of coordinated community long-term care, Berkeley Planning Associates did an extensive examination of 13 projects (Haskins et al., 1984). They included every study listed in Table 10-2 except the Nursing Home Without Walls Project and the National Channeling Demonstration, which was still underway. Second, in connection with the National Channeling Demonstration, Applebaum, Harrigan, and Kemper (1986) compared 16 studies (dropping the Texas ICF study and adding the Worcester Home Care Project, the Weissert home care/day care studies, and Channeling itself) with the particular aim of comparing their designs and findings to the National Channeling Demonstration. Third, under a project of "information synthesizing" sponsored by the Veterans Administration, Weissert, Matthews, and Pawelak (1986) prepared an exhaustive "study of the studies." Their focus was more broadly "home and community care," and thus their list grouped together twenty projects. Their review excluded only the California MSSP study from the list in Table 10-2 and added Katz's early studies of medically oriented home care (Katz et al., 1972: Papsidero et al., 1979), Hughes's Chicago home care study (Hughes, Cordray and Spiker, 1984), Weissert's own studies of home care and day care (Weissert et al., 1980a, 1980b), the Highland Heights housing study (Sherwood et al., 1981), and the demonstration of an emergency alarm system (Ruchlin and Morris, 1981).

A consensus is emerging about which studies should be used as evidence about coordinated community long-term care. The main list includes the 13

TABLE 10-2 Summary Analyses Available on Coordinated Community Care Demonstration

Project	Greenberg, Doth, and Austin (1981)[a]	Stassen & Holahan (1981)[b]	Zawadski (1983)	Haskins et al. (1984)[c]	Hughes (1985)[d]	Austin et al. (1985)[e]	Applebaum, Harrigan, and Kemper (1986)[f]	Weissert, Matthews, and Pawelak (1986)[g]
				Synthesizing Work				
Community Care Organization: Wisconsin	X	X		X	X	X	X	X
Alternative Health Services Project: Georgia	X	X	X	X	X	X	X	X
Triage: Connecticut	X	X	X	X	X	X	X	X
ACCESS: Monroe County, NY	X	X	X	X	X	X	X	X
Nursing Home Without Walls: New York State			X	X		X	X	X
Multipurpose Senior Services Project (MSSP): California				X		X	X	
New York City Home Care			X	X		X	X	X
On Lok: San Francisco	X		X	X			X	X
Project OPEN			X	X		X	X	X
South Carolina Community Long-Term Care Project			X	X		X	X	X
Florida Pentastar				X		X	X	X

Study			
Long-Term Care Project of North San Diego	X	X	X
Fig Waiver: Oregon	X	X	X
Texas ICF	X	X	
National Channeling Demonstration	X	X	X

[a]Greenberg, Doth, and Austin review four additional studies: Washington State's Community-Based Care Systems, the Weissert day care and home care studies, the Massachusetts Home Care Project, and the Highland Heights housing study.

[b]Stassen and Holahan also include Washington State's Community-Based Care System as an example of coordinated care. They review studies of home care and day care in separate categories.

[c]Haskins et al. review 13 studies selected by HCFA for a cross-cutting evaluation. The report gives most attention to South Carolina, Onlok; San Diego Home Care; New York City Home Care, and Project OPEN. Special Studies of ACCESS are forthcoming.

[d]Hughes develops three categories: traditional home care, expanded home care, and "channeling-like" projects. The four studies indicated were used to illustrate the latter group.

[e]Austin et al. focus on case management. They include the Washington State's Community-Based Care System.

[f]Applebaum, Harrigan, and Kemper review the 13 studies in Haskins et al. (plus the Massachusetts Home Care Project in Worcester and the Weissert home care/day care study) with the specific aim of comparing them to the two models of channeling.

[g]Weissert groups together 20 studies. To the 14, he adds Katz et al. (1972); Papsidero et al. (1979) (both traditional home care in Hughes' classification); Weissert et al. (1980a, 1980b); Hughes, Cordray, and Spiker (1984) (both expanded home care in Hughes' classification); a study of housing (Sherwood et al., 1981); and a study of emergency alarm systems (Ruchlin and Morris, 1981).

studies reviewed by Berkeley Planning Associates plus the National Long-Term Care Channeling Demonstration that followed.

Description of the Demonstrations

Let us now consider 13 demonstrations, characterized in more detail in Table 10-3. (In common with other synthesizers, we have considered the two models tested by the Channeling Demonstration as separate entities; our table, therefore, has 14 entries.)

Clearly the projects differed in scope, auspice, focus, and history. They were well distributed across the United States. Six projects (Triage, in a seven-town area in Connecticut; ACCESS in Rochester, New York; the San Diego Home Care Project; the New York City Home Care Project; On Lok in San Francisco; and the Florida Pentastar Project) were rather confined geographically. The Wisconsin, Georgia, South Carolina, and New York Nursing Home Without Walls projects took in more territory, but evolved into statewide programs only after the demonstration phases. California's Multipurpose Senior Services Project was in itself a multi-site project, conducted in eight parts of the state and operated under a variety of auspices. The National Channeling Demonstration took place at ten sites in ten states; the basic model was tested in Maine, eastern Kentucky, New Jersey (Middlesex County), Houston, and Baltimore, and the complex model was tested in Philadelphia, Cleveland, Massachusetts, Miami, and Rensselear County, New York. Overall the channeling site hosts were Area Agencies on Aging.

What did the programs grouped together in Table 10-3 actually do? They all provided some form of case management, and they all offered expanded public benefits for long-term care, including at least home care and homemaking services. They did differ, however, in their goals and emphases. Noting these distinctions, Austin and colleagues (1985) suggested the following classification: (1) projects designed frankly to develop an alternative long-term care system (Wisconsin, Triage, Alternative Health Services of Georgia, On Lok); (2) projects to coordinate existing long-term care delivery systems and fill alternative service gaps (California's MSSP, Florida's Pentastar Project, and the basic model of Channeling); (3) projects focused on upgrading the home care package available to clients (Project OPEN, North San Diego County Long-Term Care Project, and New York Home Care Project); and, (4) projects seeking primarily to control client access to and use of institutional services (ACCESS, South Carolina Long-Term Care Project, Nursing Home Without Walls, and the complex model of Channeling). One might quarrel with Austin's specific designations, but her scheme is useful for recognizing the diverse agendas of the projects. Moreover, a single project could have mixed agendas. Typically, a program might seek both to improve home-based services and reduce institutional use, both to control costs and to produce benefits for clients. For example, the complex model of Channeling sought to do more than control use of institutional care; it also sought to fill gaps and coordinate services.

Table 10-4 shows the targeting criteria of the 13 programs more clearly. All sought to identify those needing service by some functional criteria. In addition, 6 projects required Medicaid eligibility—3 of the 4 projects open to all adults were among this group, and 5 required Medicare eligibility for Part A, Part B, or both. Three programs approached requiring nursing home certifiability. South Carolina required that clients be processed through its preadmisison screening program, but some clients were enrolled solely on the basis of being "at risk."

The right-hand side of the table gives some indication of the projects' success in identifying clients who were impaired. Considerable inter-project variation is seen in the percentage of clients with at least one ADL impairment, though all projects supplying this data enrolled a sample of at least 50% meeting the description. In contrast, at least one IADL impairment was present for three-quarters of the clients. Impairment in one ADL function may include dressing, and impairment in IADL may include any number of complex tasks. Therefore, the presence of incontinence is a more discrete test of disability. For six projects, at least 40% of the clients were incontinent. Four sites reported that the average number of mistakes on a mental status questionnaire exceeded three, but this level of error represents only minimal cognitive impairment. The Channeling Demonstration, which used a screening tool based on the experience of most of the foregoing demonstrations, succeeded in enrolling a group that was substantially impaired.

The programs differed in the way case management was conceptualized. On the one hand, ACCESS purchased assessment and case management from community agencies. Its in-house case management resembled a tracking and approval system. In contrast, Triage, and later California's MSSP program, used teams of nurses and social workers to do a deluxe version of client-centered case management. The size of case manager caseloads is unavailable for some projects. Applebaum, Harrigan, and Kemper (1986) reported that the norm was around 50 clients per case manager, with a higher figure in South Carolina (75 to 80), and caseloads of 125 for the Triage case management teams. In MSSP, the initial assessment was done by teams of MSW social workers and health practitioners (public health nurses or nurse practitioners, assisted by case aides). The evaluators reported average caseloads of 50 to 67 for social workers and 100 to 175 for the health practitioners.

The programs also varied in the range of services offered and their emphases. For example, the San Diego Home Care Program, operated by a

TABLE 10-3 Coordinated Community Care Demonstrations—1975 to 1985

Project Title/Source[a] and Project Description	Project Goals	Selected Eligibility Criteria/ Target Characteristics	Outcomes
Community Care Organization, Wisconsin Seidl et al. (1983) *Design:* Random assignment for the Milwaukee site, only. Medicaid waivers (1975 to 1979) supported services at three county-based sites (Barron, LaCrosse, and Milwaukee counties). Services included advocacy, day care, chore service, delivered meals, homemakers, counseling, transportation, medical equipment. Host agencies, staffing patterns, and approach to care management differed among sites. Case managers did not control all services since the services were considered supplemental to the efforts of other agencies.	To test whether community-based care is less expensive than institutional care; to maximize client independence, improve quality of life, reduce inappropriate institutionalization.	Medicaid eligible adults (18+), functionally disabled, in the community or hospital at institutional risk or inappropriately placed in nursing homes.	Milwaukee site only: no positive significant impact upon level of client disability, quality of life, rate of institutionalization, nursing home days. Positive impact on hospital days. Medical and CCO costs were similar to the currently existing program.

320

Georgia Alternative Health Services Project
Skellie et al. (1982, 1984)

Design: Random assignment to experimentals and controls, pre-testing, and multiple post-tests.

AHS was administered by the Georgia Department of Medical Assistance in conjunction with county Departments of Family and Children Services. Medicaid waivers (1976 to 1981) authorized three categories of services to voluntary clients in a 17-county area: alternative living services, adult day rehabilitation, home-delivered services. Core case management functions were implemented by a team (nurse, social worker, case worker), while day-to-day tasks were handled by a case coordinator.

To test the cost-effectiveness of a comprehensive system of community-based long-term care services.

Aged 50+, Medicaid eligible, certified as eligible for SNF/ICF admission.

No significant differences between experimentals and controls regarding ADLs, IADLs, mental status, morale, mobility. Positive impact on mortality. No significant differences in nursing home days (both groups used few nursing home days). Project services supplemented rather than substituted for non-project services. At 24 months after enrollment, total per client Medicaid costs for the experimentals averaged $4,623; for the controls, $2,420.

TABLE 10-3 Continued

Project Title/Source[a] and Project Description	Project Goals	Selected Eligibility Criteria/ Target Characteristics	Outcomes
Triage, Inc., Connecticut Hicks et al. (1979); Quinn and Hodgson (1984) *Design:* Quasi-experimental with controls from a non-catchment area; attempted matching according to age, sex, living arrangement, functional ability. Triage, supported in two phases by Medicare waivers (1976–79; 1979–81), consisted of a non-profit consortium of providers and elderly consumers serving a seventown area. Case management by a multidisciplinary professional team was the core of the program. Services brokered and monitored by staff included acute and institutional care, home health care, mental health, social support, transportation, and home-delivered meals.	To develop a single-entry mechanism to coordinate care and to provide the preventive and supportive services necessary for an integrated LTC delivery system; to demonstrate cost-effectiveness.	Aged 60+, Medicare-eligible, and residing in the seven-town area. (High "risk" criteria in phase II included the need for assessment and monitoring, and an unstable informal support system.)	Different statistical tests, though varying in results, tended to support a positive impact in ADLs, IADLs, and MSQ. No differences in mortality. Within a six-month period the number of nursing home days for the experimental groups was one-third less than that of the controls (66 vs. 95 days). Total SNF and home health care costs were similar for both groups; experimentals had higher hospital/physician costs than the controls.

322

Monroe County LTC Program (ACCESS) Eggert and Brodows (1984); Price, Ripps, and Peltz (1980)

Design: Quasi-experimental design with non-catchment area controls; multiple post-testing.

ACCESS, the case management unit of MCLTCP, Inc. (freestanding, nonprofit organization) became operational in 1977 (ACCESS I) through Medicaid waivers and was expanded in 1982 (ACCESS II) through Medicare waivers. ACCESS provides "administrative" case management; all other services, including assessment, are provided by community agencies. Services include nursing home care, home nursing and home health aides, chore, respite, housing, foster care, transportation. Typically services are approved up to 75% of the institutional equivalent.

To prevent inappropriate institutionalization and to reduce the rate of increase in Medicaid costs by controlling access to and utilization of institutions and hospitals; to provide coordination and continuity of case management for clients.

All adults at risk of needing LTC (over 90 days duration); all Medicaid clients applying for nursing home admission. Clients tended to be severely impaired.

ACCESS I: positive impact upon hospital backup days; a smaller rate of non-Medicaid nursing home admissions than in the comparison counties. Medicaid expenditures increased less (20%) than in any of the comparison counties (26% to 59%) over a four-year period (pre and post ACCESS I).

TABLE 10-3 Continued

Project Title/Source[a] and Project Description	Project Goals	Selected Eligibility Criteria/ Target Characteristics	Outcomes
Nursing Home Without Walls Birnbaum et al. (1984) *Design:* Quasi-experimental with two sets of comparison groups, those within the catchment areas and those from matched, non-catchment area counties. The New York State Long-Term Home Health Care Program (Nursing Home Without Walls) began providing routine and Medicaid-waivered services in 1978, including case management and service co-ordination, nursing and home health aide, physical and occupational therapies, personal care and homemaker services, nutritional counseling, social day care, social transportation, and housing improvement. Legislation permits a mix of agencies to operate LTHHCP programs: certified home health agencies, SNFs/ICFs, hospitals. Medicaid eligibility is determined by local departments of social services. Costs are capped at 75% of the costs of a clients' appropriate level of institutional care.	To reduce fragmentation and increase the range of home care services; to promote home care awareness and to effectively forestall institutionalization; to demonstrate that home care can be provided at costs lower than institutional care.	Medicaid-eligible or otherwise eligible for institutional care according to the DSM-1 form; viable home/residence in the community; able to have service costs not exceeding 75% cap; approval by physicians and local DSS.	Upstate New York: significant positive impact on mortality; a savings of 7.8 days per month in nursing home care; total services costs were $270 per month lower for experimentals than controls. New York City: improved ADLs at 12 months; a savings of 3.0 days per month in nursing home care; total services costs were about $477 more expensive per month for the experimentals.

324

Multi-Purpose Senior Services Project, California
Miller et al. (1984)

Design: Quasi-experimental with controls from the general population matched by disability level and residence in community, hospital, or SNF.

MSSP, funded through Medicaid waivers (1979 to 1983) and administered by the state health and welfare agency, provided case management and waivered services to Medi-Cal recipients in six counties at eight sites. Case management teams (MSWs, health practitioners) brokered services on a priority basis: informal support first, then existing services, followed by 10 possible waivered services (day care, housing, in-home support, respite, meals, etc.). Total costs were capped at 70% of SNF costs, $505 per month per client.

To control costly utilization of nursing homes and acute care hospitals by providing coordinated in-home services to elders who were frail and at risk; to test a model of care as the basis for a state-wide delivery system.

Persons 65+; Medi-Cal-eligible. For each site, 50% had to be community residents (evenly divided into high, medium, and low independence ratings); 40% hospital residents; 10% recent SNF admissions. Each subgroup had "at risk" criteria. Participants tended to be moderately impaired.

A positive impact on ADLs and IALDs for certain subgroups, especially at 6 and 12 months after becoming a client. A negative impact on MSQ at 6 months. Positive impact upon longevity and nursing home days, especially for the frailest subgroups. Negative impact upon hospital days the first year, positive in the second year. Total program cost in 1982 (including administration) was $2,703 more for the experimental group, but for the frailest group there was a net savings of $322 per client.

TABLE 10-3 Continued

Project Title/Source[a] and Project Description	Project Goals	Selected Eligibility Criteria/ Target Characteristics	Outcomes
New York City Home Care Project Brill and Horowitz (1984) *Design:* Quasi-experimental design with non-catchment area controls; multiple post-testing. Medicare 222 waiver authority (1979 to 84) was used to provide case management services and to purchase services such as homemaker/personal care, transportation/escort, and prescription drugs. Two hospital-based health clinics and two social service coordinating agencies were the site-level host agencies in four New York City boroughs. Case management made extensive use of nonprofessional staff.	To upgrade home care services through case management; to promote independent living; to test a model ordered to cost-effective, appropriate care.	Persons 65+ enrolled in Medicare B with incomes too high for Medicaid but too low to afford private home care; functionally impaired with need for services such as 12 to 20 hours of homemaker/personal care per week. Participants tended to be severely disabled.	Significant improvement in MSQ at 12 months for the participants; otherwise no significant differences in ADLs and MSQ at 6 and 12 month periods. No significant difference in mortality at 12 months. Informal ADL assistance declined; informal IADL assistance declined for poorly functioning clients but increased for better functioning clients. Costs (Medicare, Medicaid, and case management) averaged $428 per client per month more than the existing system's costs.

On Lok Senior Health Services Community Care Organization for Dependent Adults, San Francisco
Ansak and Zawadski (1984)

Design: Quasi-experimental matched pair design with pre-test and multiple post-tests. However, almost half the controls were in nursing homes at baseline.

Extensive Medicare waivers (1979–83) allowed On Lok to consolidate all needed health and social services, including inpatient care, under one agency. Services included physician services, nursing, therapies, recreation, social work, meals, transportation, day health, homemaker/personal care, respite. Services such as skilled nursing inpatient care were provided by contract. Monthly payments based on a proposed capitated rate with adjustments to meet actual costs. A highly professionalized multidisciplinary staff was used for case management.

To provide, through one organization, the full range of health and social services needed to maintain elders in the community as long as possible.

Clients 55+ who resided in the catchment area and were certified at the Medicare SNF or ICF level; 90% must have been Medicare eligible. Project participants tended to be severly impaired.

Participants improved significantly in IADLs at 12 months; no other significant ADL or IADL impacts at 6 or 12 months. No significant impact upon MSQ or mortality. Participants had significant reductions in nursing home use (2.19 days per month vs. 13.08) and almost significant reductions in acute days per month (.90 vs. 1.30); total monthly payments per client were $1,240 for participants vs. $1,796 for the controls. Data supporting the findings, however, were based on a very small sample size and the reliability of the measurements is in question.

TABLE 10-3 Continued

Project Title/Source[a] and Project Description	Project Goals	Selected Eligibility Criteria/ Target Characteristics	Outcomes
Project Open, San Francisco Sklar and Weiss (1983) *Design:* Random assignment to experimentals and controls, pre-testing, and multiple post-tests. Host agency was the Geriatric Service Department of Mount Zion Hospital, in consortium with five other health and social service agencies (1979 to 1983). Case management was the only service directly provided by project staff; other services were provided by consortium agencies or contracted providers. Medicare waivers authorized a broad range of services including acute care, nursing home care, physician services, day health, home health, senior center programs, meals, homemaker-chore services, transportation. Case management was provided by service coordinators (RNs and MSWs) aided by a case conference team of physicians and geriatric specialists.	To allow clients to remain in the community and to prevent unnecessary institutionalization; to upgrade the home care intervention strategy through case management, service coordination, and the provision of services.	Persons 65+ eligible for Medicare Parts A and B and in need of assistance to live independently; meeting at least one of the criteria such as acute care hospitalization or skilled nursing hospitalization within the last 30 days; requiring assistance with personal care. Participants tended to have minor impairments.	No significant impact on ADLs, IADLs, or mortality; a positive impact on MSQ at 12 months. Positive impacts on life satisfaction/social involvement. No significant impact on acute care days, SNF days, home health visits. Both experimentals and controls used little nursing home care. Costs for the experimentals (Medicare and case management) were $163 per client per month higher than for the controls (not significant).

328

South Carolina Community Long-Term Care Project
Brown and Learner (1984)
Nocks et al. (1986)

Design: Random assignment to experimentals and controls, pre-testing, and multiple post-tests.

Mandatory preadmission screening and assessment were provided in a three-county catchment area for all Medicaid eligibles seeking nursing home care. Medicaid and Medicare waivers (1980 to 1984) authorized case management (the only service directly provided by CLTCP) and six contracted services: personal care, medical day care, respite care, home-delivered meals, medical social services, home-based therapies. Host agency was the South Carolina Department of Social Services. Waivered services were capped at 75% of the costs for a LTC facility patient for 90 days.

To control access to and use of institutional services in order to contain public nursing home costs.

Persons 18+ who were Medicaid eligible and who were dependent in at least two ADLs and/or needed care in a LTC facility as defined by Medicaid. Participants tended to be severely disabled.

No significant impact on ADLs, IADLs, and MSQ at either 6 or 12 months. No significant impact on mortality. Costs (Medicare, Medicaid, case management) per client per month were $66 lower than the existing system's total costs. There was significantly less use of acute care services for participants at both 6 and 12 months. At 12 months a significantly greater proportion of ICF controls (56%) compared to ICF experimentals (34%) entered nursing homes. An increase in the number of ADL and IADL needs not met by informal caregivers within a 12-month period but also a slight increase in units of informal care provided.

TABLE 10-3 Continued

Project Title/Source[a] and Project Description	Project Goals	Selected Eligibility Criteria/ Target Characteristics	Outcomes
Florida Pentastar Project Florida Department of Health and Rehabilitative Services (1984) *Design:* Random assignment and use of a comparison group in an outside area. The Department of Aging and Adult Services used Medicaid waivers (1980–83) to provide case management and contracted services in a five-county urban area. Services included medical/social assessment with physical exam, if needed; medical therapeutic services; personal care; specialized home management; respite; medical transportation; medical equipment; day treatment services.	To help elderly persons remain in the community through health and health-related services; to coordinate the LTC delivery system and fill in gaps in the continuum of services.	Aged 60+, Medicaid eligible, assessed as being at risk of institutionalization within 12 months; meeting at least one of such criteria as informal support not available, difficulty in performing ADLs/IADLs. Project participants tended to be moderately impaired.	No differences in ADLs; participants less impaired in IADLs at 12 months. Total monthly costs (food stamps, housing assistance, Medicare/Medicaid, other public costs) for the treatment group were $446; for the controls, $273.

Long-Term Care Project of San Diego County
Pinkerton and Hill (1984)

Design: Random assignment to experimentals and controls, pre-testing, and multiple post-tests.

Allied Home Health Assoc./Allied Community Services (1981–1984) acted as a broker of services for Medicare residents in the North County section of San Diego County, providing case management services and using contracted providers for six additional Medicare waivered services: home health, homemaker services, patient teaching and monitoring, day health care, transportation, home-delivered meals. A high proportion of advanced professionals were employed in multi-disciplinary planning teams.

To demonstrate that a home health agency can be an appropriate and cost-effective resource to administer a LTC system; to assist the frail elderly in achieving and maintaining functional independence; to reduce institutionalization.

Aged 65+, Medicare eligible clients meeting criteria such as risk of LTC placement, risk of frequent acute hospital admissions, inability to maintain self at home without ADL assistance, stable chronic health problems but education and monitoring needed to maintain stability. Participants tended to be moderately impaired.

No significant program impact upon ADLs at 6 or 12 months. The control group declined significantly more in MSQ at 12 months but not at 6 months. No significant mortality impact. Although combined Medicare and Medicaid savings were about $121 per client per month, waivered services and case management costs added $440 per month to the per client costs, resulting in $180 more than the existing system's costs. Clients used marginally more acute care; both groups used little nursing home care. Significant erosion occurred both in ADL needs and in quantities of IADL assistance met by informal caregivers.

TABLE 10-3 Continued

Project Title/Source[a] and Project Description	Project Goals	Selected Eligibility Criteria/ Target Characteristics	Outcomes
Channeling, Basic Model Kemper et al. (1986)	Tests premise that lack of information not lack of service is the main reason for a mismatch between services and needs, and that case management would rationalize system.	Aged 65+, at risk as measured by functional criteria; participants tended to be severely impaired.	No significant impact on mortality, ADLs or IADLs; higher self-reported life quality at 6 months. No significant impact on hospital or nursing home care. No impact upon type and amount of informal care; significant positive impact upon caregivers' life quality, stress, personal and employment limitations at six months.
Design: Random assignment to experimentals and controls, pre-testing, and multiple post-tests.			
Five sites in five states (1982–85) were designated as basic model projects (Maine, Kentucky, New Jersey, Texas, Maryland) in which only core channeling functions were provided: outreach, screening, assessment, case management; in addition, a specific amount was awarded for gap-filling services. Major categories of services offered included homemaker/health aide, meals, transportation, day care.			

Channeling, Complex Model
Kemper et al. (1986)

Design: Random assignment to experimentals and controls, pre-testing, and multiple post-tests.

Five sites in five states (Pennsylvania, Ohio, Massachusetts, Florida, New York) were designated as complex model projects (1982–85). In addition to case management services, these sites were authorized to provide expanded Medicare and Medicaid coverage. A maximum of 85% of Medicaid ICF and SNF rates was allowed for any individual care plan, with a cap of 60% for the aggregate. Major categories of services offered included homemaker/home health aide, skilled nursing, home-delivered meals, therapies.

Tests premise that inadequate public financing of community services leads to inappropriate use of nursing homes, and that case management with the ability to purchase services within financial constraints would reduce use of nursing homes and improve well-being for the elderly.

Aged 65+, at risk as measured by functional criteria, eligible for Medicare Part A.

No significant impact on mortality; negative impact upon ADLs at both 6 and 12 months; no impact on IADLs. Participants had a higher self-reported life quality at 6 and 12 months. Significant reduction in the percent of participants with visiting caregiver by informal supports at 6 and 12 months; positive impact upon caregivers' life quality and satisfaction with service arrangements at 6 and 12 months.

---

[a]In addition to primary sources, we used three summary treatments of the demonstrations: Haskins et al. (1984); Applebaum, Harrigan, and Kemper (1986); and Weissert, Matthews, and Pawelak (1986).

TABLE 10-4 Targeting of Clients in 13 Demonstrations

	Targeting Criteria				Characteristics of Sample[a]				
	Medicare-Eligible	Medicaid-Eligible	Nursing Home-Eligible[b]	Age	% 75+	% Impaired on 1+ ADL	% Impaired on 1+ IADL	% Incontinent	Average MSQ Errors (0 to 10)
Wisconsin	X	X		18+	37	60	unknown	unknown	unknown
Georgia	X			50+	unknown	unknown	unknown	unknown	3.1
Triage		X		60+	73	54	94	unknown	1.7
ACCESS		X		18+	80	82	99	44	2.4
Nursing Home Without Walls			X	all ages	unknown	unknown	unknown	unknown	unknown
California MSSP		X		65+	(c)	61	80	47	1.7
NYC Home Care	X (part B)			65+	68	78	100	38	2.6
On Lok			X	55+	68	85	93	60	3.2
Project OPEN	X			65+	unknown	50	81	24	.6
South Carolina		X	X	18+	55[d]	95	97	58	3.5
Florida Pentastar		X		60+	unknown	58	97	22	1.4
San Diego Home Care	X			65+	67	55	97	43	2.3
Channeling	Part A for Complex Model			65+	72	84	100	53	3.5

[a]Unless noted, these data are based on Applebaum, Harrigan, and Kemper (1986).

[b]Nursing Home Without Walls clients were eligible for nursing homes on basis of New York DSM-I but did not need to be actual applicants; On Lok clients needed to be certifiable on basis of needing 24-hour care; South Carolina clients needed to have been screened by formal preadmission screening and found "at risk."

[c]Mean age was 80.1 for the community sample, 77.7 for hospital sample, and 80.6 for nursing home sample (Miller et al., 1984).

[d]This calculation from Nocks et al. (1986) based on 284 clients during 1980 and 1981.

certified home health agency, offered upgraded home care services, as did the New York City Home Care Program. The latter sought to serve a homebound population that was ineligible for Medicaid but insufficiently well-to-do to finance home care privately. The Georgia Alternative Health Services Project, a program operated by the Medicaid agency, included alternative living programs and adult day rehabilitation as well as home care in its service repertoire. South Carolina's project, also administered by the Medicaid agency, included mandatory preadmission screening for Medicaid-sponsored nursing home care as part of its design. Project OPEN (the acronym stands for Organizations Providing for Elderly Needs) was a consortium of service agencies centered at Mount Zion, a San Francisco teaching hospital. Medicare waivers were used to provide a wide range of inpatient, outpatient, and community services for the experimental group. On Lok, another neighborhood-based program, this time in San Francisco's Chinatown area, began with a day care center and case management, gradually expanding to include a comprehensive array of all inpatient and outpatient long-term care services. The On Lok program discussed here was funded through Medicare waivers; as of 1983, On Lok began a demonstration of an at-risk capitated reimbursement system, integrating Medicare, Medicaid, and private funding. (An evaluation of this system is pending.)

The demonstrations offered expanded services, but five had cost maximums. In Georgia, the limit was 85% of the average Medicaid nursing home rate; in South Carolina and ACCESS it was 75% of the average Medicaid rates, and in Wisconsin it was $425 a month (equivalent to about 60% of the skilled nursing home rates at that time). The Channeling Demonstration Projects had limited funds for gap-filling at the basic sites, and a per client and a per program cap of 60% of the average of nursing home costs for the complex sites. Client cost-sharing was a feature of ACCESS, Florida, and the complex model of Channeling, and a discretionary component for the basic model of Channeling.

The number of persons served by the demonstrations varied. Because by design ACCESS assessed all Medicaid-eligible adults applying for nursing home care in a county of about 700,000 people, exact numbers of clients served were not readily calculated. Later the project received Medicare waivers to expand services to all elderly applying for nursing homes regardless of income. In order of size, the other programs ranged from 1,900 clients at the eight MSSP sites, 1,868 at the five complex Channeling sites, 1,632 at the five basic Channeling sites, about 1,000 each in Georgia and South Carolina, about 700 each for Nursing Home Without Walls and Florida Pentastar, about 500 each for New York City and San Diego Home Care programs, 307 for Triage, 283 in Madison, Wisconsin (the only site of the community care organization (CCO) demonstration that was systematically studied), 220 for Project OPEN, and only 70 for On Lok.

EVALUATIONS

Seven of the projects used randomized designs to compare the outcomes of their clients to those of people not receiving the benefits. These included Wisconsin CCO (for Madison only), Georgia, Project OPEN, Florida Penta-star, San Diego, South Carolina, and Channeling. This is the strongest kind of design possible because it suggests that the two groups are comparable at baseline. The most common quasi-experimental design used controls from outside the catchment area (Triage, ACCESS, New York City Home Care, and Nursing Home Without Walls). Triage did additional matching of its controls by age, sex, functional ability, and living arrangement, and Nursing Home Without Walls used controls within the target communities as well as from outside areas. (Although using a randomized design, South Carolina added a second control group from outside the experimental counties.) MSSP drew controls from the general population of the MSSP sites, matched by disability level and place of residence (community, hospital, or SNF). On Lok also drew a control group from the same community. Although clients and controls were matched on diagnosis, age, sex, and ethnicity, an important difference existed. When the first matched pairs produced a control group more functionally disabled than the experimental group, residents of nursing homes were enrolled in the control group to balance the two groups on impairment. Consequently, 44% of the control group and only 7% of the experimental group were in nursing homes at baseline (See Weissert, Matthews, and Pawelak, 1986, for a discussion of this issue.)

Most of the studies followed a panel of clients for a year or more, examining the effects of the program on outcomes like mortality, use of nursing homes and hospitals (admissions and lengths of stay), cost of care, functional status, and client well-being. There was considerable variation in the measurements used, especially for well-being. Some studies looked at cognitive functioning, psychological well-being, or contentment. There was also variation in the costs examined; only a few looked at physician care and a range of other community social services as well as the more standard nursing home, home care, and hospital care. Some studies examined the effect of the programs on the amount and type of informal care given by family, as well as the effects on the well-being of those family caregivers. The Channeling Demonstration was the most comprehensive in its effort to measure each type of outcome.

Findings

As Table 10-3 shows, some positive results have been associated with some of the demonstrations. Taken together, however, the results on mortality and quality of life are, at best, ambiguous, and the results on the use and cost of other services are discouraging.

Weissert, Matthews, and Pawelak (1986) thoroughly reviewed the methodology and findings in 20 studies of community care. Those included all those in our table (with the exception of the California MSSP) and eight others. They pointed out that the preconditions for any of these demonstrations to have shown substantial cost-savings were the following: high use and cost of institutional services in the control groups; large reductions in institutionalization rates and cost in the experimental groups; and low cost of the community care put in place for the experimental group.

Essentially, these conditions have not been met. Several of the experiments were able to show a reduction in nursing home use, but the high costs of community care offset those savings. Hospital use sometimes was higher for the experimental groups. On the whole, the control groups tended not to use nursing homes as much or stay as long in them as had been expected, considering that presumably high-risk groups were enrolled. Some investigators studied the experience of subgroups of clients to see whether cost-saving diversions from nursing homes could be achieved for particular groups, but no consistent patterns emerged. South Carolina's program stood out in its ability to identify persons at high risk of entering a nursing home. The On Lok program reported positive results, but they must be considered cautiously because the sample was tiny (70 people) and because almost half of its members were in a nursing home at the onset of the study, compared to only 7% of the On Lok clients.

Leaving aside effects on costs, does community care have beneficial results for its clientele? Again Weissert, Matthews, and Pawelak (1986) provided the most cogent summary of the findings on mortality, functional status, mental functioning, and quality of life from the 20 studies they reviewed. They pointed out that most findings on mortality, physical functioning, and mental functioning were not statistically significant, particularly in more rigorous designs with randomization and multivariate analysis. Among less rigorous studies, most statistically significant findings were positive. Disregarding statistical significance, positive tendencies were more frequent than negative, but among the six most rigorous studies, negative effects were slightly more frequent than positive effects; physical functioning seemed generally unaffected; and effects on mortality and mental functioning were tenuous, none of them having been found in the six most rigorous studies. On the other hand, benefits were found in contentment and other measures of psychological well-being. Although most of those were found in quasi experiments, the more rigorous Channeling Demonstration also found significant benefits in life satisfaction. Subgroup analyses gave tentative support to the idea that younger, less severely dependent persons with better social support were more likely to show benefits in well-being than the more severely impaired group (who were the ones more likely to enter nursing homes).

Only four of the studies in Table 10-3 attempted to estimate the effects of providing community care on informal care given by family and friends.

Here the results are quite reassuring for those who worry that formal community services will replace the volunteered assistance of family. Project OPEN, South Carolina, and the basic model of Channeling all showed no differences in type and amount of informal support. The complex model of Channeling found a significant reduction in the percentage of the experimental group who had "visiting" informal caregivers six months and twelve months later, but no differences in the number of such visits received for those who still had persons visit to give informal care. (Those visiting caregivers who stopped coming were generally friends rather than family, and the volume of care given by friends was slight to begin with.) New York City Home Care Project found no differences in the availability of informal caregivers six months later but did find that the more impaired received more informal care and that substitution seemed most likely with the less impaired. Only Channeling looked at the effects of care on the well-being of the informal caregivers, and here positive results were shown. Compared to control groups, caregivers for basic-model clients reported significantly higher quality of life six months later, and those in the complex model reported higher quality of life and greater satisfaction with service arrangements both six months and twelve months later.

Channeling Demonstration

The Channeling Demonstration is particularly important because of its careful design, large sample, and high visibility. For a social experiment, Channeling was particularly ambitious and costly. It was meant to resolve ambiguities in the results of previous demonstration projects. Essentially Channeling's two models tested two distinct hypotheses about the current problems in long-term care. Assuming that mismatches occur between the needs of the elderly and the services they receive, the basic model of Channeling tested whether lack of information and coordination was the problem. Under that model, case managers primarily provided assessment and coordination of care. The complex model took as an assumption that lack of affordable community services for functionally impaired elderly was also part of the problem, causing an overuse of nursing homes. The complex model tested the effect of giving the case managers authority to purchase services to meet that need, with the proviso that neither a per-person nor a per-program maximum be exceeded.

The evaluation contained many quality controls. A randomized design was used. Technical assistants worked with all Channeling sites to enhance consistency in the intervention within sites and across sites. A common screening tool was used at all sites to target the program to persons who met specific functional guidelines.

The benefits of both models proved modest. No effects on mortality, or nursing home or hospital use, were found. About a quarter of both the experimental and control groups in both models used nursing homes within the first year, and the average number of days of use was relatively low. In both models, the group receiving channeling had significantly fewer unmet needs (using an 8-item unmet need index) and was significantly more confident and satisfied with care arrangements a year later. Clients from both models reported higher global life satisfaction at six months, and in the complex model the difference was sustained at a year. No differences were found in other measured psychological items such as contentment, self-perceived health, and social interaction/loneliness. Any difference in functional status favored the basic model. Under that model, the experimental group had fewer restricted bed days at six months than the controls but were no different from the controls on a Katz ADL scale or an IADL measure. In contrast, the Channeling clients from the complex sites were significantly more disabled on a Katz ADL scale than the controls at both the six-month and twelve-month follow-up. Family caregivers in the demonstration group experienced significantly higher life quality than family caregivers in the control group at six months for the basic model, and yet the amount of family care given was comparable. For the complex model, the family caregivers reported significantly higher quality of life and satisfaction with care arrangements at both six months and twelve months, but at both time periods the amount of informal care given was reduced. Costs for clients in both models were higher than for the controls, but the complex model with its substantial purchase of services was much more costly than the basic model.

The rich data base of the Channeling demonstration will surely yield many more analyses than are available at this writing. The general thrust of the results, however, is unlikely to change. Among the most plausible explanations for weak effects on institutional use, and therefore costs, is that Channeling (particularly the complex model) was implemented in service-rich environments where the control group members also received case management and additional service. (In such cases the additional funding for services supplied by Channeling meant that existing services were more available for control group members.) The evaluators analyzed this phenomenon to some extent in a two-volume document discussing the implementation of the demonstration (Carcagno et al., 1986). They concluded that at least a minimum threshold of case management was widely implemented in the experimental group and much less likely to occur in the control group.

Implications

For those seeking a panacea to reduce nursing home use and lower long-term care costs, the account of these cumulative community demonstrations is disappointing. Although the individual projects were often able to produce one or more positive outcomes (expressed either as improved functioning or reduced utilization), they rarely did both. The National Channeling Demonstration represented the most careful separation of the two primary components of efforts to improve community-based long-term care: (1) the rationalization of available services through case management and (2) the addition of supplemental services. Channeling, therefore, provided the strongest basis for examining the effects of each approach. It is especially discouraging that the more comprehensive model seemed to show even fewer benefits than the basic model.

In fairness, however, all these studies must be recognized as demonstrations, with the limitations inherent in that status. They were discrete enterprises bounded by both the extent of their services under the demonstration design and the limited duration of their operation. In terms of the former, the projects rarely included activities likely to change the behavior of personnel in acute hospitals or of physicians. In terms of the latter, it is almost naive to suppose that providers of care would change their behavior markedly on the basis of a new purchaser for a limited number of people for a finite period. Some Channeling sites were able to negotiate bargain prices for their clients, but in an operational program that would be expected to include all members of a community for the indefinite future, the bargaining power of the program would be much greater.

Policy-makers are left with an inevitable dilemma. On the one hand, a demonstration imposes artificial strictures that limit its capacity to show the very effects intended. On the other hand, operational programs provide a truer test of the approach but make attribution of effects difficult.

Ironically, in several instances, the demonstrations were expanded into full-blown programs even before their results were fully ascertained. For example, South Carolina, Georgia, Wisconsin, and Florida have developed or are working on statewide programs, New York expanded Nursing Home Without Walls, and On Lok moved to a capitated risk-sharing status. In 1985, California doubled the number of MSSP sites and established them as operational programs rather than demonstrations. (MSSP now stands for Multipurpose Senior Services Program rather than "Project.")

Such growth can be attributed to at least two factors. For those operating the programs (the lead agencies, the case managers) and those participating in the system (for example, major vendors), the demonstrations created and fostered a constituency eager to preserve and expand the concept. At the same time, the tangible nature of the efforts and the apparent positive reception among consumers were politically attractive. The reaction suggests that the political viability of these community-based services may derive from factors other than their demonstrated efficacy. This is especially true when the evaluation outcomes are expressed in objective, but seemingly mechanistic indicators, whereas the programs receive rave reviews.

CASE MANAGEMENT

As we discussed in Chapter 4, case management has been hailed as the mechanism for making long-term care systems more rational, equitable, and efficient. It has also been cited as a means to coordinate services on behalf of those needing long-term care. Supposedly case management ensures that clients have accurate information needed to make decisions and advocates to assist them in negotiating a complex service structure at a time when, by definition, their functional disabilities may prevent them from acting effectively on their own behalf. Some form of case management was part of most demonstrations in long-term care (Capitman, 1986; Capitman, Haskins, and Bernstein, 1986). Indeed, the idea of "managed care" has become a staple for most planners. Even those exploring the possibility of private long-term care insurance assume that the more conventional insurance adjuster would be replaced or supplemented by a case manager, who would assess level of need and authorize benefits accordingly.

Case management is almost impossible to study in isolation from the associated service system. Nevertheless, information is urgently needed on the best way to organize case management in a long-term care system. Case management, as usually defined and as exemplified by the Channeling Demonstration, includes the functions of casefinding, assessment, care planning and implementation, and monitoring. But within this list of functions, variation is rampant, as those who compare case management have discovered (Simpson, 1982; Steinberg and Carter, 1982; Steinberg and Trejo, 1984; Austin et al., 1985). These comparisons have largely been based on program features. More recently, Austin (1987) described case management in four western states (Oregon, Washington, Idaho, and Alaska) by sampling and directly polling case managers and their supervisors. She, too, found considerable variation within agencies and across them, as well as systematic differences between the approaches taken in Oregon and in Washington, the states where most of the case management was occurring. However, her study sheds no light on the effects associated with the differences.

Regarding assessment, issues can be raised about how detailed the assessment should be, what information should be collected, who should do the assessment, and what measurements or instruments should be used. The proper frequency of monitoring and of formal reassessment is also debated. In some instances, the various functions of case management are divided. For example, one person or agency might do the assessment, with the monitoring responsibility going to someone else. Such division of labor would surely alter the relationship between case manager and client, but little agreement exists about the ideal nature of that relationship.

Furthermore, case management programs differ markedly in design features. To Austin and her colleagues (1985), the four key dimensions of program design are organizational auspice, targeting, gatekeeping, and reimbursement and financing. In terms of auspice, many different agencies do case management, including Area Agencies on Aging, home health agencies, welfare departments, hospitals, and others. Then, too, private practitioners of case management are appearing, marketing their services directly to clients and, more often, their worried adult offspring. Variation may also exist in the level of professional training and the discipline of the case manager, raising questions about whether nursing, social work, or some other preparation is most appropriate, or whether team case management is desirable. The amount of authority of the case manager to determine eligibility for benefits, to authorize services, or to purchase them directly is a key distinction in the way case management programs are designed.

Very little research is available that specifies the advantages and disadvantages of designing case management or defining its functions in a particular way. Most information is descriptive, and much has been generated from the demonstration projects just discussed. For example, time studies of case management in the California MSSP demonstration revealed that case managers were spending a large amount of time at meetings and on the telephone, doing collaborative work associated with planning care (White and Grisham, 1982). Using the same time-study data, another analysis noted that case managers became particularly active and engaged in more discretionary activities when the clients were on the brink of a transition to an institution (Miller, 1985). The evaluation of New York City's Family Support Project (Frankfather, Smith, and Caro, 1981), which was discussed in Chapter 6, shows that case managers tended not to communicate to clients the array of options from which a care plan could be constructed, or, at least, not in a way that the clients could understand sufficiently to recall later.

A technical assistance contract to Temple University was built into the Channeling Demonstration to enable preparation of manuals and other materials to train case managers and at the same time to standardize the intervention for evaluation purposes (Schneider et al., 1982; Johnson and Sterthous, 1982). Noting that case managers were reporting that they spent a great deal of time on a relatively small proportion of the clientele, Schneider and her colleagues (1984) drew a random sample of twenty-five clients from each site and studied the activity generated on their cases during the first year after the initial assessment. Twelve actions of case managers (such as changing the care plan, changing a provider, negotiating with family, or ordering an evaluation) were counted; these ranged from three to more than sixty per client during the study year. The actions of the case managers were more usually stimulated by changes in or concerns about the provider rather than events directly associated with the client (such as death of spouse, decline in functioning, admission to hospital). From a small study done at the Philadelphia Channeling site, Rickards (1985) reported that case managers' cost projections for their plans came close to the actual experience and were as likely to overstate as understate the actual expenses.

The eight MSSP and the ten Channeling sites created a laboratory for case management and yielded practical insights into the strategies that seemed acceptable and workable and the kinds of problems case managers might anticipate. Pelham and Clark (1986) edited a useful book on the MSSP experiences, which includes admonitions about the need for extra attention from case managers at a time when the client is in hospital (Peters, 1986). From Channeling, observations have been made about the tension between nurses and social workers as case managers (Amerman, 1985), the tension between case management and counseling functions (Amerman, Eisenberg, and Weisman, 1985), and efforts to enhance informal supports (Sterthous, 1986). The latter reported enthusiastically about groups arranged to bring family members of Channeling clients together for mutual support and instruction and about efforts to stimulate community voluntary activity, especially at the Houston Channeling site. However, even the anecdotal accounts suggested that few families availed themselves of the opportunity for support and instruction and that the voluntary activities seemed hard to organize for rather minimal payoff.

A few efforts are on record to test different models of case management or to separate out the effects of case management from the effects of the service given. (In some ways, the basic model of Channeling could be said to have attempted the latter, but case managers at the basic sites did have the option of purchasing gap-filling services, and presumably the services that they facilitated through brokering and coordinating activities also had effects on the clientele.) The evaluators of the California MSSP projects made an elaborate effort to define an effect of services, an effect of case management, and a combined effect, and to separate which outcomes were primarily due to which inputs. The analysis is somewhat difficult to follow, but the authors concluded that, although case managers had little effect in preventing a transition from hospital to nursing home, case managers (apart from the services they ordered) appeared to show an effect in shortening the length of time spent in nursing homes and hastening a return to the community (Miller et al., 1984). If this finding could be replicated, it would suggest a promising potential for case managers.

A study of case management grafted to the ACCESS program in Rochester, New York, suggested the efficacy of a more personal involvement of case managers with clients. The ACCESS program routinely purchases its assessments and monitoring from hospital, home health, and other personnel. ACCESS case managers are brokers of this process, and their caseloads are large. Using grant funds, ACCESS performed a randomized study comparing direct assessment to brokerage. In 1983, an experimental group began receiving more intensive, personalized services from a case management team with a vastly reduced caseload. The only analyses available at this writing compared the experiences of persons known to the ACCESS system. Considerable costs were apparently saved because the intensively case-managed group used less hospital days, home health, transportation, and other services (though more nursing home days), and these savings offset the additional costs of the case management by a wide mark. Comparisons of the experience of intensively case-managed new clients to the ACCESS program and their controls are not yet available (Monroe County Long-Term Care Program, 1984).

The only other test of how to do case management that we discovered tested the effects of conceptualizing family members of the impaired elderly as explicit partners in the case management task. Seltzer and her colleagues (Seltzer et al., 1984; Seltzer, Ivry, and Litchfield, 1985) conducted a randomized study in the Jewish Family and Children's Services agency in Boston, with the experimental group of 47 clients receiving the family-partnership model and the 50 control group families receiving case management as usual. So far, the authors have identified that families are willing to perform case management tasks (although there are some families who should not be involved in this way) and that some individual clients without families would be quite capable and willing to engage in some of these tasks themselves (such as arranging and monitoring services). Data on the outcomes of this study are not yet available.

In summary, we have been able to present only fragmentary hypotheses and insights about the effects of various case management patterns and practices rather than any solid core of evidence. Case management still has no agreed-upon meaning; some use the term to refer to the coordinating functions that are part of the casework done by all social workers, whereas others reserve it for roles analogous to those in the community long-term care demonstrations. Further study of case management per se would be helpful, but inevitably findings of such studies must be understood in the context of the particular design of the case management program and the services that the case manager can implement.

CAPITATION: SOCIAL HMOs

The social health maintenance organization (S/HMO) is a demonstration that tests the effects of consolidating fundings for acute care and long-term care and reducing the barriers to a coherent set of services to meet the needs of the functionally impaired elderly. It is a prepaid system extending the usual coverage of health maintenance organizations by adding long-term care benefits. The annual capitation paid by members (plus contractually established copayments) is expected to finance all the benefits Medicare would cover for its beneficiaries (that is, hospital care, medical care, and certain skilled nursing services in facilities and at home) plus agreed-upon additional benefits for nursing home care, home nursing and homemaking, and a wide range of other health and social services. Medicare rules about rehabilitation potential, homeboundedness, prior hospitalizations, and so on no longer apply and members waive the right to use their Medicare benefit with other fee-for-service vendors; the Health Care Financing Administration provides the S/HMO with a lump sum per enrollee on the basis of average annual Medicare expenditures.

Eventually, the S/HMOs are expected to assume full financial risk for operating within the Medicare payments, the additional enrollee premiums, and the designated copayments. Clearly, financial viability depends on the ability of S/HMOs to enroll a large group of members, many of whom will have no need for the additional long-term care services. Case management is used to identify from the larger group of enrollees those who need and are entitled to the additional long-term care benefits, to plan for their effective use and control their overuse, and to coordinate other community services on behalf of the member.

The S/HMO is now being demonstrated at four locations, each with rather different partnerships of providers. Brandeis University, where the S/HMO idea originated, served as the developer of the S/HMOs; investigators at Brandeis have written a book describing the development of the four sites (Leutz et al., 1985). The largest S/HMO program is at Kaiser Permanente in Portland, Oregon, a well-established health maintenance organization with its own hospitals, outpatient clinics, and home health agency. There, members of what is called the Medicare Plus Two program receive all the benefits of Kaiser's own Medicare Plus program, a capitated plan, and additional long-term care benefits. The case managers are actually "resource coordinators," whose main task is to activate existing parts of the Kaiser system (for example, its home care program, its discharge planners, and its social workers) on behalf of the clients as well as to coordinate purchased long-term care services at home and in nursing homes. Typically, the resource coordinators become involved after Medicare benefits no longer apply.

The other three S/HMOs required more organizational partnerships. Seniors Plus in Minneapolis is a partnership of an existing health maintenance organization, Group Health, and a voluntary agency, Ebenezer Society, which operates long-term care facilities and home health and social service programs. SCAN in Long Beach, California, is a community long-term care program that is the site of one of the MSSP projects. To produce the array of services needed for the S/HMO, SCAN entered into agreements with a group of physicians practicing in their own offices, working out ways that the physicians would be at financial risk for the effectiveness of the operation. In addition, they made agreements with a local hospital and with nursing homes; as an existing case management agency, SCAN already had working arrangements with vendors of home care in the area. Finally ELDERPLAN in Brooklyn, New York, is centered in Metropolitan Jewish Home and Hospital, a long-term care facility with an associated home health agency. To provide the medical care of a S/HMO, ELDERPLAN created its own Physician Group. Unlike the physicians at the other four sites, at ELDERPLAN primary medical care is delivered by a small group of physicians who see only ELDERPLAN members.

It is too soon to comment on advantages and disadvantages of these models. In any event, with only four programs, each in a widely different milieu, conclusive statements about optimum organization will be impossible. The benefits and costs of the S/HMO programs are currently being evaluated by the Aging Health Policy Center at the University of California, San Fransisco. Because the S/HMO is theoretically such an attractive intervention, the results of this social experiment are being eagerly awaited. It will be important to remember that the S/HMO, like the community long-term care demonstrations before it, is a demonstration project, subject to constraints and compromises in the definition of the intervention tested. For example, the long-term care benefit ultimately selected is less generous than some advocates would have preferred. Regardless of the outcome of the S/HMO evaluation, one would hope for other tests of capitated models of health and long-term care.

SYSTEM CHANGE

We have discussed the limitations of demonstrations, yet it is obvious that important learnings are derived from such projects. At some point, it becomes necessary to proceed to make systematic changes in the way long-term care is delivered. What can we say about system change in long-term care from our review of evidence?

One of the earliest and best documented efforts to change at least part of the system of care for the frail elderly was done in the early 1970s in Massachusetts. The State Unit on Aging (called in Massachusetts the Department of Elder Affairs) was authorized to create a network of home care corporations. Housed in the Area Agencies on Aging for the most part, the home care corporations used Older Americans Act, Title XX, and state funds to provide case management and other purchased services, particularly home care, to the frail elderly. According to Piktialis and Callahan (1986), the intent was to create a model of home care service delivery with the following features: lack of stigma for users; local consumer input; reduction of bureaucratic obstacles; case management; multiple funding sources; and priority for the frail elderly, to counteract documented discrimination frequently found in human service programs.

Between 1973 and 1983, the program grew from a budget of just over $1million (when the program was still only partly implemented) to $71million; by the latter date the client count was almost 40,500. The encouraging factor, however, is that the ultimate growth of the program seems limited and controllable. Based on estimations of the number of frail elderly in the community, the original goal was to serve 5% of the noninstitutionalized elderly. In fact, in 1982, the total caseload represented 4.2% of the noninstitutionalized elderly. Thus Piktialis and Callahan concluded that the fears of uncontrollable growth for this publicly funded community care program were largely unfounded. Massachusetts' experience shows it is possible to develop a universal benefit, refine its use, target it efficiently, and constrain its growth. At the same time, a program with a wide basis of public support was created. The home care corporations did not offer medically oriented home care (such as home nursing), and, therefore, their costs do not reflect the total community long-term care costs. Nevertheless, the experience points in the direction of what can be achieved by creating an operational network of state-wide programs, pooling funds, and developing a case-managed universal benefit. Our own studies in Canada (Kane and Kane, 1985) showed that it is possible to control use of community services in a case managed system. The provinces we studied experienced a sharply rising caseload initially as the program was phased in, some initial testing of the system, and then a steady state that proved affordable.

Partly with the help of waivers authorized under Section 2176 of the Omnibus Budget Reconciliation Act (see Chapter 3), individual states have made substantial efforts to rationalize long-term care and render it more efficient as well as effective. Justice and Preston (1986) profiled twelve such state efforts for the National Governors' Association. Common characteristics included pooled funds, centralized authority, and planning to effect a balance between institutional and community long-term care.

Perhaps the most striking example of change and consolidation of long-term care in the United States comes from Oregon. The state has evolved a system of long-term care that administratively combines payment for and monitoring of home-based services and nursing home services. Case management and flexibility is the hallmark of the system, which is open to people of all ages. The program purchases home care and day care, using Medicaid-waivered funds and state funds. It also purchases family foster care (defined as care in a home that houses no more than four people), a nonmedical alternative to care that is used widely in Oregon. The state purchases home care directly and also makes arrangements to partly finance live-in care; the case manager does the assessment and determines the amount of services and, therefore, the amount of money that the program will pay. These monies are provided directly to the client to defray a portion of the cost of an approved privately hired provider, but the program ensures that both the employee and employer contributions to Social Security are made. A mandatory preadmission screening program and an active reloca-tion program for persons in long-term care facilities are also features of Oregon's system. Individual monitoring of clients in nursing homes and in home care is performed, and protective service and abuse complaints are provided for both residents of the community and the nursing home.

Oregon's program is evolving faster than formal evaluation can track. However, early indications exist that the program saves money, while meeting the preferences of Oregon residents. Medicaid nursing home ex-penditures decreased in Oregon between 1979 and 1986, not only as a proportion of the elderly population, but also in absolute terms. In 1979 there were an average of 8,079 Medicaid recipients in nursing homes in Oregon, and in 1986 that number had decreased to 7,590. The average cost of maintaining a person in a nursing home rose, of course, during that period. But, taking into account all new expenditures for community pro-grams, state officials estimate that the 1986 program cost the state $13 million less than would have been the case had the system not been revised (Ladd, 1986). At the same time, a program was being created that won widespread public approval.

CONCLUDING COMMENT

This chapter has reviewed research evidence about efforts to change the way the "system" of long-term care functions, or, more aptly, efforts to move toward a more coherent system rather than a duplicative and fragmentary set of programs. As we have pointed out, the discontinuities of the status quo are many—between institutional and community long-term care, be-tween acute care and long-term care, between health and social services. Efforts to bridge those gaps seem eminently worthwhile. Strategies include preadmission screening that links acute and long-term care, especially man-datory preadmission screening that provides the same assessment to nursing home applicants regardless of whether the payor will be Medicaid, Medi-care, or themselves. Other strategies include pooling funds offering case management and modest community services to *all* who need long-term care, and capitated programs. None of the strategies applied thus far resolve all of the existing fragmentation, but each seems to make some progress toward a more coherent system.

The studies we reviewed were largely demonstration projects, probably necessarily so. The combined evidence from the demonstration projects and the few operational examples we have cited suggests it is time to move cautiously ahead with operational changes. No single approach is likely to be universally applicable. We have probably gleaned as much good informa-tion that we can from demonstrations of community-based long-term care. We know now the importance of careful targeting, the importance of maintaining informal support (but we have the reassuring information that informal support is unlikely to evaporate), and the key potential for case management. We know that providers will appear to offer home-based service if a market for them is created. Many of the remaining decisions are political not empirical. That is, we need to decide whether our policy will be to introduce community services only for those likely to enter nursing homes or for those who reach a level of functional impairment that would suggest they will benefit from such services. Advocates for the elderly will surely suggest the latter.

PART III
Conclusions

11

Synthesizing the Evidence

This book has concentrated on evidence. The lengthy reference list reflects only some of the numerous works and investigators contributing ideas to one or more aspects of this complex field. This chapter summarizes the findings, weighting their importance and suggesting some implications about the challenge of producing effective and humane long-term care systems. Without repeating all the material in the body of the book, we draw attention to selected methodological and substantive points about the evidence. For convenience, we treat the topics generally in the order they were introduced in the book.

NEED FOR LONG-TERM CARE

Evidence

Widespread agreement about the definition of long-term care has been achieved: There is general acknowledgment about the primacy of functional impairment in establishing the need for care; almost all investigators define it as health, personal care, and social services to compensate for functional impairment. Despite different ways of defining functional impairment, estimates of its prevalence have been quite consistent. Predicting the amount of service needed has been much more problematic. Key points about the state of the evidence on the need for long-term care include the following:

- One approach to estimating need is surveying levels of functional impairment. Great variation is found in the definitions and measures of impairment used and the way data are collected, even to the choice of respondent (e.g., client or proxy). Surveys are, therefore, difficult to compare. Even if functional disability were accurately measured, no agreed upon formula exists for translating disability into corresponding requirements for care.

- Projecting data on present utilization of long-term care to infer future use assumes that present patterns will continue into the future. Yet, no firm ground exists for predicting either the disability rates in the next generation or the obstacles that might interfere with family members' providing long-term care to elderly relatives in the future. Beyond that, extrapolating future need from present use introduces circular planning that assumes current arrangements are correct.

- National information about the characteristics of nursing home residents has been extremely outdated until recently. Most analysts rely heavily on the National Nursing Home Survey of 1977, which, in itself, gathered information from facility staff about residents rather than through direct observation and interview of residents. (As this book went to press, preliminary findings from the 1985 Nursing Home Survey were released.)

- Surveys of the incidence and prevalence of senile dementia, incontinence, and falls also use varying definitions. Nevertheless, we are able to produce fairly reliable estimates of these conditions. Regarding incontinence, few longitudinal studies follow the condition from its onset.

- Considerable data have been collected about long-term care given by family and friends. Because much of this is cross-sectional, we know less about how such assistance varies over time. In contrast to studies on caregiving patterns, studies of the effects of such caregiving on the family members providing the care are based only on small samples.

- Information on the public costs of long-term care in institutions and for home care is quite good. In contrast, information on the public cost of socially oriented care is available only in aggregate and cannot readily be traced to the individual. Information on the private costs of care at home is extremely limited; and even the figures on private costs of nursing homes are probably understated because expenses other than the daily rate are not easily tracked.

- The likelihood of entering a nursing home increases sharply with age. Although we cannot properly predict the fate of any individual, risk factors for a population are, in part, known. The cluster of factors associated with an increased risk of entering a nursing home include age, sex (female), and loss of functional ability. When these factors are present, the presence of social support counters the risk. In addition, the risk of admission to a nursing home is greater at times of crisis, and one reflection of such a crisis is a hospitalization. In essence, all of the indicators represent just that—indicators reflecting a set of situations rather than specific items.

Findings

- Functional dependency increases with age, although even above age 85 considerable variation in functional abilities exists. Despite this variation, those planning for a population can estimate expected levels of impairment fairly accurately. Among people aged 65 to 74, the rate of needing the help of another person in one or more ADL or IADL activity is about 70 per 1,000 (7%), whereas among persons 85 and older, the rate is 436 per 1,000 (almost 45%).
- Utilization of many health care services also increases with age. However, the utilization is uneven; at each age, a relatively small proportion of people account for the heaviest use and cost of hospital, physician, and nursing home care.
- According to the best estimates, senile dementia has a prevalence in between 5% and 7% of the elderly population in the United States. Estimations of severe dementia in persons over 65 in the United States have ranged from 1.3% to 6.2%. Prevalence of urinary incontinence is greater among women than men; studies report ranges from 18% to 23% for community-dwelling women and 7% to 17% for community-dwelling men. The rates of both incontinence and dementia are much higher for both men and women in institutions; the rates for both conditions probably approach 50%. About a third of the elderly living at home experience a fall in any year, and approximately 1 in 40 will be admitted to hospital because of a fall.
- Families have not deserted their elderly family members, but on the contrary give a heavy volume of care. Caregivers are most often women, and many women can anticipate decades of caregiving for one or another relative (perhaps a parent and spouse in sequence). No definitive information is available about the stress occasioned by such care, but it seems to be greater when the older person has senile dementia.

LONG-TERM CARE SERVICES, FINANCING, AND COSTS

Evidence

As a basis for considering changes in long-term care policies, we reviewed information about the number and characteristics of long-term care services of various types, that is, the so-called supply factors. The information base was surprisingly weak, particularly for services that are largely uncovered by third-party payments. Regarding the information, we emphasize the following:

- We can confidently assemble information about the numbers, size, and auspice of nursing home beds, and about certified home health agencies. Information about board and care homes, homemaking services, day care, meal programs, and other noncertified services is much less accurate.
- Apropos of nursing homes, we had difficulty gathering information about the profit structure of the industry, or even the growth and consolidation of chain ownership.

Findings

Findings on this topic are the commonplace statistics typically cited about long-term care services and costs. Here we would underscore the following:

- Long-term care in nursing homes is extremely expensive, having cost over $35 billion in 1985. The direct cost is equally borne by public programs and private individuals. However, private individuals expend their funds first, with widespread impoverishment of elderly nursing home residents and their spouses, who must "spend down" to Medicaid eligibility. The private costs are largely uninsured and uninsurable at this time, and are probably underestimated.
- Public expenditures for home care constitute a small fraction of those for nursing home care.
- Enormous interstate variation exists in the proportion of nursing home beds per population, ownership patterns, size of facilities, and in reimbursement rates and rules (and, therefore, per capita costs). Ownership patterns and sizes of facilities also vary by state.
- The best information about the home health industry is limited to Medicare-certified agencies. These have increased 17% between 1972 to 1982, but the growth in proprietary home health agencies has increased by almost 60% in the same time period.
- Among the trends affecting the delivery and financing of services are the rapid growth of preadmission screening programs for nursing home admission; the state initiatives developed under Section 2176 (Omnibus Budget Reconciliation Act) Medicaid waivers; moratoria and other constraints on the growth of nursing home beds within states; and the expansion of case management as a means to coordinate long-term care services in an appropriate and rational way. Private long-term care insurance has been enthusiastically studied, but the policies currently marketed have not proven attractive to large numbers of older persons or their sponsors.

PREFERENCES

Something seems amiss if the predominant form of long-term care is inconsistent with the preferences of its clients and the public. Although we need many more and better studies in the area, the existing studies provide compelling evidence that we fall short of the goal of developing services compatible with the personal preferences of the users and their families. At the least, a system should provide citizens with meaningful choices and a sense of control over their destiny. It is a moral imperative that basic civil rights of those receiving long-term care be respected.

Evidence

The material available here is quite limited. Inferences about preferences of both the elderly and the general public can be drawn from specific questions on national opinion polls. Isolated studies report what nursing home residents consider as important attributes of a good home or a good life in a facility. A few studies examine the extent to which older persons and their families plan together for expected long-term care needs. Study of preferences is methodologically difficult, requiring decisions about how to measure preferences and whom to ask. For example, people may react differently to a hypothetical condition than one they actually have, and their responses to questions of value preferences will be highly sensitive to the way questions are worded. Most of the studies we located were unsophisticated in acknowledging or addressing methodological issues.

Findings

- Older people prefer to remain in the community and, if possible, in their own homes to receive long-term care. Overwhelmingly, they prefer to avoid nursing homes.
- Seemingly, persons of all ages are willing to support services for the elderly through tax dollars.
- Few older people make advance plans for future long-term care needs, nor do they tend to discuss their preferences with family members. Perhaps this represents a fatalism about the future. It may also suggest that programs designed to provide information useful to the so-called consumer of long-term care need to provide the information closer to the time when the clients need to know enough to make a rational decision.
- Older persons, and particularly those in institutions (where this has been most studied), value privacy, freedom to exercise choice, dignified treatment, and a sense of making a meaningful contribution to society.

HOME CARE

Home care in its various forms (ranging from medical and nursing treatments to homemaking and chore services) is the bulwark of community
long-term care. Unfortunately, studies to examine the effects of home care
are few and difficult to compare.

Evidence

- Few studies of home care with comparison groups are available, and
  even fewer of these are randomized experiments. Such studies cannot be
  easily compared because the models of home care tested differ (ranging
  from highly technical post-hospital care to ongoing homemaking) and
  the outcomes sought also differ. In some studies home care is compared
  to an alternative service such as hospital care or nursing home care,
  whereas in other studies, those receiving home care are compared to
  those receiving no particular care.
- An adequate number of studies are available that describe the population receiving home care according to disability and other factors.
- Few studies test the advantages and disadvantages of organizing home
  care a particular way. Studies of the relative effects of varying auspices,
  personnel mixes, and practices would be exceedingly useful.

Findings

- Judging from available descriptive studies, home care seems to reach
  persons with severe functional impairments (some of whom are more
  disabled than some nursing home residents). Those receiving formal
  home care will likely continue to receive large amounts of informal care
  from family members. Among those receiving home care, a small percentage of clients will consume a disproportionately large share of the
  resources. Reassuring for those concerned about opening the floodgates
  by establishing home care benefits, the demand for home care in operational programs does not seem excessive and is readily controllable.
- Experimental studies examining the effect of home care on outcomes
  such as death rates, physical functioning, psychological and social
  well-being, use of other health services including nursing homes, and
  overall cost of care yield contradictory results. Despite a strong face
  validity for the advantages of home care, one cannot generalize from
  this evidence. In part, the wrong outcomes may have been measured.
  For example, expecting home care to result in improved physical
  functioning may be inappropriate; in fact, measured physical functioning may decrease if persons who previously struggled to do tasks on
  their own receive needed home care.

- Older people tend to evaluate home care programs positively, particularly the assistance with housekeeping, laundry, and other practical chores.

DAY CARE

Problems in evaluating day care are similar to those in evaluating home care, only more so. Day care may be respite care or therapy. The goals need to be clear to avoid inappropriate expectations that a particular day care program can attain a wide range of objectives for clients and their families.

Evidence

- Almost no evaluative studies of day care are available, and most are international. Only two randomized studies have been reported to date, one dealing with stroke patients over age 50 and the other limited to testing the effects of day health care as a Medicare post-hospital benefit.

Findings

- The body of evaluative data is too small and conflicting to draw conclusions about the effects of day care.
- From descriptive studies, we can generalize that day care is underutilized in the United States. Despite (or perhaps because of) the relatively few programs, day care centers report that they have difficulty filling their places. This is true even when a source of payment exists. On the other hand, those who do attend day care and their families rate the service highly.
- Among the factors that may be associated with day care's lack of broad acceptability are: transportation difficulties; problems in getting a client ready for day care; disruptiveness in routine for a demented person who attends only a few times a week; and distance from home.

OTHER COMMUNITY SERVICES
Evidence

We examined a wide variety of other services besides homes care and day care that might be considered long-term care in whole or in part. The quantity as well as the quality of evidence varied considerably from topic to topic. We identified no studies of the effects of transportation programs on individual clients and almost no studies of in-home programs, although both are staples of community long-term care provision. Similarly, we found few studies of adult protective services or guardianship, or of services in housing programs. Efforts to support family caregivers range widely (including educational and support groups) and have scarcely been evaluated. In contrast, numerous studies of geriatric assessment programs and a respectable number on adult foster care and respite services are available.

Findings

- Several quasi-experiments of adult foster care report good outcomes and high satisfaction among users. However, these studies also report high attrition rates and base their studies on small samples. Adult foster care may be particularly useful for a subset of long-term care clients without families.
- Respite care tends to be viewed positively in surveys of users, but the concept has not been subjected to any experimental designs or even quasi-experiments with control groups.
- There is ample evidence that older persons can serve reliably as volunteers in a range of programs for persons of all ages, but there is no definitive evidence that such voluntary activity postpones or reduces their own need for long-term care. As for the impact of older volunteers as deliverers of long-term care, we have virtually no information on their effectiveness in organized programs for non-relatives, nor do we know whether the role of volunteering to provide long-term care would be acceptable to many elders.
- Geriatric assessment programs (both inpatient and outpatient) have demonstrated their effectiveness in identifying remediable problems previously ignored by the acute care sector. If such programs are carefully targeted to persons with functional needs and likely to go to a nursing home, assessment and short-term treatment can actually alter the trajectory for an older person who was bound for a nursing home.
- Several tests of hospice (which have not been limited to older persons) have shown that hospice produces the same levels of pain control and psychological and social well-being as conventional care. There are some benefits in terms of client and family satisfaction. Because hospice achieves equally good results as conventional care, it represents a viable option for persons desiring it.

NURSING HOMES

Evidence

One expects to find voluminous research about nursing homes, because they are the site of most publicly supported long-term care. In fact, although material was copious, many of the most ambitious and best-designed studies have examined the quality and cost of care only in a global way. Studies examining the effects of various therapeutic efforts, programs, or environmental changes on specific residents have suffered from tiny self-selected samples, inadequate theoretical underpinnings, and poor designs. Perhaps an exception is the body of studies examining the effects of learned helplessness on nursing home residents, and the benefits of enhancing control. Here the studies do build on a theoretical framework, and though the samples tend to be small, elegant experimental and quasi-experimental designs have been reported. Overall, however, the work done on nursing homes has a mechanistic quality—the outcomes studied fail to capture matters of concern to residents.

Studies of factors associated with quality of care and quality of life in nursing homes have been marred by extremely limited definitions of quality. The tendency is to use a structural indicator such as the ratio of nursing staff to residents as a proxy for a high-quality home and to examine factors associated with a favorable ratio. The effects of various reimbursement methods and patterns have been studied only perfunctorily. To support case-mix-adjusted systems of reimbursement, considerable effort has been made to determine the actual costs of caring for residents with particular characteristics. Unfortunately, all of this work relies on time-and-motion studies based on the present patterns of staffing, yet none of these practices have been associated with desirable outcomes.

Findings

Given the limitations just discussed, findings should be viewed with caution. In that spirit, we make the following generalizations:

- Almost any intervention introduced in a nursing home seems to result in measurable benefits for the residents. This may be a reflection of the general deprivation of the environment, which makes most attention welcome.
- Notwithstanding the general positive nature of findings of studies in nursing homes, the limited data on more formal therapeutic endeavors, especially reality orientation therapy, are less positive.
- Efforts to improve choice and to enhance the sense of control in nursing home residents result in less depression, better functioning, and, sometimes, decreased morbidity and mortality.
- To the extent they have been tested, efforts to improve the nursing home environment, making it more pleasant or flexible, and efforts to bridge the gap between the facility and the community have shown positive effects.
- Little evidence is available to show that positive findings about factors associated with well-being in nursing homes have led to sustained program changes.

- Nursing home ownership has not been shown to be related to quality of care, but few studies have pursued this issue carefully.

RELATIONSHIP BETWEEN LONG-TERM CARE AND ACUTE CARE

Evidence

Information about movement of older people between hospitals and nursing homes or community long-term care programs is rather sparse. The few longitudinal studies that have been done suggest an active movement back and forth. Although states collect routine data about nursing home use under Medicaid, each readmission to a facility tends to count as a new admission. Data on nursing home residents must be read with great care to distinguish the course of new admissions from old residents. The close links between acute and long-term care call for information on full episodes of care. Better discharge planning from hospital can reduce nursing home admission rates, while some projects have demonstrated the advantages of increased medical attention in nursing homes.

Findings

- Long-term care and acute care are inextricably linked. Admission to one should not influence eligibility for the other, but actions taken in one can produce major consequences for the other. Planning should address the full episode of care, including time and effort spent in each sector. Similarly resources should be used across the sectors to permit the most efficient care. Current funding arrangements preclude such a strategy.
- About 9% of elderly persons discharged from acute hospitals go to nursing homes; this rate varies from state to state. Age is the best predictor, but certain attributes like mental status, multiple diagnoses, and functional status, where available, are crude risk factors.
- In general, once in the long-term care system, clients tend to remain in it; but there is evidence of persons leaving to return to independent care. Usually the earlier in the course of care, the greater the chance of improvement.
- Of residents admitted to a nursing home for the first time, 30% die.
- Among the survivors, about 40% go home, 45% are admitted to hospital, and the rest are transferred to other nursing homes.
- Of those admitted to hospital from the nursing home, a third die in hospital and most of the rest are readmitted to nursing homes on discharge.
- Medical care of many nursing home residents is superficial and driven mainly by the need to recertify the patients each month.

- Non-physician practitioners, like physician assistants, nurse practitioners, and even pharmacists, can assume the primary care tasks for nursing home patients with no diminution in the quality of care.

SYSTEMS OF COMMUNITY LONG-TERM CARE

Evidence

After examining various programs separately, we turned to evidence about efforts to make systems of long-term care more effective or efficient. We looked separately at preadmission screening programs designed to rationalize use of nursing homes, but here the evaluative data were weak. We also sought information about the effectiveness of case management as a tool to improve systems of care, but found it difficult to separate the effects of case management from the effects of additional services that the case managers could purchase or arrange.

The bulk of evidence on efforts to change systems of long-term care is derived from no more than twenty demonstration projects done since 1970 to examine the effects of additional entitlements to community care mediated by case management on the outcomes of older people, the informal caregiving already taking place in their families, and the use and cost of other services, including nursing homes. Many of these demonstration projects were well-designed; some, in fact, were randomized experiments. Most were attempts to demonstrate that community services might be a cost-effective alternative. Although these demonstration projects have been compared and contrasted several times, they do not lend themselves to direct comparison because they vary widely in the services allowed, the eligibility for services, the model of case management, the duration of the project, and the outcomes measured. The largest and most recent of such demonstrations, long-term care Channeling, produced only modest evidence of benefit from more extensive provision of services. However, like all demonstration projects, these studies are limited in their external generalizability; the effects on providers and consumers might have been different in operational programs than in demonstrations affecting a defined population for a limited number of years.

Findings

- The community care demonstrations yield mixed results. Although some have greater effects than others, they collectively fail to make the case that the introduction of case-managed community services will reduce nursing home use.
- For the most part, the community care programs do not identify clientele who are likely to enter nursing homes in the first place. The rate of

nursing home use is low for clients in the control groups as well as for those receiving the interventions.

- Evidence about the effects of the demonstrations on functioning, psychological well-being, and social well-being is mixed, but only a few studies show positive effects. The few studies examining effects on the well-being of family caregivers report positive outcomes.
- For the most part, family assistance continues after formal services are in place. If the family reduces its care, those reductions are modest (and perhaps highly appropriate).

CONCLUSION

What does all this research tell us about long-term care? As is so often the case, the knowledge cup is half full. We know a great deal about the nature of such care and the characteristics of those who receive it. We do not know the *best* ways to deliver it, if indeed one can truly talk about best ways in a field so full of options. We can predict the proportion of persons within a given group who are likely to need long-term care within a short period, but we cannot tell exactly which person will need the care. Nor do we have ready algorithms to convert care needs into service packages. Long-term care, like much other care, will continue to rely on people with special expertise to design programs of care.

We know that there is substantial dissatisfaction with the current state of care. The nursing home is shunned by client and provider alike. Ironically, the nursing home is also the place where an investment of effort can pay some of the greatest dividends.

We know that the course of long-term care is not inevitable. Strategic interventions can dramatically improve the lives of persons at risk of institutionalization. The right services at the right time can mean the difference between entering a dreaded institution and remaining in the community. Often careful attention to problems long overlooked can restore or preserve functional capacities.

The combination of knowing what we can reasonably expect and recognizing the variations in ways to deliver services argues for more attention to the outcomes of care. Such attention demands closer attention, too, to the preferences of the various constituencies involved in care. We know too little about how clients, families, providers, and others value the various outcomes. What we do know we tend to ignore, such as the clear preference among older persons to remain at home as long as possible.

It is equally important to appreciate what research will not tell. Research is not a substitute for commitment. It can inform policy, but it does not lead inevitably to policy. It will not show us what to do. Although it can shed light on the implications of various alternatives, great care must be taken in extrapolating too readily from the artificiality of demonstration projects. It is safe to conclude that we know enough to make some commitments about the paths of long-term care we wish to tread. Inevitably we will continue to make midcourse corrections as we refine our techniques. Similarly the nature of long-term care will continue to change as we respond to new challenges and new opportunities.

12

Improving Long-term Care: Next Steps

The demographic forecasts of growth in the elderly population, especially those over age 80, have sent shivers down the spines of health planners. One can almost hear a gerontological Paul Revere crying out, "The elderly are coming." Most of these dire predictions are based on straight line extrapolations from the current situation. In general, the age-specific rates for problems or service use are applied to the predicted numbers of older people in each category and the products calculated.

As we have emphasized, however, the present need not be a direct predictor of the future. Gerontologists are continually exhorting us to recognize differences across age cohorts. Our experience with the elderly of today compared with those of a generation ago should convince us that the next generation of older persons will likely have different physical characteristics and certainly different expectations of what they want from a service delivery system than now prevail. Probably they will be even more diverse than today's elderly.

The conflicting theories about whether disability levels among the elderly are increasing or decreasing are probably both right. More older persons will reach old age healthier than ever before, but more will also reach that stage with disabilities that would have precluded survival in years past. There is a growing set of data suggesting that the gains in survival are attributable to benefits from both preventive and curative medicine.

The goal of proposing a reasonable long-term care program for the United States requires that we consider the twin issues of cost and effectiveness. Much of this volume has, in fact, reviewed the evidence for the efficacy of various approaches. Many have been found wanting. Some of the failures can be attributed to the lack of adequate focus, some to unrealistic expectations. Sometimes the concept of appropriate users is imprecise. These frustrations have encouraged a shift of attention from effectiveness to cost, arguing that if we cannot make a difference, we might as well do it as cheaply as possible. Such a conclusion is shortsighted and misguided. There are findings to suggest that important changes in the way long-term care is delivered can make a difference. Some of these conclusions argue for across-the-board shifts, others for more focus in what we are doing well. Caution must be used in applying such information indiscriminately. An idea that is good under certain conditions may not work in other situations, just as penicillin is useful in treating some infections but is not recommended for heart disease. In considering social solutions we have a tendency to expect panaceas that will work on every occasion.

Nonetheless, there are some things that do work in long-term care. Community care—particularly home health care and homemaking—is consistently preferred over institutional care. Case management offers a means to control the expenses inherent in such care. Geriatric assessment directed toward high-risk groups can be dramatically helpful in altering the trajectory of functionally impaired persons otherwise bound for a nursing home. Nursing home care is sensitive to a wide variety of interventions, all of which improve the morale and often the functioning of residents.

FINANCING

Concern about the cost of long-term care has become so dominant that we tend to ask first, "Can we afford it?" before we decide whether it is worth buying. Over and over again, concepts have been tested to see if they will save money, when the prior issue should be whether they can improve a rather sorry situation. While there is justifiable concern over the dangers of runaway spending, first of all we need to buy something worthy. The continual obsession with cost suggests that we do not value what we have enough to pay the price and are so unsure about what we do want that we are unwilling to invest the money for it.

Nonetheless, we cannot totally avoid a discussion about the costs of long-term care. A number of creative schemes have been proposed for both private and public financing, ranging from tax-sheltered saving mechanisms (Anlyan and Lipscomb, 1985) to a lottery (Fullarton, 1981). In all these proposals, the policy analysts tend to use a dual accounting system in which public costs are totaled differently from private ones. Somehow private expenditures are seen as preferable, as though real money could be saved by shifting the burden. Such a distinction is essentially a fraud. The concern should lie with the money spent and the service purchased, not with the source of the funds. The dichotomy has been used essentially to serve a useful political purpose. The cure for public spending is thus defined as private charging. A private marketplace uses consumers' willingness to pay as the test of quality. Publicly financed services lack such a litmus test. They must rely on an external measure. The contrast helps to avoid the real problem. In truth, neither private nor public dollars can buy good long-term care in most parts of the United States. Although long-term care may indeed be underfinanced, the problem is not simply one of money.

Privately purchased long-term care insurance offers a means to tap private purses but not necessarily a way to get to the root of the problem. From a quality perspective, the private insurance policies generally proposed would not improve the delivery of long-term care. From a financing perspective, the rationale for insurance is to distribute the risks. Long-term care affects about a fifth of the elderly at present (the rate rises with age) and probably about half sometime before they die. For a subset of those needing care, the costs will be catastrophic, but others will have shorter courses with concomitantly lower costs. The risk can be quantified for large groups, although there are clear advantages to selling to those at least risk. If the goal of insurance is distributing the risk burden, the principle of universal coverage makes the most sense. Universal coverage seems to be most efficiently accomplished by some form of public financing even if the dollars are collected as part of a special tax, which may be called an insurance premium. Competitively marketed private insurance programs are more likely to spend their efforts reaching out to the most desirable markets. A little over twenty years ago that very behavior with regard to selling health insurance led to the passage of Medicare.

Any discussion of financing long-term care cannot be usefully pursued independent of similar concerns about financing acute care. The two are inextricably linked and mutually dependent. Model universal long-term care programs in Canada, for example, were added to an existing system of universal entitlement for medical care (Kane and Kane, 1985). In this country we probably cannot afford to wait for a program of universal national health insurance to diffuse the costs of long-term care. Moreover, an effective solution to long-term care financing for the elderly is unlikely unless we merge its funding with the program designed to cover the health costs for that group, namely Medicare.

Indeed, several prominent authors have recommended some form of expanded Medicare coverage to include long-term care, although the compromises they propose to generate the dollars required may impose unpalatable constraints on existing coverage for the elderly. Somers (1982) has urged that the expansion be exchanged for reductions in Social Security coverage. Davis and Rowland (1986) propose a voluntary insurance mechanism with a limited period of eligibility in exchange for heavier Medicare deductibles and copayments. The Harvard Group (Blumenthal et al., 1986) proposes a similar arrangement. Ball (1986) has urged much broader coverage but with considerable user fees for long-term care, such as a daily rent for those in facilities to cover the housing component (a variant of the Canadian arrangement).

DISTRIBUTION ISSUES

Rationing

Even under an optimistic demographic scenario, the burgeoning older population, with its increasing prevalence of disability, means that resources will be insufficient to purchase all the care that might be useful or desirable. Some system is needed to allocate care. We do not always stop to consider that the prevalent form of rationing in the United States has relied on ability to pay. Universal public coverage would represent a much needed rejection of that strategy, but it does not obviate the need to offer an alternative. The positive approach to assuring that the dollars and services reach those most likely to benefit is commonly referred to as targeting. The other strategy, involving the introduction of mechanisms to control and limit the use of services and the concomitant expenditures, is usually termed rationing. The current enthusiasm for capitated care will serve only to push back the responsibility for rationing to a local provider. The demand for some form of resource constraint will continue.

The United States is virtually unique in its inability to mount an organized approach to the care of the elderly. This does not mean that there is no care or that the care is inferior to that rendered elsewhere, but it is fragmented. Some people get a lot and some very little. There is no mechanism to assure that the distribution is appropriate to the relative needs of users. We have come to accept the idea that the supply of social and medical services is not limitless, but it is by no means clear how to ration care. The first battle is against blatant ageism.

Age is an easy basis for rationing health care. It is easy to determine and cheap to administer. It fits a stereotype that devalues the years remaining to the very old, maintaining that they have already had a fair share of life's opportunities. However, it is a misplaced prejudice that cannot go unchallenged. Its overall simplicity is at once its attraction and its curse. Gerontological evidence emphasizes the increased variability with age. It follows then that age is a poor predictor of function for any individual and hence a poor basis for any decision about the ultimate value of an investment in care. Aaron and Schwartz (1984) have described health care systems in other countries that appear to disenfranchise the elderly simply because they are old, limiting access to technologically sophisticated and expensive health services solely on the basis of age. On the other hand, in the United States eligibility for long-term care services and pensions is usually based on attaining a certain age, leading to a concern expressed in some quarters that too many social supports are provided to the elderly at the expense of other dependent groups in the population, especially children.

If we discard age as a basis for rationing, what is the appropriate basis? We argue that the place to begin is not with the recipient but with the service. If we are determined to cut back, why not reduce our investments in those activities that are least efficacious? Such an idea has a great appeal. The difficulty lies in measuring the efficacy. Especially in the case of social programs, the goals must be clearly identified and the multiple objectives specified in a manner that will permit trading off one against another. However, we need not wait until some mysterious time in the future when all the details have been worked out. We have enough information at hand to begin, even if the data are rudimentary and heavily dependent on professional judgment. Techniques are available to tap such opinion in a systematic way to ascertain those activities that appear to be least productive. If we are going to cut back, we should begin with those. Provisions can be made to reintroduce these in the context of controlled trials where their efficacy can be tested.

Certainly caution must be exercised in deciding upon the appropriate rules of evidence. There is a natural tendency to apply stringent standards to an item under examination, especially when it is proposed as a replacement or competitor for an approach already in active use. Thus a number of demonstration projects have been mounted to test the effectiveness of long-term care proposals, while much of medical care is based on untested but commonly accepted practice. We are in some danger of applying a dual standard. If the Institute of Medicine (1985) is correct in estimating that only a small proportion of health care is based on well-documented tests of efficacy, how stringent should the rules of evidence for long-term care be?

Especially in the case of long-term care, it is often very difficult to establish just which programs are effective and to develop measures for comparisons across widely disparate effects. One would not want to have to argue for decisions based solely on the evidence of absolute improvement. It might be more appropriate to consider some measure of relative benefit, compared to those not receiving the care in question.

Targeting

Many would undoubtedly argue that all this talk of rationing is unnecessary without stronger evidence that we have in fact exceeded our capacity to provide services. They would prefer instead to target services more effectively, directing them only toward those who will be helped in a significant way. Our current knowledge about risk factors permits a good discussion about the likelihood of events in general populations but far less precision about the risks assignable to a given person. We can make general statements about the increasing probability of dire events but cannot predict nearly as well for individuals. Thus the data available from current research permit statements about the relative risk of events associated with specific conditions but do not allow very accurate predictions about how these factors affect a given client. More work is needed to develop better predictive models.

The heart of any system of distribution is a gatekeeper who can control the flow of resources. The United States health sector has no system of primary care whereby each individual is the unique responsibility of an identified primary care provider. To a limited extent organized care programs like the HMOs provide such a situation, but these organizations rely on marketing to attract their clients and thus neither assure complete coverage of a population nor provide services on the basis of need.

In a socially oriented program, the gatekeeper role is filled by a case manager or care coordinator. A socially oriented case manager may potentially duplicate the effort of a primary health care provider, but the compelling argument favors the case manager. Despite difficulty in promoting the necessary medical resources and attention, case managers will likely be more responsive to social problems and better able to mobilize the relevant community services. A long-term care program appropriately directed by social services professionals will need close working support from medical care providers. Long-term care cannot afford the artificial dichotomy between the so-called medical and social models of care. Any successful models of care have been able to obtain the cooperation of the relevant medical care providers.

Although the lackluster results of the Long-term Care Channeling Demonstration have undoubtedly dampened the enthusiasm for case management somewhat, there is still a basis for optimism about its place in any comprehensive long-term care strategy. As we tried to show in Chapter 10, Channeling did not test case management per se. It is thus not an appropriate basis for an indictment. Indeed one can hardly conceive of a comprehensive long-term care program without some mechanism to monitor utilization to protect both consumers and payors.

Planning for long-term care requires a distinction between persons moderately or severely cognitively impaired and those largely cognitively intact. The latter have a right to strong opinions about their preferences for place and type of care, a right to take risks for themselves, and a right to reject imposed solutions, however benevolent. The former deserve kind and capable attention, but surely a measure of paternalism is justified for a group who cannot express opinions, implement a plan for their own survival, or even recognize where or who they are. Furthermore, we do a disservice to the mentally alert elderly by grouping their fate together with persons who are demented, and we do a disservice to family members by developing policies that exert strong pressure on them to continue caring for cognitively impaired relatives against their wishes. If we accept the principle of a separate approach to the mentally intact and the moderately or severely demented, however, we must then ensure that the assessment technology and the opportunities to use it are in place so that improper categorizations are avoided.

Reallocations from Acute Care

Acute hospital care consumes by far the largest share of the health dollar. Despite two decades of emphasis on how money saved from nursing homes might be redeployed to home care, the fairer question might be how to divert money from acute hospital care to all forms of long-term care. In the meantime, actions taken to control costs of hospitals negatively affect the frail elderly, sending them out of hospitals in frailer conditions and encouraging precipitously planned long-term care arrangements. The brevity of typical hospitalizations also leads to renewed emphasis on subacute care, or hospital aftercare. Whether this is viewed as a legitimate part of long-term care (and funded accordingly) or as part of acute care, it needs careful attention. Post-hospital rehabilitation and monitoring are critical for preservation of functioning, and functional need, in turn, dictates long-term care needs.

Conversely, better long-term care can reduce demands for hospital care. Improved attention to primary care in the nursing home and in the community as part of an organized long-term care effort can reduce hospital admissions. The potential for mutual benefits and cost savings is significantly impeded by a shortsightedness of funding. Even when the same fund stands to gain (as is the case with Medicare, where improved primary care covered under Part B might save more expensive hospital costs covered under Part A), the questions seem to be put more narrowly. Moreover, the artificial separation of acute care and long-term care has provided too easy an excuse for physicians to neglect the needs of long-term care recipients whether they live at home or in the nursing home.

One potential source of long-term care resources is the acute care dollar. In a context of resource constraint, it is appealing to seek opportunities to transfer resources laterally. The size of the acute care budget dwarfs that for long-term care. Moreover, the unit costs for social services are usually quite a bit less than those for acute care.

In fact, the lower price of social services may contribute to the misallocation. The ease of effecting such a shift is threatened by the growing appeal of acute care technology. As the cost of acute services increases, the pressure grows to pour more public resources into very expensive acute care. The more dramatic the claim for intervention, the stronger its appeal. In a political contest, it is practically quite difficult to wrest resources from the acute care sector to bolster long-term care. Thus proposals to merge the two components into a single system may represent more of a threat than an advantage, unless meticulous provisions are made to protect the long-term care interests. Certainly if the combined system is placed under the control of medical authorities, long-term care is even more likely to be slighted.

On the other hand, a long-term care system that can gain access to some of the acute care pool of resources without relinquishing control may be able to reshape the delivery system for the disabled elderly. Examples of such a reorientation can be seen in several Canadian provinces (Kane and Kane, 1985). In Manitoba and British Columbia the long-term care programs are run by provincial units based in the social services sector, but much of the funding comes from universal health insurance funds that represent a mixture of federal and provincial dollars. Formal medical services from providers like hospitals and physicians are not part of the long-term care program but are readily accessible under the universal health care benefits. At the provincial level there are opportunities for resource shifting, by controlling the flow of support into acute and long-term care.

INFORMAL CARE

Over and over again the refrain is repeated, but necessarily so: The heart of long-term care has been and will continue to be the family. Any system of long-term care must strive to recruit and retain family involvement without family exploitation. This is often a narrow line to walk. At the very least one wants to remove any disincentives to family participation in care. Thus, a system of Medicaid eligibility that penalizes the spouse caring for an older person at home is a shortsighted regulation. Careful thought must go into the process for determining assets in order not to create an incentive for family members to place relatives in institutions.

At the same time, one wants to direct resources to support family. The care is probably best given when it is offered as a partnership between the family and society. Some services are most appropriately targeted at the caregiver. Relatives of persons with Alzheimer's disease, for example, often need respite and support to handle the care burdens. Such respite can come in the form of day care or home care.

Questions are unresolved about what society should require of families or even, for that matter, of spouses. Can an equitable long-term care policy be developed with family care as the centerpiece? What, if any, negative consequences arise from the de facto demands already made of family members? Do these differ for spouses compared to adult children? We need more information about the immediate consequences of both carrot and stick policies, but we also need more careful reflection on how such policies may influence our social fabric. Are we truly prepared to reduce our social arrangements in families to a series of contractual obligations and duties?

The concern for supporting families is not incompatible with concern about possible excessive use of services in lieu of families' meeting their obligations. Some seem to fear that too generous a program of benefits could lead to excessive use, with families shirking their basic responsibilities. Certainly public benefits should be designed to meet needs decently but not luxuriously, if a program is to use a threshold that is affordable. The real dangers of excessive use seem exaggerated in the presence of a monitoring approach like case management, especially since virtually all studies to date indicate that the elderly rarely abuse their benefits; more often they are hesitant to take advantage of them. Families may alter the kinds of care and attention they provide, but these changes usually relieve them of inappropriate or excessive tasks.

HUMANE CARE

Perhaps the greatest challenge of all is to temper our passion for cost-effectiveness with a continuing concern about the purpose of the effort. The overriding goal of any long-term care program is to provide the necessary care in a humane fashion, respecting the preferences and dignity of the recipients. The ultimate test of such care is whether it is indeed decent. Is it the sort of care one would want for oneself or one's parents? Does the service come with so many strictures that more is taken away (in terms of dignity and freedom) than is given?

The emphasis on developing adequate long-term care for the elderly in their own homes does not expiate the need to continue to improve institutional care dramatically. In residential settings the distinction between care and environment is blurred. The setting is both the background and the intervention. The way things are done may be as important as which things are done. The concern and compassion of the staff may be as important as their technical expertise. These traits are not easy to monitor and often not easy to reward. They are perhaps best acknowledged in terms of the effects they produce, but the difficulty of measurement does not lessen their importance. In an era where staff look for direct response to their performance, explicit expectations and rewards are important components of a care system. Such rewards must be designed to encourage and reinforce humane care.

TOWARD SOLUTIONS

It is always easier to identify problems than to suggest solutions for them. However, some general observations can serve in lieu of easy answers to the difficult challenges posed by long-term care. The first and most obvious, but often overlooked, principle is that the solutions will very likely vary from situation to situation. No single approach to as varied and complex an undertaking can be expected to fit all the settings. As a corollary, the principle of equity must be interpreted to mean that care should be equally available, although its specific form may vary. This issue has been of great concern in the United States. The Medicaid program has been frequently cited as producing very different services in the different states. In fact, even the Medicare program, which presumably operates from a common set of national guidelines, emerges as a varied program depending on the intermediaries interpreting those guidelines.

The inability to dictate a specific system that will work in all situations makes local control a necessity. Even a cursory examination of long-term care programs in countries with better-developed systems of care confirms this need. In each country, most of which are far smaller and more homogeneous than the United States, the programs are operated by local units with varying degrees of centrally developed guidelines. In most countries this control is vested in organizations with defined geopolitical areas of responsibility. These catchment areas provide a mechanism for accountability. Certainly an important principle is that the responsibility and the authority should coincide.

Long-Term Care Needs Creative Reconfiguration

A topic so fundamental to life in later years should not be constrained by the categories of current programs, especially considering that current configurations of delivery and financing are fragmented, arbitrary, and sometimes responses to unplanned consequences of decisions made in other program sectors. Eligibility in one service sector should not foreclose options in another; we should broaden our thinking to encompass new possibilities to meet service needs better. This may require reconsideration of the concepts of housing, home care, and nursing home care to produce fresh configurations.

The more we can identify the goals we seek to achieve in a long-term care system and can specify the outcomes sought, the more leeway that can be permitted for creative solutions in individual cases. If long-term care is to move forward, it must rid itself of professional blinders. We continue to urge multidisciplinary approaches, but often this simply means that each discipline lobbies for its own stature. More opportunities for hybridization may be an answer. Certainly more thinking outside traditional compartments is vital. We must ask how professional long-term care services should be? We also must decide the extent to which we are dealing with a social service, a health service, or some composite.

Nursing Homes Belong on Continuum of Community Care

Long-term care involves care in the community and care in facilities, however the latter is designed. It is unfortunate that so much energy has been devoted to finding "alternatives to nursing home care," rather than to the developing a well-differentiated spectrum of services with facility care available in reserve when community care is impractical. Moreover, an effective long-term care system requires improvement of facility care itself, and this reform is thwarted if each nursing home admission is viewed as a failure calling for redoubled efforts on behalf of those still in the community. Nursing homes should not be viewed as being the end of the line; many thousands of people go on to live for years in nursing homes and deserve the opportunity for lives as full as possible. In fact, nursing home residents live in larger communities (cities and counties) and should be able to benefit from programs designed for the elderly or handicapped (for example, transportation, recreation, education, or volunteer opportunities).

Capitation

Fixed areas of assigned responsibility run counter to the more laissez-faire approach generally preferred in this country. Capitation appears compatible with the American philosophy and is still capable of offering flexibility together with overall direction. We use the term "capitation" here in a very general sense to refer to a method of paying for care in which the provider is paid a fixed amount per person enrolled (although not necessarily the same amount for each person) in exchange for an obligation to provide a fixed package of services as they are required. As such, the principle of capitation could be applied under the Medicare program, and indeed it is as part of the HMO benefit allowed by recent changes in the regulations.

Capitated programs then can be operated by private firms, which compete for market shares, or they can be run by governmentally sanctioned bodies that serve designated areas as monopoly utilities. Each approach presents advantages and disadvantages. For example, competition is believed by some to promote better service, but it may also rely on misleading advertising or other strategies to selectively recruit the most desirable members. A utility, on the other hand, does not have a choice about whom to serve, but neither does the consumer then have a choice about which program to join.

There is little doubt that the capitation approach is politically attractive. It moves responsibility away from the government and gives the task of making hard decisions about resource allocation to a separate group. At the same time, it permits the central government to limit its fiscal responsibility by setting a fixed overall price per person enrolled.

Although capitated care offers some very attractive advantages in terms of the flexibility it enables, this same flexibility provides the means for consumer exploitation. In a system of competing markets, the consumer does not really enjoy the protections that the advocates of free markets might assume. The older consumer is not likely or able to vote with his feet, especially if he or she is frail. To the contrary, the consumer who seeks to obtain more service than the plan is prepared to provide may be perceived as an undesirable customer, one the plan is only too happy to see depart. Nor is he likely to find more service at another plan if that plan can recruit someone else who will make fewer demands at the same capitated rate. In contrast, the plan that is held accountable for the status of all persons in a defined region is more likely to provide those services it believes will make a difference; and if the outcomes included in the accountability include consumer satisfaction, it may extend that definition to include many items of customer preference.

Assuring quality has been, and will continue to be, one of the most vexing problems in long-term care. Under the proposed capitated approach, quality is most appropriately measured in terms of population-based outcomes. The primary issue is the change in status for groups of persons, where status includes a broad range of concerns: physical, cognitive, social, and emotional functioning as well as satisfaction. Providers are held accountable for their performance across groups with appropriate correction for case mix. In essence, quality is reflected in one's batting average rather than measured with each swing of the bat, but the system also recognizes the need to adjust the measures of outcomes to accommodate the differences among clients. This sort of epidemiological approach to quality assurance is most feasible when the responsibility for care is based on populations, not selected individuals.

A group-wide approach does not vitiate, but in fact increases, the need for vigorous attention to individual expressions of dissatisfaction. Complaints from clients must be quickly attended and investigated. Because the laws of average mean that most things will usually go well most of the time, a separate mechanism is needed to identify the problem areas as quickly as possible. Averages alone will not suffice. Nor will averaging measures adequately address the important issues of humane care and ambiance.

Uniting Acute and Long-Term Care

By now it should be clear that long-term care cannot be readily disaggregated from acute care, at least for the set of acute care patients who are also long-term care users. Efforts to maintain the separation of funding seem doomed to perpetuate the inherent inefficiencies and inequities. Such a discussion is virtually unique to the United States, because most other countries begin from a system of universally covered acute health care. Above all, we need such a system in this country as well. Ironically, long-term care will be better served by universally available hospital and medical care. Once this is accomplished, appropriate attention can be directed to the multiple problems of how to coordinate the two systems. It is obvious that such interfacing is poorly served by a funding approach that puts acute care and long-term care in different streams. From the vantage point of long-term care, the principal goal should be adequate provision of social support services for those persons dependent on them and easy access to medical services needed to complement these supports or to respond to specific medical problems.

Because a number of long-term conditions are medically derived, the first and paramount question to be asked in any plan of care is, "Is this trip necessary?" There is no virtue in providing even the most humane care for a condition that is avoidable or correctable. Thus careful and competent medical attention is necessary, particularly at the outset, but it is not sufficient. The price for playing should not be owning the bat and ball. Medicine should not be allowed to dominate the game.

At an organizational level, there is a strong argument for some means of pooling funds. But here too the pooling must recognize the potential dangers of domination by the acute care sector. The size of the medical enterprise and its high unit costs equip it poorly to be a primary sponsor of a form of care that generally relies on minimally trained help working with modest technology. One would like to tap into the rich resource pool of medical services as a source of support to finance at least part of the growth of long-term care, but such transfers need to be made at a sufficient distance to allow dispassionate judgments on policy rather than on specific cases, when it will be virtually impossible to deny technology.

Similarly, the currently allocated dollars, which are provided in multiple funding streams from federal and state sources, would be more efficiently used if these streams could be pooled. At present each has its own rules of eligibility and areas of coverage. A patchwork of services and frequent gaps are the inevitable result of such an approach. Even more disservice is created by the perverse incentives promoted by the separation. Care financed from one source is not pursued if the subsequent savings are likely to accrue to another. Tasks are undertaken because they are covered rather than because they are most pressing. Many working in the field complain about spending more time and effort working with and around the systems than serving the clients. Duplication of effort and funding occurs both inadvertently and deliberately under such a regime. All of this argues persuasively that pooled funds will result in greater efficiencies.

Family Care

The family remains the cornerstone of long-term care. The goal of any program is to preserve its strength while distributing the burden of support. There is a natural temptation to acknowledge the family's central role by assigning responsibility for care on the basis of available support. Indeed one of the recurrent observations in long-term care is the importance of family support in avoiding or postponing institutionalization. However, the existence of family support should *not* cause an older person to lose eligibility for services. Nor should we conclude that the proper response to some families' failure to provide such care is to make family care compulsory. In countries with more experience with community long-term care, family care is recognized as a resource to be cultivated. As with agriculture, the harvest is greater if the soil is well tilled and fertilized. Clients with family willing and able to provide services may receive their aliquot of formal care in more indirect means, through services targeted at the supporters. Different situations will require different solutions. In some cases respite care will most effectively maintain the support. In others direct services to the caregivers in the form of support groups, therapy, or specific care may be the appropriate response.

Public policy must not penalize an elderly person because of the actions of his/her family. It would be inefficient and inhumane to deny services to someone whose family was unwilling to bear part of the burden. It is, in effect, a case of double jeopardy. In a similar vein, an equitable social policy should neither reward nor penalize older persons on the basis of the existence of a family. Practical problems come easily to mind. What is a family? Do in-laws count? Former in-laws? Do jobs, competing responsibilities, income, and place of residence matter? Should public policy assign responsibility among the relatives? Should a known abusive family be expected to provide care? These examples readily demonstrate the complexities of developing a workable, to say nothing about equitable, policy for family responsibility. The decision to provide services is more reasonably based on the client's needs and preferences. The availability and nature of family support inevitably influence the nature and type of services but not the primary decision about eligibility.

Community Care

Community care is needed! Too often this topic has been approached with the expectation that such care will substitute for institutional care. The evidence presented here and elsewhere rather clearly demonstrates that such is generally not the case. The home is the preferred site of care for many clients. Community care should be conceived as a natural response to the need for support. It is a resource in its own right, not an alternative form of care. If anything, the institution should be considered the alternative to the community, to be used when community care is no longer feasible.

Because community care can be provided in small units of service, and because it is more desired than institutional care, some policy-makers have expressed concern that granting access to such care will lead to excessive demand. Part of this misperception is based on a failure to appreciate that such care need not be given on an all-or-nothing basis. The important question is not whether or not to give community care, but rather how much to give. Again drawing upon the experience of other countries, we find that most of the efforts at controlling utilization are not directed at determining initial eligibility but at assessing the degree of impairment. Usually the initial request for assistance will be covered with a rudimentary screening to assure that the help sought is generally appropriate. Sometimes basic information is needed about which types of services are and are not provided. For a substantial group of clients, a modest package of services will suffice, and attention can be directed to the smaller subgroup who need more intensive case management and ongoing assistance.

Personnel

Long-term care is labor-intensive. People represent the major resource and the major cost of long-term care programs. Most of those people are relatively unskilled. The pool from which personnel are recruited varies from place to place. In much of the United States, and indeed in several European countries, the system relies on those at the bottom of the social scale for most of long-term care. Thus, the frail elderly depend on those with minimal education, many of whom are immigrants with poor language skills and very often of different cultural backgrounds from their clients. In the case of community care, nonprofessional caregivers are placed in situations of tremendous responsibility. They may be the only contact for vulnerable persons who are otherwise isolated and thus in danger of exploitation. A major challenge to long-term care is the need to evolve some system of accountability for the quality of community care.

Any response to the problem of assuring quality seems inevitably linked to increased costs. It is easy to visualize a complex system of supervision in which the relatively low-paid providers of most of the care are overseen by professionals. Indeed such is the case in much of contemporary home nursing. An even more direct attack on the problem may be found in paying higher wages to those delivering the basic services. Better pay should attract better workers, although this relationship is far from well established. More investment might be made in the selection, orientation, and ongoing training of such workers. At present very little attention is paid to any of these facets. More efforts might be devoted to offering a wider range of rewards for performance; unique contributions could include such approaches as differential pay scales, special bonuses, increased participation in decisions, and opportunities for career advancement. All of these are contingent of course on having some mechanism for detecting both positive and negative performance.

Another tack involves efforts to tap new pools of workers. A great deal of enthusiasm has been expressed about the desirability of using volunteers. Obviously one strong appeal is their modest cost, but the indirect costs need to be considered along with the direct costs. Long-term care is just that—long-term. It must be reliable and sustained. Many of the tasks involve basic care with substantial amounts of manual labor and unpleasant work. Often the clients are not communicative and, if expressive, may not show gratitude. These are hardly the conditions to attract a corps of volunteers. Indeed the costs of maintaining volunteers are too often overlooked. They need supervision, encouragement, satisfaction, recognition, and engagement. In some instances people may be willing to provide menial services to strangers, but it remains to be proven whether such care can form the backbone of a system of long-term care.

One variation on the volunteer theme has been the idea of work credits. Essentially, this approach relies on a form of nonmonetary currency whereby credits are accrued that are later redeemable for similar or equivalent services. Aside from the bookkeeping problems, this sort of bartering approach dramatically changes the nature of the voluntary social contract. The same problems that haunted the original dilemma pertain here. The absence of money will not obviate the need for supervision and incentives.

New Forms of Service

One prediction about long-term care seems safe—it will not look the same in the future. Any discussion about new directions needs to recognize the opportunity to find new ways to package services. One of the most fruitful places to look for new modes of care is in the nursing home. Nursing homes per se are not destined to last. The paradigm of separate approaches to community-based care and institutionally delivered services should give way to a synthesis in which elements of both are combined. Clearly for some long-term care clients, supervision and shelter are essential components of a service package. But these need not be combined into what we currently know as a nursing home. It should be possible to separate the functions and thereby gain more degrees of freedom.

For example, a corporation operating a housing program might contract for nursing services, in essence combining sheltered housing and home nursing. Such an arrangement would permit greater flexibility in organizing services. It would allow a clearer distinction between the primary goal of providing a supportive living situation and the secondary role of providing medical services as needed. By combining services in this way, providers may be more able to avoid the regulatory pressures that push for a uniform management of all clients.

The flexibility facilitated under these arrangements offers advantages at the risk of exploitation. As we move to more creative ways of combining services, the pressure intensifies for developing better methods of accountability. More freedom can be allowed in terms of structure and process when providers are held accountable for the outcomes of their care. The goal of long-term care should indeed be care in the least restrictive environment. The protection of consumers and payors comes from a system of responsibility for achieving defined outcomes, identified as reasonable expectations of what good care can produce.

The links between specific interventions and outcomes do not support a clear prescription about precisely what to do in a given situation. Instead the evidence argues for encouraging flexibility and creativity of approach, while pushing for accountability of results. The expectations for the results should be realistic; that is, they should be derived from empirical data that indicate the art of the possible. The incentives should be directed toward achieving these ends. Premature closure on orthodoxies should be avoided. Of course, an outcome-based approach cannot be used as an excuse to violate civil rights or basic human dignity.

Long-term care has been too long viewed as a static phenomenon with fixed approaches. The expectation for clients has been for unchanging courses. The error in this area is matched by a similar failure to appreciate the dynamic nature of the problem. Clients move in and out of the system. They get better and worse. So too should the system change as new opportunities emerge and as changes occur in the nature of the clients served. It is naive to think that the future will bring the same, only more of it. Planners for long-term care must position themselves and their programs to respond in creative ways to meet the daily needs of persons with functional impairment.

CONCLUDING COMMENT

In our discussions of long-term care we work from the abstract notion of a care system treating hypothetical persons. In the end, the true test of our ideas is how they work in reality. Despite the difficulty in defining it, long-term care is known when it is given and missed when it is not. It comes down to someone answering the call button, the difference between friendly assistance and sullen attention. Long-term care is born out of dependency. It is best provided when it is offered by persons who believe in what they are doing and take pride and pleasure in helping others. These are not necessarily traits derived from training. Nor are they likely to be found by shopping for the lowest bidder. If we are going to truly improve long-term care in this country, we must be prepared to invest in it. The real question is not whether we are willing to pay more for better care but how care can be made better. Long-term care comes down to people caring for people. Whatever we may think of corporations and institutions, the success of any reform in this area will depend on the ability to populate the caring cadres with persons who are motivated to help others. Their performance will be measured not by major analyses but by very small events—Is there someone there when I call? Do they make me feel like a person? Can I maintain my dignity and self-respect? These are the issues by which our measure will be taken.

References

Aaron, HJ & WB Schwartz. *The Painful Prescription: Rationing Hospital Care.* Washington, DC: Brookings Institution, 1984.

ACTION. *Descriptive Evaluation of RSVP and FGP Volunteers Working with Head Start: Final Report.* Washington, DC: Office of Policy and Planning Evaluation Division, 1984a.

ACTION. *The Effect of Foster Grandparents on Juvenile Offenders in Georgia Youth Development Centers.* Washington, DC: Office of Policy and Planning Evaluation Division, 1984b.

ACTION. *Impact Evaluation of the Foster Grandparent Program on the Foster Grandparents: Final Report.* Washington, DC: Litigation Support Services, 1984c.

ACTION. *National Retired Senior Volunteer Program Participant Impact Evaluation. Final Report.* Bethesda, MD: Booz, Allen, and Hamilton, Inc., 1985a.

ACTION. *Senior Companion Program Impact Evaluation: Final Report.* Alexandria, VA: SRA Technologies, Inc., 1985b.

Aiken, LH, MD Mezey, JE Lynaugh & CR Buck, Jr. Teaching Nursing Homes: Prospects For Improving Long-Term Care. *Journal of the American Geriatrics Society,* 33: 196-201, 1985.

Allan, C & H Brotman. *Chartbook on Aging in America.* Washington, DC: The White House Conference, 1981.

Allen, CM, PM Becker, LJ McVey, C Saltz, JR Feussner & HJ Cohen. A Randomized Controlled Clinical Trial of a Geriatric Consultation Team: Compliance with Recommendations. *Journal of the American Medical Association,* 255: 2617-2621, 1986.

American Association of Retired Persons. *Long-Term Care Survey.* Washington, DC: American Association of Retired Persons, 1984.

American Board of Family Practice. *Rights and Responsibilities. A National Survey of Healthcare Opinions,* Lexington, KY: The American Book of Family Pratice, 1985.

Amerman, E. The Nurse/Social Worker Dyad in Community-Based Long-Term Care. In Austin, CD, J Low, EA Roberts & K O'Connor (eds.), *Case Management: A Critical Review.* Seattle: Pacific Northwest Long-Term Care Gerontology Center, University of Washington, 1985.

Amerman, E, D Eisenberg & R Weisman. Case Management and Counseling: A Service Dilemma. In Austin, CD, J Low, EA Roberts & K O'Connor (eds.), *Case*

Management: A Critical Review. Seattle: Pacific Northwest Long-Term Care Gerontology Center, University of Washington, 1985.

Anderson, NN, SK Patten & JN Greenberg. *A Comparison of Home Care and Nursing Home Care for Older Persons in Minnesota. Volume III—Summary.* Minneapolis: University of Minnesota, 1980.

Anlyan WG, Jr. & J Lipscomb. The National Health Care Trust Plan: A Blueprint for Market and Long-Term Care Reform. *Health Affairs,* 4: 5-31, 1985.

Ansak, M & R Zawadski. On Lok CCODA: A Consolidated Model. In Zawadski, R (ed.), *Community-Based Systems of Long-Term Care,* (147–194), New York: Haworth, 1984.

Applebaum, R, M Harrigan & P Kemper. *The Evaluation of the National Long-Term Care Demonstration: Tables Comparing Channeling to Other Community Demonstrations.* Princeton, NJ: Mathematica Policy Research, Inc., 1986.

Applegate, WB, D Akins, R Vanderzwagg, K Thoni & MG Baker. A Geriatric Rehabilitation and Assessment Unit in a Community Hospital. *Journal of the American Geriatrics Society,* 31: 206-210, 1983.

Arling, G, EB Harkins & M Romaniuk. Adult Day Care and the Nursing Home. The Appropriateness of Care in Alternative Settings. *Research on Aging,* 6: 225-242, 1984.

Arling, G & WJ McAuley. The Feasibility of Public Payments for Family Caregiving. *The Gerontologist,* 23: 300-306, 1983.

Austin, CD. *Improving Access for Elders: The Role of Case Management: Final Report.* Seattle: University of Washington Institute on Aging, 1987.

Austin, CD, J Low, EA Roberts & K O'Connor. *Case Management: A Critical Review.* Seattle: Pacific Northwest Long-Term Care Gerontology Center, University of Washington, 1985.

Baker, M. *A Study of Home Health Care in Arizona.* Tucson: Arizona Long-Term Care Gerontology Center, 1983a.

Baker, M. *The 1982 Sun City Area Long Term Care Survey: A Statistical Profile of Resident Characteristics, Attitudes and Preferences.* Tucson: Arizona Long-Term Care Gerontology Center, 1983b.

Ball, R. *Priority Issues in Long-Term Care and Retirement Income Security in the United States.* Paper presented at the US/Canadian Expert Group Meeting on Policies for Midlife and Older Women (sponsored by the American Association of Retired Persons), Washington, DC, October 1986.

Baltes, MM & MB Zerbe. Independence Training in Nursing-Home Residents. *The Gerontologist,* 16: 428-432, 1976.

Bang, A, JH Morse & EW Campion. Transition of VA Acute Care Hospitals into Acute and Long Term Care. In Wetle, T & JW Rowe (eds.), *Older Veterans: Linking VA and Community Resources* (69-92). Cambridge, MA: Harvard University Press, 1984.

Banziger, G & S Roush. Nursing Homes for the Birds: A Control-Relevant Intervention with Bird Feeders. *The Gerontologist,* 23: 527-531, 1983.

Barker, WH, TF Williams, JG Zimmer, C Van Buren, SJ Vincent & SG Pickrel. Geriatric Consultation Teams in Acute Hospitals: Impact on Back-Up of Elderly Patients. *Journal of the American Geriatrics Society,* 33: 422-428, 1985.

Barney, JL. *Nursing Home Community Councils Project: Final Report.* Ann Arbor, MI: Institute of Gerontology, University of Michigan, 1981.

Barresi, CM & DJ McConnell. *Discriminators of Adult Day Care: Participation Among Impaired Elderly.* Paper presented at the annual meeting of the Gerontology Society of America, San Antonio, TX, November 1984.

Barton, EM, MM Baltes & MJ Orzech. Etiology of Dependence in Older Nursing Home Residents During Morning Care: The Role of Staff Behavior. *Journal of Personality and Social Psychology*, 38: 423-431, 1980.

Bass, D. *Planning to Meet Lifecare Needs*. Washington, DC: National Association of Social Workers, 1986.

Bass, SA & R Rowland. *The Elderly Have Spoken: Is Anybody Listening? The Impact of Fuel Costs on the Elderly*. Boston: Gerontology Program, College of Public and Community Service, the University of Massachusetts/Boston, 1980.

Bass, SA & RH Rowland. *Client Satisfaction of Elderly Homemaker Services—An Evaluation*. Boston: Gerontology Program, College of Public and Community Service, the University of Massachusetts/Boston, 1983.

Becker, PM, LJ McVey, C Saltz, JR Feussner & HJ Cohen. *A Randomized Controlled Clinical Trial of a Geriatric Consultation Team: Impact on Hospital-Acquired Complications*. Durham, NC: Geriatric Research, Education, and Clinical Center, VA Medical Center, 1986.

Beland, F. Who Are Those Most Likely to Be Institutionalized, the Elderly Who Receive Comprehensive Home Care Services or Those Who Do Not? *Social Science & Medicine*, 20: 347-354, 1985.

Bell, WG & JS Revis. *Transportation for Older Americans. Issues and Options for the Decade of the 1980's*. DOT-1-83-42. Washington, DC: Department of Transportation, 1983.

Bennett, RG. *Institutional Innovative Programs Survey. Executive Summary of Final Report*. New York: Columbia University Faculty of Medicine and New York State Office of Mental Health, 1983.

Bennett RG, E Killefer, M Sharron & G Gruer. *Some Issues in Group and Individual Psychotherapy and Psychosocial Programs for the Elderly, 1970-80*. New York: Columbia University Long-Term Care Gerontology Center, mimeo, n.d.

Berger, RM & SD Rose. Interpersonal Skill Training with Institutionalized Elderly Patients. *The Gerontologist*, 32: 346-353, 1977.

Berghorn, FJ & DE Schafer. Reminiscence Intervention in Nursing Homes: What and Who Changes? *International Journal of Aging and Human Development*, 24: 113-127, 1986-87.

Birkel, RC. *Sources of Caregiver Strain in Long-Term Home-Care: Executive Summary*. Grant No. 05002. Washington, DC: National Center for Health Services Research, 1984.

Birnbaum, H, G Gaumer, F Pratter & R Burke. *Nursing Home Without Walls: State Long-Term Home Health Care Program*. Cambridge, MA: Abt Associates, Inc., 1984.

Birnbaum, HG & D Kidder. What Does Hospice Cost? *American Journal of Public Health*, 74: 689-697, 1984.

Bishop, CE, AL Plough & TR Willemain. Nursing Home Levels of Care: Problems and Alternatives. *Health Care Financing Review*, 2: 33-45, 1980.

Blackman, DK, M Howe & EM Pinkston. Increasing Participation in Social Interaction of the Institutionalized Elderly. *The Gerontologist*, 16: 69-76, 1976.

Blenkner, M, M Bloom & M Nielson. A Research Demonstration Project of Protective Services. *Social Casework*, 52: 483, 1971.

Blumenthal, D, M Schlesinger, P Brown Drunheller & Harvard Medicare Project. The Future of Medicare. *New England Journal of Medicine*, 314: 722-728, 1986.

Borup, JH & DT Gallego. Mortality as Affected by Interinstitutional Relocation. Update and Assessment. *The Gerontologist*, 21: 8-16, 1981.

Borup, JH, DT Gallego & PG Heffernan. Relocation and Its Effect on Mortality. *The Gerontologist*, 19: 135-146, 1979.

Borup, JH, DT Gallego & PG Hefferman. Relocation: Its Effect on Health Functioning and Mortality. *The Gerontologist*, 20: 468-479, 1980.

Branch, LG. *Understanding the Health and Social Service Needs of People Over Age 65*. Boston: Center for Survey Research, 1977.

Branch, LG. *Panel Study of Massachusetts Elders: Third Wave, Executive Summary*. Boston: Division on Aging, Harvard Medical School, 1982.

Branch, LG. Relative Risk Rates of Nonmedical Predictors of Institutional Care Among Elderly Persons. *Comprehensive Therapy*, 10: 33-40, 1984.

Branch, LG. Health Practices and Incident Disability Among the Elderly. *American Journal of Public Health*, 75: 1436-1440, 1985.

Branch, LG & AM Jette. The Framingham Disability Study: I. Social Disability Among the Aging. Framingham Disability Study: II. Physical Disability Study Among the Aged. *American Journal of Public Health*, 71: 1202-1212, 1981.

Branch, LG & AM Jette. A Prospective Study of Long Term Care Institutionalization Among the Aged. *American Journal of Public Health*, 72: 1373-79, 1982.

Branch, LG & AM Jette. Elders' Use of Informal Long-Term Care Assistance. *The Gerontologist*, 23: 51-56, 1983.

Branch, LG & AM Jette. Personal Health Practices and Mortality Among the Elderly. *American Journal of Public Health*, 74: 1126-1129, 1984.

Branch, L, S Katz, K Kniepmann & J Papsidero. A Prospective Study of Functional Status Among Community Elders. *American Journal of Public Health*, 74: 266-268, 1984.

Branch, L & K Nemeth. When Elders Fail to Visit Physicians. *Medical Care*, 23: 1256-1275, 1985.

Braun, K & C Rose. The Hawaii Geriatric Foster Care Experiment: Impact Evaluation and Cost Analysis. *The Gerontologist*, 26: 516-523, 1986.

Brickel, CM. Depression in the Nursing Home: A Pilot Study Using Pet-Facilitated Psychotherapy. In Anderson, RK, BL Hart & LA Hart (eds.), *The Pet Connection: Its Influence on Our Health and Quality of Life*. Minneapolis: Center for the Study of Animal-Human Relationships and Environments, 1984.

Brickner, PW, JF Janeski, G Rich, Sister T Duque, L Starita, R LaRocco, T Flannery & S Werlin. Home Maintenance for the Home-Bound Aged. *The Gerontologist*, 16: 25-29, 1976.

Brill, R & A Horowitz. The New York City Home Care Project: A Demonstration of Health and Social Services. In Zawadski, R (ed.), *Community-Based Systems of Long-Term Care*. New York: Haworth Press, 1984.

Brocklehurst JC. *Incontinence in Old People*. Edinburgh, Scotland: Livingstone, 1951.

Brocklehurst, JC, JB Dillane, L Griffiths & J Fry. The Prevalence and Symptomatology of Urinary Infection in Aged Population. *Gerontologia Clinica*, 10: 242, 1968.

Brody, EM. The Aging of the Family. *Annals of the American Academy of Political and Social Science*, 438: 13-27, 1978.

Brody, EM. "Women in the Middle" and Family Help to Older People. *The Gerontologist*, 21: 471-480, 1981.

Brody, EM. Parent Care as a Normative Family Stress. *The Gerontologist*, 25: 19-29, 1985.

Brody, EM & MH Kleban. Physical and Mental Health Symptoms of Older People: Who Do They Tell? *Journal of the American Geriatrics Society*, 24: 442-449, 1981.

Brody, EM, MH Kleban & PT Johnsen. *Women Who Provide Parent Care: Characteristics of Those Who Work and Those Who Do Not*. Paper presented at the annual meeting of the Gerontological Society of America, San Antonio, TX, November 1984.

Brody, EM, MH Kleban & B Liebowitz. Intermediate Housing for the Elderly: Satisfaction of Those Who Moved In and Those Who Did Not. *The Gerontologist,* 15: 350-356, 1975.

Brody, EM, MH Kleban, MS Moss & F Kleban. Predictors of Falls Among Institutionalized Women with Alzheimer's Disease. *Journal of the American Geriatrics Society,* 32: 877-886, 1984.

Brody, EM & CB Schoonover. Patterns of Parent Care When Adult Daughters Work and When They Do Not. *The Gerontologist,* 26: 372-381, 1986.

Brody, SJ & N Persily. *Hospitals and the Aged: The New Old Market.* Rockville, MD: Aspen, 1984.

Brody, SJ, S. Poulshock & C Masciocchi. The Family Caring Unit: A Major Consideration in the Long-Term Support System. *The Gerontologist,* 18: 556-561, 1978.

Brooks, CH & K Smyth-Staruch. Hospice Home Care Cost Savings to Third Party Insurers. *Medical Care,* 8: 691-703, 1984.

Brown, T & RM Learner. The South Carolina Community Long Term Care Project. In Zawadski, R (ed.), *Community-Based Systmes of Long-Term Care* (73-90). New York: Haworth, 1984.

Buford, AD. *Advocacy for the Nursing Home Resident: An Examination of the Ombudsman Function and Its Relationship to Licensing and Certification Activities in Insuring Quality of Care.* Los Angeles: Center for the Public Interest, Inc., 1984.

Bursac, K. *An Analysis of a Nationwide Survey of Respite Care Services.* Tucson: University of Arizona Long Term Gerontology Center, 1983.

Buschman, M & J Sainer. The National Supports Program: A Service Model to Strengthen Families' Care for Their Older Relatives. In Community Service Society of New York, *Strengthening Informal Supports for the Aging* (25-34). New York: Community Service Society of New York, 1981.

Cairl, RE, E Pfeiffer & DM Keller. *The Florida Pre-Nursing Home Assessment Project: A Capsule Summary of Findings, Policy Issues, and Recommendations.* Tampa: Suncoast Gerontology Center, College of Medicine, University of South Florida, 1984.

Callahan, JJ Jr. Elder Abuse Programming: Will it Help the Elderly? *Urban and Social Change Review,* 15: 15-16, 1982.

Callahan, JJ, LD Diamond, JZ Giele & R Morris. Responsibility of Families for Their Severely Disabled Elders. *Health Care Finacing Review,* 1:29-48, 1980.

Cameron, JM. Case Mix and Resource Use in Long-Term Care. *Medical Care,* 23: 296-309, 1985.

Campion, EW, A Jette & B Berkman. An Interdisciplinary Geriatric Consultation Service: A Controlled Trial. *Journal of the American Geriatrics Society,* 31: 792-796, 1983.

Cantor, M. Neighbors and Friends. *Research on Aging,* 1: 434-463, 1979.

Cantor, M. The Extent and Intensity of the Informal Support System Among New York's Inner City Elderly-Is Ethnicity a Factor. In Community Service Society of New York, *Strengthening Informal Supports for the Aging: Theory, Practice, Ond Policy Implications* (1-11). New York: Community Service Society of New York, 1981.

Capitman, JA. *Evaluation of Adult Day Health Care Programs in California.* Sacramento: Office of Long Term Care and Aging, Department of Health Services, 1982.

Capitman, JA. Community-Based Long-Term Care Models, Target Groups, and Impacts on Service Use. *The Gerontologist,* 26: 389-397, 1986.

Capitman, JA, B Haskins & J Bernstein. Case Management Approaches in Community-Oriented Long-Term Care Demonstrations. *The Gerontologist*, 26: 398-404, 1986.

Carcagno, G, R Applebaum, J Christianson, B Phillips, C Thornton & J Will. *The Evaluation of the National Channeling Demonstration: Planning and Operational Experience of the Channeling Projects.* Princeton, NJ: Mathematica Policy Research, Inc., 1986.

Chappell, NL. *An Evaluation of Adult Day Care, Phase I, A Summary.* Winnipeg: Department of Social & Preventive Medicine, University of Manitoba, 1982.

Chappell, NL. *Adult Day Care and Change in the Utilization of Medical and In-Patient Hospital Services, Final Report.* Winnipeg: Centre on Aging, University of Manitoba, 1984.

Chappell, NL. Social Support and the Receipt of Home Care Services. *The Gerontologist*, 25: 47-54, 1985.

Chappell, N & B Havens. Who Helps the Elderly Person: A Discussion of Informal and Formal Care. In Peterson, W and J Quadagho (eds.), *Social Bonds in Later Life.* Beverly Hills: Sage Publications, 1985.

Cheah, K & O Beard. Psychiatric Findings in the Population of a Geriatric Evaluation Unit: Implications. *Journal of the American Geriatrics Society*, 29: 398-401, 1980.

Christensen, B, J Mistarz & J Riffer (eds.). Trends, Home Care Wrap-Up. *Hospitals*, 58: 33-40, 1984.

Cicirelli, V. *Helping Elderly Parents.* Boston: Auburn Publishing Company, 1981.

Clark, MM, JR Corbisiero, ME Procidano & SA Grossman. The Effectiveness of Assertive Training with Elderly Psychiatric Outpatients. *Community Mental Health Journal*, 20: 262-268, 1984.

Clauser, S. Comments on the 222 Adult Day Care and Homemaker Service Experiments. *Home Health Care Services Quarterly*, 1: 103-106, 1980.

Cohen, RG. Team Service To The Elderly. *Social Casework: The Journal of Contemporary Social Work*, 64: 555-560, 1983.

Cohen, S. *Adult Residential Day Care.* Boise, ID: Mountain States Health Corporation, 1984.

Colen, JN & DL Soto. *Service Delivery to Aged Minorities: Techniques of Successful Programs.* Sacramento: California State University School of Social Work, 1979.

Colvez, A & M Blanchet. Disability Trends in the United States Population 1966-76: Analysis of Reported Causes. *American Journal of Public Health*, 71: 464-471, 1981.

Community Council of Greater New York. *Dependency in the Elderly of New York City.* New York: Community Council of Greater New York, 1978.

Community Service Society of New York. *Strengthening Informal Supports for the Aging: Theory, Practice, and Policy Implications.* New York: Community Service Society of New York, 1981.

Cornoni-Huntley, JC, DJ Foley, LR White, R Suzman, LF Berkman, DA Evans & RB Wallace. Epidemiology of Disability in the Oldest Old: Methodologic Issues and Preliminary Findings. *Health and Society*, 63: 350-376, 1985.

Cross, P & B Gurland. *The Epidemiology of Dementing Disorders.* A report on work performed for and submitted to the U.S. Congress, Office of Technology Assessment, Washington, DC, draft, 1985.

Crossman, L, C London & C Barry. Older Women Caring for Disabled Spouses: A Model for Supportive Services. *The Gerontologist*, 21:464-470, 1981.

Cummings, V, JF Kerner, S Arones & C Seinbock. *An Evaluation of a Day Hospital*

Service in Rehabilitation Medicine. Washington, DC: National Center for Health Services Research, 1980.

Currie, CT, JT Moore, SW Friedman, & GA Warshaw. Assessment of Elderly Patients at Home: A Report of Fifty Cases. *Journal of the American Geriatrics Society,* 29: 398-401, 1981.

Daiches, S. *Protective Services Risk Assessment Guide (PRS): Version II.* New York: Human Resources Administration of the City of New York, 1984.

Davis, J, M Shapiro & RL Kane. Level of Care and Complications Among Geriatric Patients Discharged from the Medical Service of a Teaching Hospital. *Journal of the American Geriatrics Society,* 32: 427-430, 1984.

Davis, K & D Rowland. *Medicare Policy, New Directions for Health and Long-Term Care.* Baltimore: The Johns Hopkins University Press, 1986.

Day-Lower, D, D Bryant & JW Mullaney. *National Policy Workshop on Shared Housing. Findings & Recommendations.* HUD-0003567. Philadelphia: Shared Housing Resource Center, Inc., 1982.

Deimling, GT, & DM Bass. *Mental Status Among the Aged: Effects on Spouse and Adult-Child Caregivers.* Paper presented at the annual meeting of the Gerontological Society of America, San Antonio, TX, November, 1984.

Dobrof, R. *Community Involvement: An Approach to Enhancement of Quality of Life in Nursing Homes.* Paper prepared for the Institute of Medicine Committee on Nursing Home Regulation, Fredericksburg, VA 1984.

Dorosin, E & J Phillips. *Share A Fare: A User-Side Subsidy Transportation Program for Elderly and Handicapped Persons in Kansas City, Missouri.* Washington, DC: Department of Transportation, 1979.

Dudley, CJ & GA Hillery, Jr. Freedom and Alienation in Homes for the Aged. *The Gerontologist,* 17: 140-145, 1977.

Duke University. *Multidimensional Functional Assessment: The Oars Methodology.* Durham, NC: Center for the Study of Aging and Human Development, Duke University, 1978.

Dunkle, RE, SW Poulshock, B Silverstone & GT Deimling. Protective Services Reanalyzed: Does Casework Help or Harm? *The Social Casework.* 64: 195-199, 1983.

Ebersole, P. Problems of Group Reminiscing with the Institutionalized Aged. *Journal of Gerontological Nursing,* 2: 23-27, 1976.

Eggert, GM & B Brodows. Five Years of ACCESS: What Have We Learned? In Zawadski, R (ed.), *Community-Based Systems of Long-Term Care* (27-48). New York: Haworth, 1984.

Eggert, GM, CV Granger, R Morris & SF Pendleton. *Community Based Maintenance Care for the Long-Term Patient.* Waltham, MA: Florence Heller Graduate School, Brandeis University, 1976.

Elwell, F. The Effects of Ownership on Institutional Services. *The Gerontologist,* 24: 77-83, 1984.

Emling, DC. *Adult Chore Services: A Profile of In-Home Assistance.* (Studies in Welfare Policy, No. 10), Lansing: Department of Social Services, State of Michigan, 1976.

Engler, M. *Home-Delivered Meals Survey, Fourth Report: Participants' Satisfaction with the Home-Delivered Meals Program.* (Research & Evaluation Report, No. 41). New York: Department for the Aging, 1983.

Engler, M & MJ Meyer. *Home-Delivered Meals Survey. Third Report: Description Of and Comparisons Between Black and White Elderly Receiving Home-Delivered Meals with Respect to Functional Ability, Sources of Support and Demographics.* (Research & Evaluation Report, No. 5). New York: Department for the Aging, 1982.

Epstein, WM. A Comparison Between the Veteran Administration's Long-Term Nursing Home Care Program and Three Examples of Similar Care Outside of the V.A. *International Journal on Aging and Human Development*, 13: 61-69, 1981.

Estes, CL. *The Aging Enterprise*. San Francisco: Jossey-Bass, 1979.

Estes, CL & JB Wood. A Preliminary Assessment of the Impact of Block Grants on Community Mental Health Centers. *Hospital and Community Psychiatry*, 35: 1125-1129, 1984.

Eustis, N, J Greenberg & S Patten. *Long-Term Care for Older Persons: A Policy Perspective*. Monterey, CA: Brooks/Cole Publishing Company, 1984.

Evans, JG. Prevention of Age-Associated Loss of Autonomy: Epidemiological Approaches. *Journal of Chronic Diseases*, 37: 353-363, 1984.

Evashwick, CJ, T Rundall & B Goldiamond. Hospital Services for Older Adults. *The Gerontologist*, 25: 631-637, 1985.

Exton-Smith, AN. Clinical Manifestations. In Exton-Smith, AN and G Evans (eds.), *Care of Elderly: Meeting the Challenge of Dependency*. London: Academic Press, 1977.

Fackelmann, K(ed.). *Washington Report on Medicine and Health—Perspectives*. Washington, DC: McGraw-Hill, 1986.

Family Survival Project for Brain-Damaged Adults. *Annual Report of Fourth Year Progress, Findings and Conclusions of a State Pilot Project to Assist Families in Securing Services, Information and Counseling Necessary for the Care of Brain-Damaged Family Members*. Contract 83-74017, California Department of Mental Health. San Francisco: Family Survival Project, 1983/1984.

Faulkner, LR. Mandating the Reporting of Suspected Cases of Elder Abuse: An Inappropriate, Ineffective and Ageist Response to the Abuse of Older Adults. *Family Law Quarterly*, 16: 69-91, 1982.

Feder, J & W Scanlon. Regulating the Bed Supply in Nursing Homes. *Milbank Memorial Fund Quarterly/Health and Society*, 58: 54-88, 1980.

Federal Council on the Aging. *House Rich, But Cash Poor. Home Equity Conversion Options for Older Homeowners. A Sale-Leaseback Fact Finding Session*. Washington, DC: Federal Council on the Aging, 1983.

Feller, BA. Americans Needing Help to Function at Home. *Advanced Data from Vital and Health Statistics*. No. 92, DHHS Publ. No. (PHS) 83-1250. Washington, DC: National Center for Health Statistics, 1983.

Ferguson, GD & MJ Holin. *Establishing a Home Maintenance Program for Elderly Homeowners: A Guidebook*. Cambridge, MA: Urban Systems Research & Engineering, Inc., 1983.

Ferguson, GD, MJ Holin & WG Moss. *An Evaluation of the Seven City Home Maintenance Demonstration for the Elderly: Final Report. Volume I*. Cambridge: MA: Urban Systems Research & Engineering, Inc., 1983.

Fitting, M, P Rabins, J Lucas & J Eastham. Caregivers for Dementia Patients: A Comparison of Husbands and Wives. *The Gerontologist*, 26: 248-252, 1986.

Flemming, AS, JG Buchanan, JF Santos & LD Rickards. *Mental Health Services for the Elderly: Report on a Survey of Community Mental Health Centers. Volume I*. Washington, DC: Action Committee to Implement the Mental Health Recommendations of the 1981 White House Conference on Aging, 1984a.

Flemming AS, JG Buchanan, JF Santos & LD Rickards. *Mental Health Services for the Elderly: Report on a Survey of Community Mental Health Centers. Volume II*. Washington, DC: Action Committee to Implement the Mental Health Recommendations of the 1981 White House Conference on Aging, 1984b.

Florida Department of Health and Rehabilitative Services. *Nursing Home Evalua-*

tive Study. E-80-8, Tallahassee: Office of Evaluation and Management Review, 1981.

Florida Department of Health and Rehabilitative Services. *An Evaluation of the District XI Long Term Care Unit.* E-83-6. Tallahassee: Office of Evaluation and Management Review, 1983.

Florida Department of Health and Rehabilitative Services. *Final Report and Evaluation of the Florida Pendastar Project, Tallahassee, Florida.* Tallahassee: Florida Department of Health and Rehabilitative Services, 1984.

Food and Beverage Trades Department, AFL-CIO. *Beverly Enterprises in Michigan: A Case Study of Corporate Takeover.* Washington, DC: Beverly Employees Cooperative Action and Reform Effort, 1983.

Fottler, MD, HL Smith & WL James. Profits and Patient Care Quality in Nursing Homes: Are They Compatible? *The Gerontologist,* 21: 532-538, 1981.

Foundation for Long Term Care. *Respite Care for the Frail Elderly: A Summary Report on Institutional Respite Research.* Albany, NY: Center for the Study of Aging, 1983.

Fox, M & M Lithwick. Groupwork with Adult Children of Confused Institutionalized Patients. *Long-Term Care & Health Services Administration Quarterly,* 2: 121-131, 1978.

Frankfather, DL, MJ Smith, & FG Caro. *Family Care of the Elderly: Public Initiatives and Private Obligations.* Lexington, MA: D.C. Heath, 1981.

Frenkel, ER, ES Newman & SR Sherman. Classification Decisions Within Psychogeriatric Day Care. *Community Mental Health Journal,* 19: 279-289, 1983.

Friedman, S. The Resident Welcoming Committee: Institutionalized Elderly in Volunteer Services to Their Peers. *The Gerontologist,* 15: 362-367, 1975.

Fries, BE & LM Cooney. Resource Utilization Groups: A Patient Classification System for Long-Term Care. *Medical Care,* 23: 110-122, 1985.

Fries, JF. Aging, Natural Death, and the Compression of Morbidity. *New England Journal of Medicine,* 303: 130-135, 1980.

Fries, JF. The Compression of Morbidity: Miscellaneous Comments About a Theme. *The Gerontologist,* 24: 354-359, 1984.

Fries, JF & LM Crapo. *Vitality and Aging: Implications of the Rectangular Curve.* San Francisco: WH Freeman, 1981.

Fullarton, WD. Finding the Money and Paying for Long-Term Care Services—The Devil's Briar Patch. In Meltzer, J, F Farrow & H Richman, *Policy Options in Long-Term Care.* Chicago: University of Chicago Press, 1981.

Gardiner, JA & KL Maloc. *Policy Issues in Nursing Home Regulatory Enforcement.* Report prepared for the Institute of Medicine Committee on Nursing Home Regulation of the National Academy of Sciences, Washington, DC, 1984.

Gaumer, GL & TL Williams. *Home Health Agency Prospective Payment Demonstration.* Cambridge, MA: Abt Associates Inc., 1984.

Gayton, DC, S Wood-Dauphinee, JA Hanley & M DeLorimier. *An Interdisciplinary Geriatric Team in an Acute Care Setting.* Paper presented at the annual meeting of the American Public Health Association, Washington, DC: November 1985.

Gehrke, JR & SH Wattenberg. Assessing Social Services in Nursing Homes. *Health & Social Work,* 6(2): 14-25, 1981.

General Accounting Office. *The Well-Being of Older People in Cleveland, Ohio.* HRD-77-70. Washington, DC: U.S. General Accounting Office, 1977.

General Accounting Office. *Problems in Auditing Medicaid Nursing Home Chains.* HRD-78-158. Washington, DC: U.S. General Accounting Office, 1979.

General Accounting Office. *Medicare Home Health Services: A Difficult Program to Control,* HRD-81-155. Washington, DC: U.S. General Accounting Office, 1981.

General Accounting Office. *The Elderly Should Benefit from Expanded Home Health Care but Increasing These Services Will Not Insure Cost Reductions.* GAO/IPE-83-1. Washington, DC: U.S. General Accounting Office, 1982b.

General Accounting Office. *The Elderly Remain in Need of Mental Health Services.* GAO/HRD-82-112. Washington, DC: U.S. General Accounting Office, 1982a.

General Accounting Office. *Status of Special Efforts to Meet Transportation Needs of the Elderly and Handicapped.* CED-82-66. Washington, DC: U.S. General Accounting Office, 1982c.

General Accounting Office. *Medicaid and Nursing Home Care: Cost Increases and the Need for Services are Creating Problems for States and the Elderly.* GAO/IPE-84-1. Washington, DC: U.S. General Accounting Office, 1983.

General Accounting Office. *States Use Several Strategies to Cope with Funding Reductions Under Social Services Block Grant.* GAO/HRD-84-68. Washington, DC: U.S. General Accounting Office, 1984.

George, L & L Gwyther. Caregiver Well-Being: A Multidimensional Examination of Family Caregivers of Demented Adults. *The Gerontologist,* 26: 253-259, 1986.

German, PS, S Shapiro & M Kramer. Nursing Home Study of the Eastern Baltimore Epidemiological Catchment Area Study. In Harper, M & B Lebowitz (eds.), *Mental Illness in Nursing Homes. Agenda for Research.* Washington, DC: U.S. Government Printing Office, 1986.

Gerson, L & AF Berry. Psychosocial Effects of Home Care: Results of a Randomized Trial. *International Journal of Epidemiology,* 5: 159-165, 1976.

Gerson, L & OP Hughes. A Comparative Study of the Economics of Home Care. *International Journal of Health Services,* 6: 543-563, 1976.

Gibbins, FJ, M Lee, PR Davison, P O'Sullivan, M Hutchinson, DR Murphy & CN Ugwu. Augmented Home Nursing as an Alternative to Hospital Care for Chronic Elderly Invalids. *British Medical Journal,* 284: 330-333, 1982.

Gilleard, CJ. Predicting the Outcome of Psychogeriatric Day Care. *The Gerontologist,* 25: 280-285, 1985.

Glosser, G & D Wexler. Participants' Evaluation of Educational/Support Groups for Families of Patients with Alzheimer's Disease and Other Dementias. *The Gerontologist,* 25: 232-236, 1985.

Gooding, BA. *Choice and Effects of Participation in Home Health Care.* Unpublished doctoral dissertation, University of Michigan, Ann Arbor, 1984.

Gordon, W, RL Kane & R Rothenberg. Acute Hospitalization in a Home for the Aged. *Journal of the American Geriatrics Society,* 33: 519-523, 1985.

Greenberg, JN, DS Doth & CD Austin. A Comparative Study of Long-Term Care Demonstrations. Minneapolis: University of Minnesota Center for Health Services Research, 1981.

Greenberg, JN & A Ginn. A Multivariate Analysis of the Predictors of Long-Term Care Placement. *Home Health Care Services Quarterly,* 1: 75-99, 1979.

Greenberg, JN, MP Schmitz & KC Lakin. *An Analysis of Responses to the Medicaid Home- and Community-Based Long-Term Care Waiver Program. (Section 2176 of PL 97-35).* Washington, DC: State Medicaid Information Center, 1983.

Greene, VL & DJ Monahan. Structural and Operational Factors Affecting Quality of Patient Care in Nursing Homes. *Public Policy,* 29: 399-415, 1981.

Greene, VL & DJ Monahan. The Impact of Visitation on Patient Well-Being in Nursing Homes. *The Gerontologist,* 22: 418-423, 1982.

Greer, DS, V Mor, JN Morris, S Sherwood, D Kidder & H Birnbaum. An Alternative in Terminal Care: Results of the National Hospice Study. *Journal of Chronic Diseases,* 39: 9-26, 1986.

Grey, C. Moving 137 Elderly Residents to a New Facility. *Journal of Gerontological Nursing,* 4: 34-38, 1978.

Grier, MR. Living Arrangements for the Elderly. *Journal of Gerontological Nursing,* 3: 19-22, 1977.

Grimaldi, PL. RUGs and "Medi-Cal" Systems for Classifying Nursing Home Patients. *Health Progress,* 66: 50-57, 1985.

Groth-Juncker, A. *Home Health Care Team: Randomized Trial of a New Team Approach to Home Care.* Executive summary of research grant from National Center for Health Services Research (NCHSR No. HS03030). Rochester, NY: University of Rochester School of Medicine and Dentistry, 1982.

Groth-Juncker, A & J McCusker. Where Do Elderly Patients Prefer To Die? *Journal of the American Geriatrics Society,* 3l: 457-461, 1983.

Gruchow, HW & KA Sobocinski. *Need For Help With Basic Physical Activities Among Wisconsin's Elderly.* Milwaukee, WI: The Milwaukee Long-Term-Care Gerontology Center, 1984.

Gryfe, CI, A Amies & MJ Ashley. A Longitudinal Study of Falls in an Elderly Population. I. Incidence and Mobility. *Age and Aging,* 6:201-210, 1977.

Gryfe, CI & S Proctor. *The Effect on Hospitalization and Death Rates of Increased Frequency of Physicians' Visits to a Nursing Home for the Aged.* Toronto: Baycrest Centre for Geriatric Care, 1984.

Gubrium, JF & M Ksander. On Multiple Realities and Reality Orientation. *The Gerontologist,* 15: 142-145, 1975.

Gurian, B. Mental Health Outreach and Consultation Services for the Elderly. *Hospital & Community Psychiatry,* 33: 142-147, 1982.

Gurland, B, R Bennett & D Wilder. Reevaluating the Place of Evaluation in Planning for Alternatives to Institutional Care for the Elderly. *Journal of Social Issues,* 37: 51-70, 1981.

Gurland, B, L Dean, R Gurland & D Cook. Personal Time Dependency in the Elderly of New York City: Findings from the U.S.-U.K. Cross-National Geriatric Community Study. In Community Council of Greater New York, *Dependency in the Elderly of New York City* (9-45). New York: Community Council of Greater New York, 1978.

Gurland, BJ & A Mann. *A Comparison of the Frail Elderly in Day Treatment to Those in Long-Term Institutional Care in New York City and London, England.* New York: Faculty of Medicine, Columbia University Center for Geriatrics and Gerontology, 1982.

Hackman, H. Day Care for the Frail Elderly: An Alternative. *Public Welfare,* 34: 36-44, 1978.

Halbur, BT. Nursing Personnel in Nursing Homes. A Structural Approach to Turnover. *Work and Occupations,* 10: 381-411, 1983.

Hammond, J. Home Health Care Cost Effectiveness: An Overview of the Literature. *Public Health Reports,* 94: 305-311, 1979.

Hannan, EL & JF O'Donnell. Adult Day Care Services in New York State: A Comparison with Other LTC Providers. *Inquiry,* 21: 75-83, 1984.

Hansen, M. *Single-Entry Long-Term Care Programs: A Review of Options.* Seattle: Long-Term Care Gerontology Center, University of Washington, 1981.

Hanson, SM & WJ Sauer. Children and Their Elderly Parents. In Sauer, WJ & RT Coward, *Social Support Networks and the Care of the Elderly.* New York: Springer Publishing, 1985.

Harel, Z. Nutrition Site Service Users: Does Racial Background Make a Difference? *The Gerontologist,* 25: 286-310, 1985.

Harel, Z & B Harel. On-Site Coordinated Services in Age-Segregated and Age-Integrated Public Housing. *The Gerontologist,* 18: 153-158, 1978.

Harel, Z & L Noelker. Social Integration, Health, and Choice. Their Impact on the Well-Being of Institutionalized Aged. *Research on Aging,* 4: 97-111, 1982.

Harkins, EB & CA Bowlenz. *Virginia Nursing Home Pre-Admission Screening Program: Final Report.* Richmond, VA: Virginia Center on Aging, Virginia Commonwealth University, 1982.

Harmon, C. *Board and Care: An Old Problem, A New Resource for Long Term Care.* Washington, DC: Center for the Study of Social Policy, 1982.

Harrill, I, M Bowski, A Kylen & R Wemple. The Nutritional Status of Congregate Meal Recipients. *Aging,* No. 311-312: 36-41, 1980.

Harrington, C & J Swan. Institutional Long-Term Care Services. In Harrington, C, R Newcomer, C Estes and Associates, *Long-Term Care of the Elderly. Public Policy Issues* (153-176). Beverly Hills: Sage Publications, 1985.

Harris, R & S Harris. Therapeutic Uses of Oral History Techniques in Medicine. *International Journal on Aging and Human Development,* 12: 27-34, 1980/81.

Harris, CS & PBCB Ivory. An Outcome Evaluation of Reality Orientation Therapy with Geriatric Patients in a State Mental Hospital. *The Gerontologist,* 16: 496-503, 1976.

Harris & Associates. *Aging in America: Myths & Reality.* Washington, DC: National Council on Aging, 1975.

Harris & Associates. *Priorities and Expectations for Health and Living Circumstances. A Survey of the Elderly in Five English-Speaking Countries.* New York: The Commonwealth Fund, 1982.

Haskins, B, J. Capitman, J. Bernstein, et al. *Final Report. Evaluation of Coordinated Community-Oriented Long-Term Care Demonstration Projects.* Berkeley, CA: Berkeley Planning Associates, 1984.

Hawes, C & CD Phillips. The Changing Structure of the Nursing Home Industry and the Impact of Ownership on Quality, Cost, and Access. In Institute of Medicine, *For-Profit Enterprise in Health Care.* Washington, DC: Academy Press, 1986.

Hay, DG. Health Care Services in 100 Superior Nursing Homes. *Long-Term Care & Health Services Administration Quarterly,* 1: 300-313, 1977.

Hay, JW. *An Incentive Reimbursement Plan for Medicaid Home Health Care Services.* Paper presented at the annual meeting of the American Public Health Association, Anaheim, CA, November 1984.

Hayslip, B Jr., ML Ritter, RM Oltman & C McDonnell. Home Care Services and the Rural Elderly. *The Gerontologist,* 20: 192-199, 1980.

Health Care Financing Administration. *Directory of Adult Day Care, 1980.* Department of Health and Human Services (HCFA-30040). Washington, DC: U.S. Government Printing Office, 1980.

Hedrick, SC. *Evaluation of Effectiveness and Costs of Adult Day Health Care.* Investigator-initiated grant application to the Veterans Administration Central Office. Unpublished document available from author at the Veterans Administration Medical Center, Tacoma, WA, 1985.

Hedrick, S & T Inui. The Effectiveness and Cost of Home Care: An Information Synthesis. *Health Services Research,* 20: 851-880, 1986.

Hedrick, S, J. Papsidero & C Maynard. Analysis of Alternative Definitions of Function in Studies of Long-Term Care. In Scanlon, W (ed.), *Project to Analyze Existing Long-Term Care Data.* (Appendix). Washington, DC: The Urban Institute, 1984.

Hendriksen, C, E Lund & E Stromgard. Consequences of Assessment and Intervention Among Elderly People: A Three Year Randomized Controlled Trial. *British Medical Journal,* 289: 1522-1524, 1984.

Hendy, HM. Effects of Pets on the Sociability and Health Activities of Nursing

Home Residents. In Anderson, RK, BL Hart & LA Hart (eds.), *The Pet Connection: Its Influence on Our Health and Quality of Life*. Minneapolis: Center to Study Animal-Human Relationships and Environments, 1984.

Henkleman-Kelly, J. *Caregiver Support Programs: Development and Implementation*. Paper presented at Respite Care: New Opportunities Conference, Phoenix, AZ, June 1983.

Hicks, B, H Raisz, J Segal & N Doherty. The Triage Experiment in Coordinated Care for the Elderly. *American Journal of Public Health*, 71: 991-1003, 1981.

Hicks, B, J Segal, J Quinn & H Raisz. *Triage: Coordinated Delivery of Services to the Elderly. Final Report*. Hartford: Connecticut State Department on Aging, 1979.

Hing, E. Use of Nursing Homes by the Elderly: Preliminary Data from the 1985 National Nursing Home Survey. NCHS Advance Data From Vital and Health Statistics, DHHS Pub. No. (PHS) 87-1250. Hyattsville, MD: National Center for Health Statistics, No. 135. May 14, 1987.

Hinzpeter, DA & AK Fischer. *Graying in the Shadows. A Study of the Aged on Manhattan's West Side*. New York: New York Service Program for Older People, Inc., 1983.

Hirsch, CS. Integrating the Nursing Home Resident into a Senior Citizens Center. *The Gerontologist*, 17: 227-234, 1977.

Hodges, SJ & EG Goldman. *Allowing Accessory Apartments. Key Issues for Local Officials*. Washington, DC: Office of Policy Development and Research, U.S. Department of Housing and Urban Development, 1983.

Hogan, DB & RD Cape. A Geriatric Assessment Unit in a Long-Term Care Facility. *Canadian Journal of Public Health*, 75: 301-303, 1984.

Hogue, C. Injury in Late Life: Part I-Epidemiology. *Journal of the American Geriatrics Society*, 30: 183-190, 1982a.

Hogue, CC. Injury in Late Life: Part II-Prevention. *Journal of the American Geriatrics Society*, 30, 276-280, 1982b.

Holahan, J. *How Should Medicaid Programs Pay for Nursing Home Care?* Washington, DC: The Urban Institute, 1985.

Holahan, J & J Cohen. *Nursing Home Reimbursement Systems and Cost Containment Quality and Access: A Summary of Interim Findings*. Washington, DC: The Urban Institute, 1984.

Holahan, J, J Cohen & W Scanlon. *Nursing Home Costs and Reimbursement Policy: Evidence from the 1977 National Nursing Home Survey*. Washington, DC: The Urban Institute, 1983.

Horen, JH. The Labor Supply Question. In Vogel, RJ & HC Palmer (eds.), *Long-Term Care. Perspectives from Research and Demonstrations*. Health Care Financing Administration, U.S. Department of Health and Human Services, (0-391-955). Washington, DC: U.S. Government Printing Office, 1983.

Horowitz A & L Shindelman. Reciprocity and Affection: Past Influences on Current Caregiving. *Journal of Gerontological Social Work*, 5: 5-21, 1983.

Horowitz, MJ & R Schulz. The Relocation Controversy: Criticism and Commentary on Five Recent Studies. *The Gerontologist*, 23: 229-234, 1983.

Howe, E, B Robins & D Jaffe. *Evaluation of: Homeshare Program*. Madison, WI: Independent Living, Inc., 1984.

Howells, D. *Reallocating Institutional Resources: Respite Care as a Supplement to Family Care of the Elderly*. Paper presented at the annual meeting of the Gerontological Society of America, San Diego, November 1980.

Hughes, SL. Apples and Oranges: A Critical Review of Evaluations of Community-Based Long Term Care. *Health Services Research*, 20: 461-488, 1985.

Hughes, SL, DS Cordray & VA Spiker. Evaluation of a Long-Term Home Care Program. *Medical Care,* 22: 460-475, 1984.

Huttman, E. *Social Services for the Elderly.* New York: The Free Press, 1985.

Hyerstay, BJ. The Political and Economic Implications of Training Nursing Home Aides. *Journal of Nursing Administration,* 8: 22-24, 1978.

Institute of Medicine. *Assessing Medical Technologies.* Washington, DC: National Academy Press, 1985.

Institute of Medicine. *Improving the Quality of Care in Nursing Homes,* Washington, DC: Academy Press, 1986.

Institute on Aging, University of Washington. *Improving Access for Elders: The Role of Case Management. Final Report.* Seattle: Institute on Aging, University of Washington, 1987.

Inui, TS, KM Stevenson, D Plorde & I Murphy. Need Assessment for Hospital-Based Home Care. *Research in Nursing and Health,* 3: 101-106, 1980.

Isaacs, B & FA Walkey. A Survey of Incontinence in the Elderly. *Gerontologia Clinica,* 6: 367, 1964.

Isaacs, MR & SK Goldman. *State Initiatives in Long-Term Care. Report of a Survey of 32 States.* HRP-0905897. Washington, DC: Office of Health Planning, Bureau of Health Maintenance Organizations and Resources Development, 1984.

Iverson, LH. *A Description and Analysis of State Preadmission Screening Programs.* Minneapolis, MN: InterStudy, Center for Aging and Long-Term Care, 1986.

Jacobs, B & W Weissert. Home Equity Financing of Long-Term Care for the Elderly. In Feinstein, P, M Gornick, & J Greenberg (eds.), *Long-Term Care Financing and Delivery Systems: Exploring Some Alternatives. Conference Proceedings* (82-94). Washington, DC: Health Care Financing Administration, 1984.

Jette, AM & LG Branch. Targeting Community Services to High-Risk Elders: Toward Preventing Long-Term Care Institutionalization. *Aging and Prevention,* 3: 53-69, 1981.

Jette, AM, LG Branch, RA Wentzel, WF Carney, DL Dennis & MM Heist. Home Care Service Diversification: A Pilot Investigation. *The Gerontologist,* 21: 572-579, 1981.

Johnson, ML & LM Sterthous. *A Guide to Memorandum of Understanding Negotiation and Development for Long Term Care Case Management Agencies.* Philadelphia: Temple University Institute on Aging, 1982.

Johnson, SH. *Evaluation of the Use of Intermediate Sanctions by the States and Recommendations for State and Federal Enforcement Policies.* Report submitted to the Committee on Nursing Home Regulation, Institute of Medicine, National Academy of Sciences, Washington, DC, 1985.

Jones, BJ & MR Meiners. Nursing Home Discharges: The Results of an Incentive Reimbursement Experiment. Hyattsville, MD: National Center for Health Services Research, 1984.

Jost, TS. *Enforcement of Quality Nursing Home Care in the Legal System.* Report prepared under contract for the Committee on Nursing Home Regulation, Institute of Medicine, National Academy of Sciences, Washington, DC, 1984.

Justice, D & B Preston. *State Long Term Care Programs: Summary Profiles of Twelve States.* Washington, DC: National Governors' Association, 1986.

Kahana, EF & HA Kiyak. Attitudes and Behavior of Staff in Facilities for the Aged. *Research On Aging,* 6: 395-416, 1984.

Kane, RA & RL Kane. *Assessing the Elderly: A Practical Guide to Measurement.* Lexington, MA: DC Heath, 1981.

Kane, RA, RL Kane, D Kleffel, R Brook, C Eby, G Goldberg, L Rubenstein & J

VanRyzin. *The PSRO and the Nursing Home. Volume I—An Assessment of PSRO Long-Term Care Review.* Santa Monica, CA: The Rand Corporation. 1979a.

Kane, RA, RL Kane, D Kleffel, R Brook, C Eby, G Goldberg, L Rubenstein & J VanRyzin. *The PSRO and the Nursing Home. Volume II—Ten Demonstration Projects in Long-Term Care Review.* Santa Monica, CA: The Rand Corporation, 1979b.

Kane, RL, RM Bell & SZ Riegler. Value Preferences for Nursing Home Residents. *The Gerontologist,* 26: 303-308, 1986.

Kane, RL, R Bell, S Reigler, A Wilson & RA Kane. Assessing the Outcomes of Nursing-Home Patients. *Journal of Gerontology,* 38: 385-393, 1983a.

Kane, RL, R Bell, S Reigler, A Wilson & E Keeler. Predicting the Outcomes of Nursing-Home Patients. *The Gerontologist,* 23: 200-206, 1983b.

Kane, RL, L Bernstein, J Wales & R Rothenberg. Hospice Effectiveness in Controlling Pain. *Journal of the American Medical Association,* 253: 2683-2686, 1985b.

Kane, RL, M Hammer & N Byrnes. Getting Care to Nursing Home Patients: A Problem and a Proposal. *Medical Care,* 15: 174-180, 1977.

Kane, RL, LA Jorgenson, B Teteberg & J Kuwahara. Is Good Nursing Home Care Feasible. *Journal of the American Medical Association,* 235: 516-519, 1976.

Kane, RL & RA Kane (eds.). *Values and Long-Term Care.* Lexington, MA: DC Heath, 1982.

Kane, RL & RA Kane. *A Will and A Way: What the United States Can Learn from Canada About Care of the Elderly.* New York: Columbia University Press, 1985.

Kane RL, SJ Klein, L Bernstein & R Rothenberg. The Role of Hospice in Reducing the Impact of Bereavement. *Journal of Chronic Diseases,* 39: 735-742, 1986.

Kane RL, SJ Klein, L Bernstein, R Rothenberg & J Wales. Hospice Role in Alleviating the Emotional Stress of Terminal Patients and Their Families. *Medical Care,* 23: 189-197, 1985a.

Kane, RL & R Matthias. From Hospital to Nursing Home: The Long-Term Care Connection. *The Gerontologist,* 24: 604-609, 1984.

Kane, RL, R Matthias & S Sampson. The Risk of Placement in a Nursing Home After Acute Utilization. *Medical Care,* 21: 1055-1061, 1983.

Kane, RL, DH Solomon, JC Beck, E Keeler & RA Kane. *Geriatrics in the United States: Manpower Projections and Training Considerations.* Lexington, MA: DC Heath, 1981.

Kane, RL, J Wales, L Bernstein, A Liebowitz & S Kaplan. A Randomized Controlled Trial of Hospice Care. *Lancet,* 1: 890-894, 1984.

Katz, S, AB Ford, Adams & Rusky. *Effects of Continued Care: A Study of Chronic Illness in the Home.* DHEW Publ. No. (HSM) 73-3010. Washington, DC: U.S. Government Printing Officer, 1972.

Katz, S, AB Ford, RW Moskowitz, BA Jackson & MW Jaffe. Studies of Illness in the Aged: The Index of ADL. A Standardized Measure of Biological Function. *Journal of the American Medical Association,* 185:914-919, 1963.

Kay, DWK, K Bergmann, EM Foster, AA McKechnie & M Rath. Mental Illness and Hospital Usage in the Elderly: A Random Sample Followed Up. *Comprehensive Psychiatry,* 11: 26-35, 1970.

Kaye, LW. The Adequacy of the Older Americans Act Home Care Mandate: A Front Line View from Three Programs. *Home Health Care Services Quarterly,* 5: 75-87, 1984.

Kemper, P, RS Braun, GJ Carcagno et al. *The Evaluation of the National Long-*

Term Care Channeling Demonstration. Princeton, NJ: Mathematica Policy, Inc., 1986.

Kempler, D & L Gallup. *An Evaluation of the Growing Younger Health Promotion Program for Older Adults.* Boise, ID: Healthwise, Inc., 1984.

Kepferle, L. Projects and Demonstrations. In Yokie, J & P Ebersole (eds.), *Training and Practice of the Geriatric Nurse Practitioner.* Special issue of the *Journal of Long-Term Care Administration,* 11: 54-57, 1983.

Kirschner, R et al. *An Evaluation of the Nutrition Services for the Elderly.* Albuquerque, NM: Kirschner Associates, Inc., 1983.

Klapfish, A. Problems with the Weissert Reports Conclusion About Adult Day Health Services. *Home Health Care Services Quarterly,* 1: 112-114, 1980.

Knowles, DH. Exploration of the Emotional Feelings of the Elderly Confined to a Nursing Home. *Nursing Homes,* 24: 8-13, 1975.

Knowlton, J, S Clauser & J Fatula. Nursing Home Pre-Admission Screening: A Review of State Programs. *Health Care Financing Review,* 3: 75-87, 1982.

Koger, LJ. Nursing Home Life Satisfaction and Activity Participation. *Research On Aging,* 2: 61-72, 1980.

Kramer, M. Trends of Institutionalization and Prevalence of Mental Disorders in Nursing Homes. In Harper, M & B Lebowitz (eds.), *Mental Health in Nursing Homes. Agenda for Research.* Washington, DC: U.S. Government Printing Office, 1986.

Kraus, AS, RA Spasoff, EJ Beattie, DEW Holden, JS Lawson, M Rodenburg & GM Woodcock. Role and Value of Foster Homes for the Elderly. *Canadian Journal of Public Health,* 68: 32-38, 1977.

Krout, JA. *The Organization, Operation, and Programming of Senior Centers: A National Survey.* Final report prepared for the AARP Andrus Foundation, Fredonia, NY: State University of New York-College at Fredonia, 1983.

Kulys, R. Future Crises and the Very Old: Implications for Discharge Planning. *Health and Social Work,* 8: 182-195, 1983.

Kulys, R & SS Tobin. Older People and Their Responsible Others. *Social Work,* 25: 138-145, 1980.

Ladd, RC. Oregon's Long-Term System for the Elderly and Physically Disabled. Paper presented at the conference on Building Affordable Long Term Care Alternatives (a working conference for senior state officials sponsored by the National Governor's Association Center for Policy Research), Portland, OR, July 1986.

Lalonde, B & N Hooyman. *Evaluation of Long-Term Effectiveness of a Health Promotion Program for the Elderly: The Wallingford Wellness Project.* Paper presented at annual meeting of Gerontological Society of America, San Antonio, TX, November 1984.

Lamont, C, S Sampson, R Mathias & RL Kane. The Outcome of Hospitalization for Acute Illness in the Elderly. *Journal of the American Geriatrics Society,* 31: 282-288, 1983.

Langer, E & J Rodin. The Effects of Choice and Enhanced Personal Responsibility for the Aged. A Field Experiment in an Institutional Setting. *Journal of Personality & Social Psychology,* 34: 191-198, 1976.

Langley, A. *Abuse of the Elderly.* (Human Services Monograph Series, No. 27) Washington, DC: Aspen Systems Corporation, 1981.

Larson, EB, BV Reifler, HJ Featherstone & DR English. Dementia in Elderly Outpatients: A Prospective Study. *Annals of Internal Medicine,* 100: 417-423, 1984.

Laurie, W. The Cleveland Experience: Functional Status and Service Use. *Multi-*

dimensional Functional Assessment: The OARS Methodology. Durham, NC: Center for the Study of Aging & Human Development, Duke University, 1978.

LaViolette, S. Nursing Home Chains Scramble for More Private-Paying Patients. *Modern Healthcare,* 13: 130-138, 1983.

Lawton, MP. *Social and Medical Services in Housing for the Aged.* DHHS Publication No. (ADM)80-861. Washington, DC: U.S. Government Printing Office, 1980.

Lee, JT & MA Stein. Eliminating Duplication in Home Health Care for the Elderly: The Guale Project. *National Association of Social Workers,* 5: 29-36, 1980.

Lefton, E, S Bonstelle & JD Frengley. Success with an Inpatient Geriatric Unit: A Controlled Study of Outcome and Follow-up. *Journal of the American Geriatrics Society,* 31: 149-155, 1983.

Lesser, J, LW Lazarus, R Frankel & S Havasy. Reminiscence Group Therapy with Psychotic Geriatric Patients. In Tobin, SS (ed.), *Current Gerontology: Long Term Care.* Washington, D.C.: Gerontological Society of America, 1982.

Leutz, WN, JN Greenberg, R Abrahams, J Prottas, LM Diamond & L Gruenberg. *Changing Health Care for an Aging Society.* Lexington, MA/Toronto: Lexington Books, 1985.

Levit, K, H Lazenby, D Waldo & L Davidoff. National Health Expenditures, 1984. *Health Care Financing Review,* 7: 1-35, 1985.

Lewis, M, S Cretin & RL Kane. The Natural History of Nursing Home Patients. *The Gerontologist,* 25: 382-388, 1985.

Lewis, M, RL Kane, S Cretin & V Clark. The Immediate and Subsequent Outcomes of Nursing Home Care. *American Journal of Public Health,* 75: 758-761, 1985.

Lichtenstein, H & CH Winograd. Geriatric Consultation: A Functional Approach. *Journal of the American Geriatrics Society,* 32: 356-361, 1984.

Liem PH, R Chernoff & W Carter. Geriatric Rehabilitation Unit: A 3-Year Outcome Evaluation. *Journal of Gerontology,* 41: 45-50, 1986.

Lind, SD. *Visiting Nurse Association Risk Reduction Project.* Paper presented at the annual meeting of the Gerontological Society of America, San Antonio, TX, November, 1984.

Linn, M, E Caffey, J Klett & G Hogarty. Hospital vs. Community (Foster) Care for Psychiatric Patients. *Archives of General Psychiatry.* 34: 78-83, 1977.

Linn, MW, L Gurel & BS Linn. Patient Outcome as a Measure of Quality of Nursing Home Care. *American Journal of Public Health,* 67: 337-344, 1977.

Linn, M, J Klett & E Caffey. Foster Home Characteristics and Psychiatric Patient Outcome. *Archives of General Psychiatry,* 37: 129-132, 1980.

Lowy, L. *Services to Maintain Elderly Homeowners in Their Own Homes. United South End Settlements Housing and Living Assistance Program. Final Report. October 1, 1980 - September 30, 1983.* Boston: School of Social Work, Boston University, 1984.

Lubitz, J & R Prihoda. The Use and Costs of Medicare Services in the Last Two Years of Life. *Health Financing Review,* 3: 117-131, 1984.

Lyons, M & GA Steele. Evaluation of a Home Health Aide Training Program for the Elderly. *Evaluation Quarterly,* 1: 609-620, 1977.

MacDonald, ML & JM Settin. Reality Orientation Versus Sheltered Workshops as Treatment for the Institutionalized Aging. *Journal of Gerontology,* 33: 416-421, 1978.

Mace, NL & PV Rabins. *A Survey of Day Care for the Demented Adult in the United States.* Washington, DC: The National Council on the Aging, 1984.

Manton, KG. Changing Concepts of Morbidity and Mortality in the Elderly Population. *Milbank Memorial Fund Quarterly/Health and Society,* 60: 183-244, 1982.

Manton, KG. *Changing Health Status and the Need for Institutional and Noninstitutional Long-Term Care Services.* Report prepared for Subcommittee on Reimbursement and Other Factors Affecting Quality, Institute of Medicine Panel on Nursing Home Regulations, National Academy of Sciences, Washington, DC, 1984.

Manton, KG & B Soldo. Dynamics of Health Change in the Oldest Old: New Perspectives and Evidence. *Milbank Memorial Fund Quarterly/Health and Society,* 63: 206-285, 1985.

Margulec, I, G Libroch & M Schadel. Epidemiological Study of Accidents Among Residents of Home for the Aged. *Journal of Gerontology,* 25: 342-346, 1970.

Master, R, M Feltin, J Jainchill, R Mark, W Kavesh, M Rabkin, B Turner, S Bachrach & S Lennox. A Continuum of Care for the Inner City. *New England Journal of Medicine,* 302: 1434-1440, 1980.

Mather, J. An Overview of the Veterans Administration and Its Services for Older Veterans. In Wetle, T and J Rowe (eds.), *Older Veterans: Linking VA and Community Resources* (35-48). Cambridge: Harvard University Press, 1984.

McAuley, WJ & G Arling. Use of In-Home Care by Very Old People. *Journal of Health and Social Behavior,* 25: 54-64, 1984.

McCall, N, T Rice & J Sangl. Consumer Knowledge of Medicare and Supplemental Health Insurance Benefits. *Health Services Research,* 20: 633-657, 1986.

McCall, N & HS Wai. An Analysis of the Use of Medicare Services by the Continuously Enrolled Aged. *Medical Care,* 21: 567-581, 1983.

McCaslin, R. Next Steps in Information and Referral for the Elderly. *The Gerontologist,* 21: 184-193, 1981.

McCoy, JL & BE Edwards. Contextual and Sociodemographic Antecedents of Institutionalization Among Aged Welfare Recipients. *Medical Care,* 19: 907-921, 1981.

Meiners, MR. The Case for Long-Term Care Insurance. *Health Affairs.* 2: 55-79, 1983.

Meiners, MR. *The State of the Art in Long-Term Care Insurance.* Washington, DC: National Center for Health Services Research, 1984.

Meiners, MR, P Thorburn, PC Roddy & BJ Jones. Nursing Home Admissions: The Results of an Incentive Reimbursement Experiment. Washington, DC: National Center for Health Services Research, 1984.

Meltzer, JW. *Respite Care: An Emerging Family Support Service.* Washington, DC: The Center for the Study of Social Policy, 1982.

Mercer, SO & JD Garner. Social Work Consultation in Long-Term Care Facilities. *Health and Social Work,* 6(2): 5-13, 1981.

Mercer, S & RA Kane. Helplessness and Hopelessness Among the Institutionalized Aged: An Experiment. *Health & Social Work,* 4: 90-116, 1979.

Merriam, S. The Concept and Function of Reminiscence: A Review of the Research. *The Gerontologist,* 20: 604-608, 1980.

Meyer, M, M Engler & B Lepis. *Home Delivered Meals Survey. Second Report: The Support Systems of Participants in Home-Delivered Meal Programs in New York City.* New York: New York City Department for the Aging, 1982.

Miller, DB & JT Barry. The Relationship of Off Premises Activities to the Quality of Life of Nursing Home Patients. *The Gerontologist,* 16: 61-64, 1976.

Miller, LS. *Multi-Purpose Senior Services Project. The Comparative Evaluation of the Multipurpose Senior Services Project—1981-1982: Final Report.* U.S. Department of Health and Human Services (Grant 11-P-97553/9-04—MSSP). Berkeley, CA: University of California at Berkeley. 1984.

Miller, LS, ML Clark, LJ Walter et al. *The Comparative Evaluation of the Multipurpose Senior Services Project, 1981-82. Final Report*. Berkeley, CA: University of California at Berkeley, 1984.

Miller, MG. Manageable Caseload Size for Clients on the Threshold of Institutionalization. In Austin, CD, J Low, EA Roberts & K O'Connor (eds.), *Case Management: A Critical Review*. Seattle: Pacific Northwest Long-Term Care Gerontology Center, University of Washington, 1985.

Mitchell, JB. Patient Outcomes in Alternative Long-Term Care Settings. *Medical Care*, 16: 439-52, 1978.

Mitchell, JB & H Hewes. Medicare Access to Physician Services in Nursing Homes. Boston, MA: Center for Health Economics Research, 1982.

Mitchell, J & JC Register. An Exploration of Family Interaction with the Elderly by Race, Socioeconomic Status, and Residence. *The Gerontologist*, 24: 48-54, 1984.

Monk, A, LW Kaye & H Litwin. *Resolving Grievances in the Nursing Home: A Story of the Ombudsman Program*. New York: Columbia University Press, 1984.

Monroe County Long-Term Care Program. *Direct Assessment vs. Brokerage: A Comparison of Case Management Models. Final Report*. Rochester, NY: ACCESS, mimeo, 1984.

Moon, M. *Private Capacity to Finance Long Term Care* (rev.). Washington, DC: The Urban Institute, 1983.

Mor, V, S Sherwood & C Gutkin. A National Study of Residential Care for the Aged. *The Gerontologist*, 26: 405-417, 1986.

Morales-Martinez, F, AJ Carpenter & J Williamson. The Dynamic of a Geriatric Day Hospital. *Age and Aging*, 13:34-41, 1984.

Morris, J & S Sherwood. Informal Support Resources for Vulnerable Elderly Persons: Can They Be Counted On, Why Do They Work? *International Journal of Aging and Human Development*, 18: 81-99, 1983/84.

Morris, J, S Sherwood & E Bernstein. *Quality of Life Standards in Long-Term Care Institutions*. Boston: Hebrew Rehabilitation Center for Aged, mimeo, 1984.

Mortimer, JA. Alzheimer's Disease and Senile Dementia: Prevalence and Incidence. In Reisberg, B (ed.), *Alzheimer's Disease: The Standard Reference* (141-148). New York: Free Press, 1983.

Mortimer, JA & JT Hutton. Epidemiology and Etiology of Alzheimer's Disease. In Hutton T & A Kenny (eds.), *Senile Dementia of the Alzheimer Type* (177-196). New York: Alan R. Liss, Inc., 1985.

Mortimer, JA, LM Schuman & LR French. Epidemiology of Dementing Illness. In Mortimer, JA & LM Schuman (eds.), *Epidemiology of Dementia* (3-23). Oxford and New York: Oxford University Press, 1981.

Moscovice, I. Preadmission Screening, Case Management, and Community Services for the At-Risk Elderly: Evaluation Issues from the Minnesota Experience. Paper presented at the annual meeting of the American Public Health Association, Washington, DC, November 1985.

Mossey, J, B Haves, N Roos & E Shapiro. The Manitoba Longitudinal Study on Aging: Description and Methods. *The Gerontologist*, 21: 551-558, 1981.

Mossey, J & E Shapiro. Self-Rated Health: A Predictor of Mortality Among the Elderly. *American Journal of Public Health*, 72: 800-805, 1982.

Mossey, J & E Shapiro. Physician Use by the Elderly Over an Eight-Year Period. *American Journal of Public Health*, 75: 1333-1334, 1985.

Myers, P. *Aging in Place. Strategies to Help the Elderly Stay in Revitalizing Neighborhoods*. Washington, DC: The Conservation Foundation, 1982.

Nagi, SZ. An Epidemiology of Disability Among Adults in the United States. *Health and Society,* 54: 439-468, 1976.

National Association of State Units on Aging. *A Profile of State and Area Agencies on Aging, 1981.* Washington, DC: National Association of State Units on Aging, 1982.

National Center for Health Statistics. *The National Nursing Home Survey: 1977 Summary for the United States.* DHEW Publ. No. (PHS) 79-1794. Washington, DC: U.S. Department of Health and Human Services, 1979.

Nelson, JR. *Tax Subsidies for Elderly Care.* Washington, DC: Center for the Study of Social Policy, 1982.

Nestle, M, PR Lee & J Fullarton. *Nutrition Policy and the Elderly.* San Francisco: Aging Health Policy Center, University of California at San Francisco, 1983.

Netting, FE & LN Kennedy. Project RENEW: Development of a Volunteer Respite Care Program. *The Gerontologist,* 25: 573-583, 1985.

Newman, S, LW Lyons & R Onawola. The Development of an Intergenerational Service-Learning Program at a Nursing Home. *The Gerontologist,* 25: 130-133, 1985.

New York City Department for the Aging. Bureau of Research, Planning, and Policy Analysis. *Home-Delivered Meal Participants Survey. First Report: An Overview of Patient Characteristics and Their Relation to Criteria for Program Participation.* (Research & Evaluation Report, No. 3). New York: Department for Aging, 1982.

Nickens, H. Intrinsic Factors in Falling Among the Elderly. *Archives of Internal Medicine,* 145: 189-196, 1985.

Nielson, M, M Blenkner, M Bloom, T Downs & H Beggs. Older Persons After Hospitalization: A Controlled Study of Home Aide Service. *American Journal of Public Health,* 62: 1094-1101, 1972.

Nocks, BC, M Learner, D Blackman & TE Brown. The Effects of a Community-Based Long-Term Care Project on Nursing Home Utilization. *The Gerontologist,* 26: 151-157, 1986.

Noelker, LS. *Incontinence in Elderly Cared for by Family.* Paper presented at the annual meeting of the Gerontological Society of America, San Francisco, November, 1983.

Nurick, L. *Respite Care Services in the Nursing Home: Findings from a Study Conducted in New York State.* Paper presented at Respite Care: New Opportunities, (sponsored by the Arizona Department of Health Services and the Arizona Long Term Care Gerontology Center), Phoenix, AZ, June 1983.

Oktay, J. *A Community Program for the Elderly.* Paper presented at the symposium of the National Association of Social Workers, Washington, DC, September 1984.

Oktay, JS & PJ Volland. Community Care Program for the Elderly. *Health and Social Work,* 6: 41-48, 1981.

Orr, LL, J Williams & S Bell. *AFDC-Homemaker-Home Health Aide Demonstration: First Operational Year.* Second Annual Report to the Health Care Financing Administration. Cambridge, MA: Abt Associates, 1984.

Oster, C & WH Kibat. Evaluation of a Multidisciplinary Care Program for Stroke Patients in a Day Care Center. *Journal of the American Geriatrics Society,* 23: 63-69, 1975.

Ouslander, JG. Urinary Incontinence in the Elderly. *The Western Journal of Medicine,* 136: 482-491, 1981.

Ouslander, JG & RL Kane. The Costs of Urinary Incontinence in Nursing Homes. *Medical Care,* 22: 69-79, 1984.

Ouslander, JG, RL Kane & IB Abrass. Urinary Incontinence in Elderly Nursing Home Patients. *Journal of the American Medical Association,* 248: 1194, 1982.

Ovrebo, B, P Liljestrand & M Minkler. *The Health and Social Service Needs of Elderly Residents of Single Room Occupancy (SRO) Hotels in the United States.* (Policy Paper, No. 12). San Francisco: Aging Health Policy Center, University of California, San Francisco, 1984.

Packwood, T. Supporting the Family: A Study of the Organization and Implications of Hospital Provision of Holiday Relief for Families Caring for Dependents at Home. *Social Science and Medicine,* 14A: 613-620, 1980.

Padula, H. *Developing Adult Day Care.* Washington, DC: The National Institute on Adult Day Care, Inc., 1985.

Palmer, HC. Adult Day Care. In Vogel RV & HC Palmer (eds.), *Long-Term Care: Perspectives From Research and Demonstrations.* Washington, DC: Health Care Financing Administration, 1983.

Palmore, E. Total Chance of Institutionalization Among the Aged. *The Gerontologist,* 16: 504-507, 1976.

Papsidero, JA, S Katz, S Kroger & C Apkom. *Community Care: The Chronic Disease Service Model.* East Lansing: Michigan State University Press, 1979.

Patten, S. *An Evaluation of the Wilder Caregiver Support Program. Executive Summary.* Minneapolis: Hubert H. Humphrey Center for Public Affairs, University of Minnesota, 1984.

Pelham, AO & WF Clark. *Managing Home Care for the Elderly. Lessons from Community-Based Agencies.* New York: Springer Publishing, 1986.

Perry, BC. Falls Among the Elderly: A Review of the Methods and Conclusions of Epidemiologic Studies. *Journal of the American Geriatrics Society,* 30: 367-371, 1982.

Peters, B. The Ten Commandments of Case Management During Hospitalization: A Practice Perspective. In Pelham, AO & WF Clark (eds.), *Managing Home Care for the Elderly.* New York: Springer Publishing, 1986.

Peters, R, WC Schmidt Jr. & KS Miller. Guardianship of the Elderly in Tallahassee, Florida. *The Gerontologist,* 25: 532-538, 1985.

Pies, H. Life Care Communities for the Aged: An Overview. In Feinstein, P, M Gronick & J Greenberg (eds.), *Long-Term Care Financing and Delivery Systems: Exploring Some Alternatives. Conference Proceedings* (41-52). Health Care Financing Administration Publ. No. 03174. Washington, DC: Health Care Financing Administration, 1984.

Piktialis, DS & J Callahan. Organization of Long-Term Care: Should There be a Single or Multiple Focal Points for Long-Term Care Coordination. In Grana, JM & DB McCallum (eds.), *The Impact of Technology on Long-Term Care.* Millwood, VA: Project HOPE Center for Health Affairs, 1986.

Pinkerton, A & D Hill (Allied Home Health Association). *Long-Term Care Demonstration Project of North San Diego County: Final Report.* Report prepared for the Health Care Financing Administration. Springfield, VA: National Technical Information Service, U.S. Department of Commerce, 1984.

Polich, CL. *Quality Assurance for Long-Term Care Options for Minnesota.* Minneapolis: Center for Health Services Research, University of Minnesota, 1983.

Polich, CL. *Home Care in Minnesota: Issues and Future Directions.* Minneapolis: Health Policy Analysis Group, Center for Health Services Research, University of Minnesota, 1985.

Poliquin, N & M Straker. A Clinical Psychogeriatric Unit: Organization and Function. *Journal of the American Geriatrics Society,* 25: 132-137, 1977.

Poulshock, SW & G Deimling. Families Caring for Elders in Residence: Issues in the Measurement of Burden. *Journal of Gerontology,* 39: 230-239, 1984.

Price, LC, HM Ripps & DM Peltz. *Second Year Evaluation of the Monroe County Long-Term Care Program.* Silver Spring, MD: Macro Systems, Inc., 1979.

Quinn, J & J Hodgson. Triage: A Long-Term Care Study. In Zawadski, R (ed.), *Community-Based Systems of Long-Term Care* (171-194). New York: Haworth, 1984.

Quinn, MJ & SK Tomita. *Elder Abuse and Neglect: Causes, Diagnosis, and Intervention Strategies.* New York: Springer Publishing Co., 1986.

Rainey LC, LA Crane, DM Breslow & PA Ganz. Cancer Patients' Attitudes Toward Hospice Services. *CA/A Cancer Journal for Clinicians,* 34: 191-201, 1984.

Ralston, PA. *Senior Center Research: Concept, Programs And Utilization.* Paper presented at the annual meeting of the Gerontological Society of America, San Antonio, TX, November 1984.

Ranii, D. Meals On Wheels: How to Turn Victory Into Defeat—and Back Into Victory. *National Journal,* 10: 522-524, 1980.

Reger, D, JK Meyers, M Kramer, L Robins, D Blazer, R Hough, W Eaton & B Locke. The NIMH Epidemiologic Catchment Area Program. Historical Context, Major Objectives, and Study Population Characteristics. *Archives of General Psychology,* 41: 934-941, 1984.

Reichstein, KJ & L Bergofsky. Domiciliary Care Facilities for Adults: An Analysis of State Regulations. *Research on Aging,* 5: 25-43, 1983.

Reifler, BV, E Larson, G Cox & H Featherstone. Treatment Results at a Multi-Specialty Clinic for the Impaired Elderly and Their Families. *Journal of the American Geriatrics Society,* 29: 579-582, 1981.

Reiger, AJ & D Engel. *Granny Flats: An Assessment of Economic and Land Use Issues.* HUD-0003030. Washington, DC: Office of Policy Development and Research, U.S. Department of Housing and Urban Development, 1983.

Retsinas, J & P Garrity. Nursing Home Friendship. *The Gerontologist,* 25: 376-381, 1985.

Rickards, S. Cost Projections in the Channeling Care Planning Process. In Austin, CD, J Low, EA Roberts & K O'Connor (eds.), *Case Management: A Critical Review.* Seattle: Pacific Northwest Long-Term Care Gerontology Center, University of Washington Institute on Aging, 1985.

Rickards, SW, MK Galper, LM Sterthous, C Hirsch & BW Schneider. Client Couples in the National Long Term Care Channeling Demonstration. In Austin, CD, J. Low, EA Roberts & K O'Connor (eds.), *Case Management: A Critical Review.* Seattle: Pacific Northwest Long-Term Care Gerontology Center, University of Washington, 1985.

Rinehart, BH. *Day Care for the Psychogeriatric Population. What Works and for Whom?* Paper presented at the annual meeting of the Gerontological Society of America, San Antonio, TX, November 19, 1984.

Romaniuk, M, WJ McAuley & G Arling. An Examination of the Prevalence of Mental Disorders Among the Elderly in the Community. *Journal of Abnormal Psychology,* 92: 458-467, 1983.

Roos, NP & E Shapiro. The Manitoba Longitudinal Study on Aging. Preliminary Findings on Health Care Utilization of the Elderly. *Medical Care,* 19: 644-657, 1981.

Rosenblum, RW. Out-of-Pocket Health Care Expense and the Elderly: An Economic Analysis. *Health Care Management Review,* 8: 77-87, 1983.

Rosenfeld, AS. *Factors Affecting Home Health Agency Behavior: An Interactionist View.* Waltham, MA: Levinson Policy Institute, Brandeis University, 1980.

Rubenstein, LZ. Falls in the Elderly: A Clinical Approach. *Western Journal of Medicine,* 138: 273-75, 1983.

Rubenstein, LZ, IB Abrass, & RB Kane. Improved Care for Patients on a New Geriatric Evaluation Unit. *Journal of the American Geriatrics Society,* 29: 531-536, 1981.

Rubenstein, LZ, K Josephson, GD Wieland, PA English, J Sayre & RL Kane. Effectiveness of a Geriatric Evaluation Unit. *The New England Journal of Medicine,* 311: 1664-1670, 1984.

Rubenstein, LZ, L Rhee & RL Kane. The Role of Geriatric Assessment Units in Caring for the Elderly: An Analytic Review. *Journal of Gerontology,* 37: 513-521, 1982.

Ruchlin, HS & JN Morris. Cost-Benefit Analysis of an Emergency Alarm and Response System: A Case of a Long-Term Care Program. *Health Services Research,* 16: 65-80, 1981.

Ruchlin, H & J Morris. Pennsylvania's Domiciliary Care Experiment: II. Cost-Benefit Implications. *American Journal of Public Health,* 73: 654-660, 1983.

Rue, VM. Retooling Information Systems for Aging. *International Journal on Aging and Human Development,* 4: 361-374, 1973.

Sager, AP. *Planning Home Care with the Elderly. Patient, Family, and Professional Views of an Alternative to Institutionalization.* Cambridge, MA: Ballinger Publishing Company, 1983a.

Sager, AP. A Proposal for Promoting More Adequate Long-Term Care for the Elderly. *The Gerontologist.* 23: 13-17, 1983b.

Salend, E, M Shatz, RA Kane & J Pynoos. Elder Abuse Reporting: The Limitations of Statutes. *The Gerontologist,* 24: 61-69, 1984.

Sauer, WJ & RT Coward(eds.). *Social Support Networks and the Care of the Elderly.* New York: Springer Publishing Co., 1985.

Scanlon, WJ (ed.). *Project to Analyze Existing Long-Term Care Data. Volumes I-VI and Appendix.* (Volume I.—*Summary and Conclusion.* Volume II.—*Definition and Measurement.* Volume III.—*Long-Term Care Service Utilization and Outcomes.* Volume IV.—*Financing Long-Term Care.* Volume V.—*Long-Term Care Service Supply: Levels and Behavior.* Volume VI.—*Long-Term Care Costs.* Appendix.—*Long-Term Care Instrument and Definition Review.*) Washington: The Urban Institute, 1984.

Scanlon, W & C Hamcke. *Long-Term Care Needs, Resources and Service Use Among Aged Community Residents: Evidence from Four Local Surveys.* Washington, DC: The Urban Institute, 1983.

Schlenker, RE. Expanding Home Health Services: Evaluation of the Federal Grant Program. *Home Health Care Services Quarterly,* 1: 49-64, 1980.

Schlenker, RE. *Case Mix Reimbursement Nursing Homes. Journal of Health, Politics, Policy and Law,* 11: 445-461, 1986.

Schneider, B, M Galper, L Gottesman, P Kohn, B Morrell, L Staroscik & L Sterthous. *The Channeling Case Management Manual.* Philadelphia, PA: Temple University Center on Aging, 1982.

Schneider, BW, C Hirsch, MK Galper, SW Rickards & LM Sterthous. *A Year in the Lives of Clients and Case Managers.* DHEW Contract 90-AR-0004A/01. Philadelphia: Temple University Institute on Aging, 1984.

Schneider, EL & JA Brody. Aging, Natural Health and the Compression of Morbidity: Another View. *New England Journal of Medicine,* 309: 854-856, 1983.

Schneider, MJ, DD Chapman & DE Voth. Senior Center Participation: A Two Stage Evaluation. *The Gerontologist,* 25: 194-200, 1985.

Scholen, K & Y-P Chen. *Unlocking Home Equity for the Elderly.* Cambridge, MA: Ballinger Publishing Company, 1980.

Schulz, R. Effects of Control and Predictability on the Physical and Psychological Well-Being of the Institutionalized Aged. *Journal of Personality & Social Psychology,* 33: 563-573, 1976.

Schulz, R & G Brenner. Relocation of the Aged: A Review and Theoretical Analysis. *Journal of Gerontology,* 32: 323-333, 1977.

Schulz, R & M Horowitz. Meta-Analytic Biases and Problems of Validity in the Relocation Literature: Final Comments. *The Gerontologist,* 23: 460-461, 1983.

Schuman, JE, EJ Beattie, DA Steed, JE Gibson, GM Merry, WD Campbell & AS Kraus. The Impact of a New Geriatric Program in a Hospital for the Chronically Ill. *Canadian Medical Association Journal,* 118: 639-643, 1978.

Segal, JL, JF Thompson & RA Floyd. Drug Utilization and Prescribing Patterns in a Skilled Nursing Facility: The Need for a Rational Approach to Therapeutics. *Journal of the American Geriatrics Society,* 27: 117-122, 1979.

Seidl, FW, R Applebaum, C Austin & K Mahoney. *Delivering In-Home Services to the Aged and Disabled: The Wisconsin Experiment,* Lexington, MA: Lexington Books, 1983.

Seltzer, MM, J Ivry & LC Litchfield. *Family Members as Case Managers: Partnership Between the Formal and Informal Support Networks.* Paper presented at the annual meeting of the Gerontological Society of America, New Orleans, November 1985.

Seltzer, MS, K Simmons, J Ivry & L Litchfield. Agency-Family Partnerships: Case Management of Services for the Elderly. *Journal of Gerontological Social Work,* 7: 57-71, 1984.

Shadish, WR Jr & RR Bootzin. Nursing Homes and Chronic Mental Patients. *Schizophrenia Bulletin,* 7: 488-498, 1981.

Shanas, E. *The Health of Older People: A Social Survey.* Cambridge, MA: Harvard University Press, 1962.

Shanas, E. Social Myth as Hypothesis: The Case of the Family Relations of Older People. *The Gerontologist,* 19: 169-174, 1979.

Shapiro, E. Impending Death and the Use of Hospitals by the Elderly. *Journal of the American Geriatrics Society,* 31: 348-351, 1983.

Shapiro, E & R Tate. Predictors of Long Term Care Facility Use Among the Elderly. *Canadian Journal on Aging,* 4: 11-19, 1985.

Shapiro, E & LM Webster. Nursing Home Utilization Patterns for All Manitoba Admissions, 1974-1981. *The Gerontologist,* 24: 610-615, 1984.

Sherwood, S, DS Greer, JN Morris & V Mor. *An Alternative to Institutionaliztion. The Highland Heights Experiemnt.* Cambridge, MA: Ballinger Publishing Company, 1981.

Sherwood, S & JN Morris. *A Study of the Effects of an Emergency Alarm and Response System for the Aged: A Final Report.* Boston: Hebrew Rehabilitation Center for the Aged, 1980.

Sherwood, S & J Morris. *Pennsylvania Domiciliary Care Pilot Program. A Digest of Key Findings Concerning Program Effectiveness and Operations.* Boston: Hebrew Rehabilitation Center for the Aged, 1981.

Sherwood, S & J Morris. The Pennsylvania Domiciliary Care Experiment: I. Impact on Quality of Live. *American Journal of Public Health,* 73: 646-653, 1983.

Simmons, KH, J Ivry & MM Seltzer. Agency-Family Collaboration. *The Gerontologist,* 25: 343-346, 1985.

Simpson, DF. *Case Management in Long-Term Care Programs.* Washington, DC: Center for the Study of Social Policy, 1982.

Simson, S, LB Wilson & SS Henry. Creating Comprehensive Gero-Psychiatric Care in the Community. *Social Work in Health Care,* 7: 53-65, 1982.

Skellie, A, F Favor, C Tudor & R Strauss. *Alternative Health Services Project Final Report.* Atlanta: Georgia Department of Medical Assistance, 1982.

Skellie, A, F Favor, C Tudor & R Strauss. The Georgia Alternative Health Services Project: Cost Effectiveness Depends on Population Selection. In Zawadski, R (ed.), *Community-Based Systems of Long-Term Care* (49-72). New York: Haworth, 1984.

Skinner, JH. *Improving the Use of Scarce Resources in Long-Term Care by Targeting Services More Appropriately.* Paper presented at the annual meeting of the Gerontological Society of America, San Antonio, TX. 1984.

Sklar, BW & LJ Weiss. *Project OPEN (Organization Providing for Elderly Needs): Final Report.* San Francisco: Mt Zion Hospital and Medical Center, 1983.

Sloane, P. Nursing Home Candidates: Hospital Inpatient Trial to Identify Those Appropriately Assignable to Less Intensive Care. *Journal of the American Geriatrics Society,* 28: 511-514, 1980.

Smits, HL, J Feder & W Scanlon. Medicare's Nursing-Home Benefit: Variations in Interpretation. *The New England Journal of Medicine,* 307: 855-862, 1982.

Snipes, G. Analyses and Prevention of Falls. *Geriatric Consultant,* 1: 22-25, 1983.

Snyder, B & K Keefe. The Unmet Needs of Family Caregivers for Frail and Disabled Adults. *Social Work in Health Care,* 10: 1-15, 1985.

Snyder, LH, P Rupprecht, J Pyrek, S Brekhus & T Moss. Wandering. *The Gerontologist.* 20: 656-660, 1980.

Soldo, B. Supply of Informal Care Services: Variations and Effects on Service Utilization Patterns. In Scanlon, W (ed.), *Project to Analyze Existing Long-Term Care Data. Volume III* (56-97). Washington, DC: The Urban Institute, 1984.

Soldo, BJ. In-Home Services for the Dependent Elderly. *Research on Aging,* 7: 281-304, 1985.

Soldo, B & K Manton. Health Status and Service Needs of the Oldest Old: Current Patterns and Future Trends. *Milbank Memorial Fund Quarterly/Health and Society,* 63: 286-319, 1985.

Solon, JA, RP Amthor, MY Rabb & JC Shelley Jr. Linking Young and Old Institutionalized People. *Public Health Reports,* 92: 57-64, 1977.

Solon, J & L Greenawalt. Physicians' Participation in Nursing Homes. *Medical Care,* 12: 486-495, 1974.

Somers, AR. Long-Term Care for the Elderly and Disabled: A New Health Priority. *New England Journal of Medicine,* 307: 221-226, 1982.

Sonberg, P & L Emrich. Training Family and Friends as Caregivers. Mid-Atlantic Long Term Care Gerontology Center, Philadelphia, PA: Temple University, 1982.

Spalding, J. *A Consumer Perspective on Quality Care: The Residents' Point of View.* Washington, DC: Coalition for Nursing Home Reform, 1985.

Sparer, G, MA Cahn, K Robbins & N Sharp. The Paid Aide Demonstration: Summary of Operational Experiences. *AANNT Journal,* 10: 19-29, 1983.

Spitz, B. States' Options for Reimbursing Nursing Home Capital. *Inquiry,* 19: 246-254, 1982.

Spivack, S. An Appraisal of the Current State of Long Term Care Health and Social Planning. Philadelphia: National Health Care Management Center, University of Pennsylvania, 1981.

Stark, AJ & GM Gutman. Client Transfers in Long-Term Care: Five Years' Experience. *American Journal of Public Health,* 76: 1312-1316, 1986.

Stark, AJ, G Gutman & B McCashin. Acute Care Hospitalizations and Long-Term Care. *Journal of the American Geriatrics Society,* 30: 509-515, 1982.

Stark, A, E Kliewer, G Gutman & B McCashin. Placement Changes in Long-Term Care: Three Years Experience. *American Journal of Public Health,* 74: 459-463, 1984.

Stassen, M & J Holahan. *Long-Term Care Demonstration Projects: A Review of Recent Evaluations.* (Working Paper 1227-02). Washington, DC: The Urban Institute, 1981.

Stein, S, MW Linn & EM Stein. Patients' Anticipation of Stress in Nursing Home Care. *The Gerontologist,* 25: 88-94, 1985.

Steinberg, R & G Carter. *Case Management and the Elderly.* Lexington, MA: DC Heath, 1982.

Steinberg, RM & L Trejo. *Front-Line Practitioners' Views of Long-Term Care in Los Angeles County.* Los Angeles: Andrus Gerontology Center, University of Southern California, 1984.

Stephens, SA & JB Christianson. *Informal Financial Assistance to the Impaired Elderly.* Paper presented at the annual meeting of the Gerontological Association of America, San Antonio, TX, November 1984.

Sterthous, LM. *Informal Services and Supports in the Long-Term Care Channeling Demonstration: A Collection of Practice-Oriented Papers.* Philadelphia: Temple University Institute on Aging, draft mimeo, 1986.

Stoller, EP & LL Earl. Help with Activities of Everyday Life: Sources of Support for the Noninstitutionalized Elderly. *The Gerontologist,* 23: 64-70, 1983.

Stone, R & R Newcomer. The State Role in Board and Care Housing. In Harrington, C, R Newcomer, C Estes & Associates, *Long Term Care of the Elderly, Public Policy Issues* (177-196). Beverly Hills: Sage Publications, 1985.

Stone, R, RJ Newcomer & M Saunders. *Descriptive Analysis of Board and Care Policy Trends in the 50 States.* San Francisco: Aging Health Policy Center, University of California, 1982.

Strahan, G. Nursing Home Characteristics. Preliminary Data from the 1985 National Nursing Home Survey. *NCHS Advance Data from Vital and Health Statistics.* DHHS Pub. No. (PHS) 87-1250. Hyattsville, MD: National Center for Health Statistics, No. 131. March 27, 1987.

Strain, LA & NL Chappell. Rural-Urban Differences Among Adult Day Care Participants in Manitoba. *Canadian Journal on Aging,* 2: 197-209, 1980.

Struyk, RJ & BJ Soldo. *Improving the Elderly's Housing. A Key to Preserving the Nation's Housing Stock and Neighborhoods.* Cambridge, MA: Ballinger Publishing Company, 1980.

Stryker, R. The Effect of Managerial Interventions on High Personnel Turnover in Nursing Homes. *The Journal of Long-Term Care Administration,* 10: 21-33, 1982.

Thomas, TM, KR Plymat, J Blannin & TW Meade. Prevalence of Urinary Incontinence. *British Medical Journal,* 281: 1243-1245, 1980.

Thompson, JF, WF McGhan, RL Ruffalo, DA Cohen, B Adamcik & JL Segal. Long-Term Care. Clinical Pharmacists Prescribing Drug Therapy in a Geriatric Setting: Outcome of a Trial. *Journal of the American Geriatrics Society,* 32: 154-159, 1984.

Thorburn, P & MR Meiners. *Nursing Home Patient Outcomes: The Results of an Incentive Reimbursement Experiment.* National Center for Health Services Research (DID/PTNZ5YA7). Hyattsville, MD: National Center for Health Services, November 1984.

Tobin, S. Old People. In Maas, H (ed.), *Social Service Research: Reviews of Studies.* Washington, DC: National Association of Social Workers, 1978.

Toff, GE. *Alternatives to Institutional Care for the Elderly: An Analysis of State Initiatives.* Washington, DC: Intergovernmental Health Policy Project, George Washington University, 1981.

Tomlinson, BE, G Blessed & M Roth. Observations on the Brains of Demented Old People. *Journal of Neurological Science,* 11: 205-242, 1970.

Townsend, A & SW Poulshock. Intergenerational Perspectives on Impaired Elders' Support Networks. *Journal of Gerontology,* 41: 101-109, 1986.

Travelers Employee Caregiver Survey: A Survey on Caregiving Responsibilities for Older Americans. Hartford: The Travelers, mimeo, 1985.

Tulloch, AJ & V Moore. A Randomized Controlled Trial of Geriatric Screening and Surveillance in General Practice. *Journal of the Royal College of General Practitioners,* 29: 733-742, 1979.

Turner, L & E Mangum. *Report on the Housing Choices of Older Americans. Summary of Survey Findings and Recommendations for Practitioners.* Bryn Mawr, PA: The Graduate School of Social Work & Social Research, Bryn Mawr College, 1982.

Tydeman, A. *Nursing Home Projects for Area Agencies on Aging.* Washington, DC: National Citizens' Coalition for Nursing Home Reform, 1981.

United States Department of Health, Education, and Welfare, Office of Human Development, Administration on Aging, National Clearinghouse on Aging. *No. 2, Human Resources Issues in the Field of Aging, Homemaker-Home Health Aide Services.* DHEW Publication No. (OHD) 77-20086. Washington, DC: U.S. Government Printing Office, 1978.

United States Senate Special Committee on Aging. *Developments in Aging: 1984.* Report 99-5. Washington, DC: U.S. Government Printing Office, 1985.

United States Senate Special Committee on Aging. *Aging America, Trends and Projections, 1985-86.* Washington, DC: United States Government Printing Office, 1986a.

United States Senate Special Committee on Aging. *Developments in Aging: 1985.* Report 99-242. Washington, DC: U.S. Government Printing Office, 1986b.

Urban Systems Research and Engineering, Inc. *Evaluation of the Effectiveness of Congregate Housing for the Elderly. Final Report.* Cambridge, MA: Urban Systems Research and Engineering, 1976.

Vandivort, R, GM Kurren & K Braun. Foster Family Care for Frail Elderly: A Cost-Effective Quality Care Alternative. *The Journal of Gerontological Social Work* 7: 101-114, 1984.

Veterans Administration. *Caring for the Older Veteran.* Washington, DC: U.S. Government Printing Office, 1984.

Veterans Administration. *The VA's Home Health Care Program: Hospital Based Home Care.* Washington, DC: Department of Medicine, Veterans Administration, mimeo, 1985.

Vetter, NJ, DA Jones, & CR Victor. Urinary Incontinence in the Elderly at Home. *Lancet,* 2: 1275, 1981.

Vetter, NJ, DA Jones & CR Victor. Effect of Health Visitors Working With Elderly Patients in General Practice: A Randomised Controlled Trial. *British Medical Journal,* 288: 369-372, 1984.

Vicente, L, JA Wiley & RA Carrington. The Risk of Institutionalization Before Death. *The Gerontologist.* 19: 361-367, 1979.

Vicente, L, JA Wiley & RA Carrington. Duration of Stay and Other Aspects of Nursing Home Use. *International Journal of Aging and Human Development,* 12: 301-312, 1980/81.

Wachtel, TJ, C Derby & JP Fulton. Predicting the Outcome of Hospitalization for Elderly Persons: Home Versus Nursing Home. *Southern Medical Journal,* 77: 1283-1285, 1984.

Waldo, DR, KR Levit & H Lazenby. National Health Expenditures, 1985. *Health Care Financing Review*, 8: 1–21, 1986.

Wallace, J. *Factors Contributing to Low Retention Rates in Adult Day Care Centers*. Presented at the annual meeting of the Gerontological Society of America, San Antonio, TX, November 1984.

Wallace, J. *Day Care Centers: Not Just for Kids Anymore*. Cedar Falls IA: Department of Psychology, University of Northern Iowa, n.d.

Wallace, R & L Noelker. *The Quality of Marital Relationships in Later Life: The Impact of Caring for an Impaired Older Spouse*. Paper presented at the National Council on Family Relations, St. Paul, MN, October 1983.

Wallach, HF, F Kelley & JP Abrahams. Psychosocial Rehabilitation for Chronic Geriatric Patients: An Intergenerational Approach. *The Gerontologist*, 19: 464-470, 1979.

Waller, J. Falls Among the Elderly: Human and Environmental Factors. *Accident Analysis and Prevention*, 10: 22-23, 1978.

Wan, T & WG Weissert. Social Support Networks, Patient Status, and Institutionalization. *Research on Aging*, 3: 240-256, 1981.

Wasylenki, DA, MK Harrison, J Britnell & J Hood. A Community-Based Psychogeriatric Service. *Journal of the American Geriatrics Society*, 32: 213-218, 1984.

Waxman, HM & EA Carner. Physicians' Recognition, Diagnosis, and Treatment of Mental Disorders in Elderly Medical Patients. *The Gerontologist*, 24: 593-597, 1984.

Waxman, HM, EA Carner & G. Berkenstock. Job Turnover and Job Satisfaction Among Nursing Home Aides. *The Gerontologist*, 24: 503-509, 1984.

Weiland, D, L Rubenstein, J Ouslander & S Martin. Organizing an Academic Nursing Home. Impacts on Institutionalized Elderly. *Journal of the American Medical Association*, 255: 2622-2627, 1986.

Weiler, P. Response to the Study: Effects and Costs of Day Care and Homemaker Services for the Chronically Ill: A Randomized Experiment. *Home Health Care Services Quarterly*, 1: 97-99, 1980.

Weiler, P, RR Fine, & ML Reid. *Adult Day Health Care Development in California: Unfinished Task*. Davis, CA: Center for Aging and Health, University of California at Davis, 1982.

Weiler, P, P Kim & L Pickard. Health Care for Elderly Americans: Evaluation of an Adult Day Care Center. *Medical Care*, 14: 700-708, 1976.

Weiler, P & E Rathbone-McCuan. *Adult Day Care: Community Work with the Elderly*. New York: Springer Publishing, 1978.

Weinrobe, M. Home Equity Conversion: Its Practice Today. In Feinstein, P, M Gornick & J Greenberg (eds.), *Long Term Care Financing and Delivery Systems: Exploring Some Alternatives. Conference Proceedings* (95-96). Washington, DC: Health Care Financing Administration, 1984.

Weissert, WG. *Adult Day Care in the United States. A Comparison Study*. Washington, DC: Transcentury Corporation, 1975.

Weissert, WG. *Size and Characteristics of the Noninstitutionalized Long-Term Care Population*. Washington, DC: The Urban Institute, 1982.

Weissert, WG. *Source Book on Long-Term Care Data*. Washington, DC: The Urban Institute, 1983.

Weissert, WG, CL Matthews & JE Pawelak. *Home and Community Care: Two Decades of Findings*. Paper prepared for the Veterans Administration Project on Information Syntheses in Long-Term Care. Chapel Hill, NC: University of North Carolina, mimeo, 1986.

Weissert, WG & WJ Scanlon. *Determinants of Nursing Home Discharge Status*. Washington, DC: The Urban Institute, 1984a.

Weissert, WG & WJ Scanlon. Estimating the Long-Term Care Population: National Prevalence Rates and Selected Characteristics. In Scanlon, W (ed.), *Project to Analyze Existing Long-Term Data. Volume II* (129-163). Washington, DC: The Urban Institute, 1984b.

Weissert, WG & W Scanlon. Determinants of Institutionalization of the Aged. In Scanlon, W (ed.), *Project to Analyze Existing Long-Term Care Data. Volume III*. Washington, DC: The Urban Institute, 1984c.

Weissert, WG, WJ Scanlon, TTH Wan & DE Skinner. Care for the Chronically Ill: Nursing Home Incentive Payment Experiment. *Health Care Financing Review*, 5:41-49, 1983.

Weissert, WG, TTH Wan & BB Livieratos. *Effects and Costs of Day Care and Homemaker Services for the Chronically Ill: A Randomized Experiment.* DHEW Publication No. (PHS) 79-3258. Office of Health Research, Statistics, and Technology, National Center for Health Services Research, Department of Health, Education, and Welfare. Hyattsville, MD: National Center for Health Services Research, 1980.

Weissert, WG, T Wan, B Livieratos & S Katz. Effects and Costs of Day-Care Services for the Chronically Ill. *Medical Care*, 18: 567-584, 1980a.

Weissert, WG, TTH Wan, BB Livieratos & J Pellegrino. Cost-Effectiveness of Homemaker Services for the Chronically Ill. *Inquiry*, 17: 230-243, 1980b.

Wells, T. Promoting Urine Control Among Older Adults, the Scope of the Problem. *Geriatric Nursing*, 1: 236-240, 1980.

White, M & M Grisham. *The Structure and Processes of Case Management in California's Multipurpose Senior Services Project*. Berkeley, CA: University of California at Berkeley, 1982.

White, M & RM Steinberg. *Conservatorship Care Planning and Monitoring Formats*. Los Angeles: Andrus Gerontology Center, 1984.

Widmer, G, R Brill & A Schlosser. Home Health Care: Services and Cost. *Nursing Outlook*, 26: 488-493, 1978.

Wiley, JA. *Two Studies of Family Structure and Dependency in Old Age*. Berkeley, CA: Survey Research Center, National Center for Health Services Research, mimeo, 1983.

Willemain, TR. A Comparison of Patient-Centered and Case-Mix Reimbursement for Nursing Home Care. *Health Services Research*, 15: 365-377, 1980.

Willemain, TR. Beyond the GAO Cleveland Study: Client Selection for Home Care Services. *Home Health Care Services Quarterly*, 1: 65-83, 1980.

Willemain, TR. *Designing Quality Incentive Systems for Nursing Homes*. Final report prepared for the National Center for Health Services Research, Washington, DC, 1983a.

Willemain, TR. Survey-Based Indices for Nursing Home Quality Incentive Reimbursement. *Health Care Financing Review*, 4: 83-90, 1983b.

Willemain, TR & R Mark. The Distribution of Intervals Between Visits as a Basis for Assessing and Regulating Physician Services in Nursing Homes. *Medical Care*, 18: 427-441, 1980.

Williams, C. Teaching Nursing Homes: Their Impact on Public Policy, Patient Care, and Medical Education. *Journal of the American Geriatrics Society*, 33: 189-195, 1985.

Williams, J, G Gaumer & M Cella. *Home Health Services: An Industry in Transition. Home Health Agency Prospective Payment Demonstration*. Cambridge, MA: Abt Associates, 1984.

Winograd, IR & MM Mirassou. A Crisis Intervention Service: Comparison of Younger and Older Adult Clients. *The Gerontologist*, 23: 370-377, 1983.

Wood, JB & C Estes. Private Nonprofit Organizations and Community-Based

Long-Term Care. In Harrington, C, R Newcomer, C Estes and Associates (eds.), *Long Term Care of the Elderly, Public Policy Issues* (213-232). Beverly Hills: Sage Publications, 1985.

Wood, JB, CL Estes, PR Lee & PJ Fox. *Public Policy, the Private Nonprofit Sector and the Delivery of Community-Based Long Term Care Services for the Elderly*. San Francisco: Aging Health Policy Center, University of California, 1983.

Worthy, EH, C Eisman & R Wood. *Voluntary Action and Older People: An Annotated Bibliography*. Washington, DC: National Policy Center on Education, Leisure and Continuing Opportunities for Older Americans, National Council on the Aging, 1982.

Yarnell, JWG & A Stilegar. The Prevalence, Severity and Factors Associated with Urinary Incontinence in a Random Sample of the Elderly. *Age and Aging*, 8: 81, 1979.

Yocom, B. *Respite Care Options for Families Caring for the Frail Elderly*. Seattle: Pacific Northwest Long-Term Care Center, University of Washington, 1982.

Yocom, B & W Graff. *Utilization of Sheltered Housing by the Elderly*. Seattle: Pacific Northwest Long-Term Care Center, University of Washington, 1983.

Zarit, SH & CR Anthony. Interventions with Dementia Patients and Their Families. In Gilhooley, M, J Birren & S Zarit (eds.), *The Dementias: Policy & Management*. Englewood Cliffs, NJ: Prentice-Hall, 1986.

Zarit, S, P Todd & J Zarit. Subjective Burden of Husbands and Wives as Caregivers: A Longitudinal Study. *The Gerontologist*, 26: 260-266, 1986.

Zawadski, R. Methodological Constraints of the Medicare 222 Day Care/ Homemaker Demonstration Project. *Home Health Care Services Quarterly*, 1: 109-112, 1980.

Zawadski, RT (ed.). *Community-Based Systems of Long Term Care*, New York: Haworth Press, 1983.

Zimmer, A & J Sainer. Strengthening the Family as an Informal Support for the Aged: Implications for Social Policy and Planning. In Community Service Society of New York, *Strengthening Informal Supports for the Aging* (44-51). New York: Community Services Society of New York, 1981.

Zimmer, JG, A Groth-Juncker & J McCusker. Effects of a Physician-Led Home Care Team on Terminal Care. *Journal of the American Geriatrics Society*, 32: 288-292, 1984.

Zimmer, JG, A Groth-Juncker & J McCusker. A Randomized Controlled Study of a Home Health Care Team. *American Journal of Public Health*, 75: 134-144, 1985.

Zimmer, JG, N Watson & A Treat. Behavioral Problems Among Patients in Skilled Nursing Facilities. *American Journal of Public Health*, 74: 1118-1121, 1984.

Zimmerman, D, JR Egan, D Guftason, C Metcalf & F Skidmore. *Evaluation of the State Demonstrations in Nursing Home Quality Assurance Programs*. Princeton, NJ: Mathematica Policy Research, 1984.

Index

Aaron, HJ, 369
Abuse, elder, 97, 206–207; *see also* Protective social services
Access, 83–84, 89–92, 93, 269–270, 271, 316, 318–319, 323, 334–335, 343–344
ACTION, 185–189
Acute care and long-term care, 103–105, 279–281, 362, 372–373, 377–378
transition from acute to long-term care, 281–285, 304–305, 343
transition from long-term to acute care, 285–295, 300, 302, 304–305
Activities of Daily Living, 4, 16–19, 21, 25, 27–32, 38, 46–47, 66, 187, 200, 233, 241, 270, 272, 289, 292, 294; *see also* Functional status, Functioning
day care, 145, 148, 157, 158, 161
foster care, 172–174, 177
geriatric assessment, 190–197
home care, 119, 124–125, 126, 139
long-term care demonstrations, 319, 321–322, 324–333, 339
mental health, 203–205
ADLs, *see* Activities of Daily Living
Administration on Aging, 71, 91, 188
Adult day care, 58, 60, 143–164
auspices of, 59
costs of, 145–146, 149–150, 156–158, 161
day health versus social day care, 104–105, 143–144, 145, 146
definition of, 58–59, 143
descriptive studies, 145–155
hospital-based, 144, 150–151, 157
long-term care demonstrations, 164, 314–315, 321, 327–329, 331
respite in, 60, 61
studies of effectiveness, 155–162, 356
Adult foster care, 65–66, 108, 163–164, 168–175, 347–348, 360
costs of, 169, 171–174
hospital-based, 169
AFDC Homemaker–Home Health Aide Demonstration, 142
Aiken, LH, 259, 266
Alameda County, 26

Alaska, 341
Allen, CM, 196, 197
Alternative Care Grant, 311, 312
Alternative Health Services Project, 91, 316, 317, 321, 334–335
Alzheimer's disease, 45, 60, 181, 373; *see also* Senile dementia
Ambulation, *see* Mobility
Ambulatory care, 290, 291–292
and home care, 111, 115, 128, 133, 299
American Association of Retired Persons, 76, 96, 98, 99
American Board of Family Practice, 98
Amerman, E, 343
Anderson, NN, 120, 126
Anlyan, WG, 367
Ansak, M, 327
Applebaum, R, 315, 316, 319, 333, 334
Applegate, WB, 191, 193
Area Agencies on Aging, 91, 181, 202, 204, 237, 318, 342, 346
Arizona, 261
Arling, G, 97, 148, 154
Assessment, 13, 20; *see also* Geriatric assessment services
Austin, CD, 315, 316, 318, 341, 342

Baker, M, 99
Ball, R, 368
Baltes, MM, 229, 230
Banzinger, G, 235, 238
Barker, WH, 192, 193
Barney, JL, 258, 266
Barresi, CM, 151, 154
Barton, EM, 241, 244
Bass, D, 97
Bass, SA, 140, 142, 217
Becker, PM, 196, 197
Behavioral therapy, 229, 230
Beland, F, 124
Bell, WG, 164
Benjamin Rose Institute, 42, 49–50, 130
Bennett, RG, 205, 206, 238
Berger, RM, 229, 230
Berghorn, FJ, 229, 231
Beverly Enterprises, 56
Birkel, RC, 41, 50

Birnbaum, HG, 201, 324
Bishop, CE, 271
Blackman, DK, 232, 236
Blenkner, M, 207
Blumenthal, D, 368
Board and care homes, 61, 65, 108, 284, 356; see also Adult foster care
Borup, JH, 239
Branch, LG, 16, 17, 22, 28, 31, 35, 46, 293, 294
Braun, K, 169, 173
Brickel, CM, 229, 231
Brickner, PW, 118, 127
Brill, R, 326
British Columbia, 289–290, 373
British Columbia Long-Term Care Program, 287–288, 289
Brody, EM, 33, 43, 51, 99, 209, 211, 280, 305
Brody, SJ, 26
Brooks, CH, 199
Brown, T, 329
Buford, AD, 87
Bursac, K, 60
Buschman, M, 181, 183

Cairl, RE, 310, 312
California, see Multipurpose Senior Citizens Project
Callahan, JJ, 33, 207
Cameron, JM, 274
Campion, EW, 193, 194
Cantor, M, 37, 47
Capitation, 369, 376–377; see also Social HMOs
Capitman, JA, 159, 161, 341
Carcagno, G, 339
Case management, 164, 184, 307, 314
    and access to care, 90–92
    definition of, 91
    and long-term care systems, 315, 319, 322–326, 328–333, 340–344, 348, 356, 363
Case managers, 117, 140, 149, 371
Case mix, see Reimbursement
Certificate of Need (CON), 92, 93
Certification of facilities, 54, 55, 85–87, 251
Chain ownership, 55–56
Channeling, see National Long-Term Care Channeling Demonstration
Chappell, NL, 39, 48, 125, 126, 146, 155, 160, 161
Cheah, K, 190
Chore services, 112, 123, 214, 359
Cicirelli, V, 50. 99
Clauser, S, 389
Cleveland, 15, 34, 47
Client satisfaction, 167, 200, 204, 219
    with day care, 159
    with foster homes, 170–171, 173
    with home care, 129, 133, 138, 140
    with housing, 209, 210–212
    with nursing homes, 227, 242, 301, 302, 303
    with respite care, 176–178, 180

Coalition for Nursing Home Reform, 99
Cognitive status, see Mental status
Cohen, RG, 219, 221
Cohen, S, 148, 155
Colen, JN, 216, 222
Colvez, A, 20
Community Care Organizations Project, 91, 316, 318, 334, 335–336, 340
Community Development Block Grants, 210; see also Omnibus Budget Reconciliation Act
Community mental health clinics (CMHCs), 201–202, 203–204
Community Service Society of New York, 181, 183
Congregate housing, 145
Congregate meals, see Meals, congregate
Connecticut, see Triage
Conservatorship, see Protective social services
Cost-effective services, 108, 366–367
Costs of long-term care, 53, 70–71 83–84, 92, 106–107, 366–367, 378; see also Reimbursement, Adult day care, costs of, Adult foster care, costs of, Home care, costs of
    in long-term care demonstrations, 309, 311, 312, 319, 320–333, 335–336, 337–339, 344
Contentment, client, 129, 130, 132, 207
Cornoni-Huntley, JC, 14, 19, 23
Crisis intervention, 202, 203, 205
Crossman, L, 175, 177, 181
Cummings, V, 155, 157
Currie, CT, 190, 193

Daiches, S, 206
Davis, J, 283, 284
Davis, K, 368
Day care, see Adult day care
Deimling, GT, 42, 49
Demonstration projects, 25, 84, 142, 155, 272, 365, 370
    and systems of long-term care, 306–349, 363–364
Depression, 190–191, 193, 200, 203, 229, 231, 243, 361
Diagnosis-related groups (DRGs), see Reimbursement
Dialysis, 136, 139
Dobrof, R, 236
Domiciliary care, see Adult foster care
Dorosin, E, 216, 221
Dudley, CJ, 239, 240
Dunkle, RE, 207

Ebenezer Society of Minnesota, 345
Effectiveness of long-term care
    criteria for, 105–108
    difficulties in demonstrating, 103–105
    nature of evidence for, 109–110
Eggert, G, 52, 323
ELDERPLAN, 346
Elwell, F, 249, 260
Emergency alarm system, 215, 217, 315
Emling, DC, 117, 118

Engler, M, 166, 167
Epstein, WM, 248, 260
Estes, CL, 69, 202, 203
Eustis, N, 13
Evashwick, CJ, 305
Expenditures, 76–80; *see also* Costs of
    long-term care, Reimbursement
  Medicaid, 76–77
  Medicare, 75–76
  Older Americans Act, 78
  Out-of-pocket, 78–80
  Title XX, 77
  Veterans Administration, 78

Family, *see* Informal caregivers, Social sup-
    port
Family Support Program, 181, 183
Feder, J, 92
Federal Council on Aging, 67
Ferguson, GD, 68, 213, 215
Financial help, 20
Financing long-term care, 70–81
Fitting, M, 44, 50
Flemming, AS, 202, 204
Florida, 142; *see also* Florida Pentastar
    Project
Florida Department of Health and Reha-
    bilitative Services, 247, 260, 330
Florida Pentastar Project, 310, 316, 330,
    334–336, 340
Food stamps, 71
Foster care, *see* Adult foster care
Foster Grandparent Program, 185
Fottler, MD, 247, 260
Fox, M, 181, 182
Fractures, 104, 113, 130, 289
Frankfather, DL, 181, 183, 342
Friedman, S, 231, 236
Friendly visiting, 99, 112, 118, 134,
    185, 189, 237; *see also* Volunteer
    programs
Fries, BE, 20, 274
Functional status, *see also* Activities of
    Daily Living, Instrumental Activities
    of Daily Living, Functioning
  in adult foster care, 169–171, 173, 179
  as a long-term care goal, 104, 107–108
  and long-term care need, 353–355, 372
  in day care, 146, 147, 149, 151, 153–
    154, 156–157, 159
  in home care, 114–115, 119–120, 127,
    128, 129, 130–133, 358
  and housing, 208, 212, 215
  in long-term care demonstrations, 309,
    310, 312, 320, 337–339, 364
  in nursing homes, 226–227, 234, 236,
    238, 246, 276, 299, 301, 302
  in protective services, 207
  and transitions between acute and long-
    term care, 280, 281–282, 283, 286,
    289–290, 292
  in volunteer programs, 187–189
Functioning, *see also* Functional status
  components of independent, 4
  goal for, 7
Fullarton, WD, 367

Gardiner, JA, 250, 261
Gaumer, GL, 94
Gayton, DC, 193, 195
Gehrke, JR, 254, 265
General Accounting Office, 16, 34, 47, 77,
    94, 95, 122, 127, 185, 201, 218, 221,
    266, 273
George, L, 44, 50
Georgia, *see* Alternative Health Services
    Project
Geriatric assessment services, 150, 163–
    164, 189, 279, 360
  experimental studies, 193–197
  uncontrolled studies of, 190–193
Geriatric day hospitals, 150, 155
Geriatric nurse practitioners, 301–302
Geriatric specialists, 133, 264
Gerson, L, 116
Gibbins, FJ, 136, 139
Gilleard, CJ, 153, 154
Glosser, G, 181, 182
Gordon, W, 287, 289
Grade of membership, 19, 32
Greenberg, JN, 80, 314, 316
Greene, VL, 241, 244, 248, 260
Greer, DS, 200, 201
Grey, C, 234, 238
Grier, MR, 100
Grimaldi, PL, 274
Groth-Juncker, A, 129, 133, 135
Group Health, Inc., 345
Growing Younger Health Promotion Pro-
    ject, 219, 221
Gryfe, CI, 300, 303
Guardianship, *see* Abuse, elder
Gubrium, JF, 229, 230
Gurland, BJ, 36, 47, 155, 159

Hackman, H, 155
Halbur, BT, 257, 265
Hammond, J, 128
Hannan, EL, 145, 149
Hanson, SM, 50
Harel, Z, 165, 209, 211, 239, 242
Harkins, EB, 308, 309
Harmon, C, 61, 66
Harrill, I, 165, 166
Harrington, C, 266, 267, 269
Harris & Associates, 39, 98
Haskins, B, 315, 316, 333
Hawes, C, 56
Hay, DG, 246, 261
Hay, JW, 94
Hayslip, B, 122, 127
HCFA, *see* Health Care Financing Adminis-
    tration
Health and Human Services, U.S. Depart-
    ment of, 91
Health Care Financing Administration, 10,
    86, 91, 310, 315
Health clinics, *see* Ambulatory care
Health education, 112, 218–219, 221
Health, Education and Welfare (HEW), De-
    partment of, 187
Health Interview Survey, 18, 20, 24, 35,
    46

Health maintenance organizations (HMOs), 95, 371, 376; *see also* Social HMOs
Health status, 133, 148, 167, 233–234, 291–293
Hebrew Rehabilitation Center for Aging, 275
Hedrick, SC, 13, 128, 129, 131, 162, 185
Hendriksen, C, 193, 195
Hendy, HM, 242, 244
Henkleman-Kelly, J, 175, 181
Hicks, B, 322
Highland Heights Study, 212, 314
Hillhaven, 56
Hirsch, CS, 232, 236
HMOs, *see* Health maintenance organizations
Hogan, DB, 190, 193
Holahan, J, 267, 268, 269, 271
Home care, 20, 39, 99, 104, 105, 111, 198, 284, 285, 288, 290, 347, 358–359; *see also* Home-delivered services and long-term care demonstrations
   costs of, 76, 77, 94–95, 112, 114, 116, 118–120, 125, 126–127, 128, 131–134, 136, 138, 183, 299, 315
   definitional problems, 112–115
   descriptive studies, 117–128
   evaluation studies, 128–143
   hospital-based, 117, 118, 121–122, 125, 127, 134
   targeting, 115–117
Home care corporations, 138, 140, 142, 347
Home companions, 136
Home-delivered services and long-term care demonstrations, 318–336, 344
Home equity conversion, 61, 63, 67
Home health agencies, 56–58, 94, 112, 127, 137, 342, 346, 356
Home health aides, 58, 104, 113, 114, 120, 130–131, 134, 136, 137, 139, 142, 143, 185; *see also* Home health agencies
Home maintenance/repair, 61, 64, 68, 163, 208, 213–214, 215
Home-share Program, 68, 214
Homemaker/Home health aide, 123, 138, 199, 207
Homemakers, 20, 104, 112, 114, 116, 123, 124, 126, 129, 134, 136, 138; *see also* Home-delivered services and long-term care demonstrations
Homemaking, 118, 120, 125, 127, 132, 140, 142, 145, 164, 183, 314, 356; *see also* Home-delivered and long-term care demonstrations
Horowitz, A, 40, 51
Horowitz, MJ, 239
Hospice care, 112, 163, 164, 197–201, 279, 360
   costs, 198–199, 201
   reimbursement, 149

Hospital admissions/discharges, 22, 24, 299; *see* Acute care and long-term care
Hospital costs, 76, 77
Housekeeping, 112–113, 117, 118, 130, 138, 210–211
Housing, 61–69, 163–164, 208–213; *see also* Home maintenance/repair
   congregate housing, 61, 63, 65, 164, 209, 210
   ECHO housing, 64, 67, 68
   public housing, 63, 65, 210, 211–212
   Section 8, 62, 65, 71, 210
   Section 202, 62, 65, 71, 210, 212
   Section 312, 210, 212
   Shared housing, 61, 64, 68, 164, 215
Howe, E, 68, 214, 215
Howells, D, 176, 180
Hughes, SL, 129, 134, 135, 136, 315, 316, 317
Huttman, E, 59, 69

IADLs, *see* Instrumental Activities of Daily Living
ICF, *see* Intermediate Care Facilities
Illinois, 271, 274
Incontinence, 50, 173, 194, 354–355
Informal caregivers, 33–52, 117, 125, 133, 148, 153, 169, 172, 178, 183, 206, 329, 338, 358, 360, 364, 373–374, 378; *see also* Social supports
   burden, 40–45, 49–52, 108, 177, 179, 182, 184, 331–334, 355
   children as, 34, 35, 37, 38, 39, 46–51
   daughters as, 36, 46, 51
   friends as, 37, 38, 47
   grandchildren as, 39
   satisfaction, 133, 169–170, 176, 331–334, 349
   spouses as, 37, 44, 45, 47, 48, 51
Information and Referral Programs, 69, 70, 89, 237
Institute of Medicine, 54, 56, 86, 87, 88, 253, 262, 370
Institutionalization, 203–204, 302, 303–304, 362
   day care, effect on, 147–148, 151, 152, 156–158, 159
   foster care, effect on, 169, 171, 178, 180
   geriatric assessment, effect on, 192, 195–197
   home care, effect on, 130–132, 134, 139
   housing, effect on, 209, 211, 212, 214
   long-term care demonstrations, effect on, 310–311, 319, 320–333, 335–336, 337–340, 344, 363
Instrumental Activities of Daily Living, 4, 16, 19, 25, 28, 30–32, 38, 47
   in day care, 157
   in foster care, 66, 172
   in geriatric assessment, 191, 193–197
   in home care, 119

in long-term care demonstrations, 319,
321–322, 325–330, 332–333, 334,
389
Insurance for long-term care, 79–80, 96,
341, 356, 368,
and universal benefits, 125, 126, 373
Intermediate Care Facility (ICF), 54, 55,
88, 93, 104, 120, 126–127, 149,
159, 169, 176, 178, 267, 269, 289,
297
Inui, TS, 121, 127
Isaacs, MR, 54, 60, 61, 93
Iverson, LH, 90, 311

Jacobs, B, 68
Jette, AM, 136, 138
Johns Hopkins University Hospital, 169,
172
Johnson, ML, 342
Johnson, SH, 252, 262
Jones, BJ, 270, 272
Jost, TS, 251, 261
Justice, D, 347

Kahana, EF, 258, 266
Kaiser Permanente, 345
Kane, RA, 85, 225, 302
Kane, RL, 28, 53, 93, 100, 200, 201, 224,
276, 277, 280, 281, 282, 295, 296,
299, 302, 304, 313, 347, 368, 373
Katz, S, 13, 17, 18, 129, 130, 135, 315,
317,
Kaye, LW, 123, 127
Kemper, P, 307, 332, 333
Kempler, D, 219, 221
Kepferle, L, 303
Kirschner, R, 167, 168
Klapfish, A, 162
Knowles, DH, 99
Knowlton, J, 308, 310
Koger, LJ, 232, 236
Kramer, M, 201
Kraus, AS, 169, 170
Krout, JA, 69
Kulys, R, 46, 47, 96, 99

Ladd, RC, 174, 348
Lalonde, B, 218, 221
Lamont, C, 283, 284
Langer, E, 234, 237
Langley, A, 206
Larson, EB, 192, 193
Laundry, 138, 140, 358
Laurie, W, 15
Lawton, MP, 209, 212
Learned helplessness, 237, 238
Lee, JT, 136, 138
Lefton, E, 193, 194
Legal services, 207
Leutz, WN, 96, 279, 307, 345
Levit, K, 78
Lewis, M, 277, 285, 286, 289
Lexington, KY, 132, 157–158
Licensing of facilities, 85, 87, 168, 250–
251
Lichtenstein, H, 190, 193

Liem, PH, 192, 193
Life care community, 61, 67, 93, 99
Life-care planning, 97
Life expectancy, 20, 21
Lifeline, 215, 217
Life satisfaction, 146, 172, 231–233, 236,
242, 337–339
Lind, SD, 141, 142
Linn, MW, 168, 170, 246, 260
Long-term care
definition of, 4–6, 103, 353
goals of, 104, 105–108
nature of, 6–9
Lowy, L, 213, 215
Lubitz, J, 198
Lyons, M, 137, 142

MacDonald, ML, 229, 231
Mace, NL, 59, 60, 150, 154
Master, R, 299, 302
Manitoba, 23, 25, 30, 48, 125, 126, 146,
155, 160–161, 290, 292, 294, 313,
373
Manton, K, 19, 20
Maryland, 274
Massachusetts, 51, 121, 138, 145, 290,
293, 308, 310, 346, 347
Massachusetts Health Care Panel Study,
22, 35, 46, 293, 294
McAuley, WJ, 124, 126
McCall, N, 76
McCoy, JL, 27
Meals, 108, 164, 181, 356
congregate 69, 70, 99, 163–164, 164–
168, 207–208
and day care, 148, 158
and home care, 113, 126, 130, 136, 138,
140
home-delivered, 99, 129, 134, 163–164,
165–168
on wheels, 122, 185
Medicaid, 53, 54, 55, 65, 71, 73, 76, 81,
94, 95, 96, 116, 121, 166, 173, 280,
284, 285, 296, 373; see also Expenditures, Reimbursement
day care, 145, 147, 149, 154, 162
eligibility, 90
long-term care demonstrations, 307–312,
313, 319, 320–323, 325, 329–330,
334–335, 348
nursing homes, 247, 260, 302, 303,
356
waivers, 61, 164, 208, 313–314
1115 waivers, 90
2176 waivers, 56, 80
Medical care evaluation (MCE), 225
Medi-Cal, 270
Medical care in nursing homes, 295–304,
362–363; see also Physicians
Medicare, 54, 58, 71, 72, 76, 78, 79,
81, 94, 95–96, 98, 280, 295–296,
298, 303, 359, 368, 372, 375–376;
see also Expenditures, Reimbursement
222 waivers, 90, 313
day care, 158, 161

home care, 113, 116, 121–122, 127, 129, 132, 136, 356
hospice, 164, 199, 200–201
long-term care demonstrations, 307, 313–314, 315, 322, 326–331, 333–335, 348
Medication, 29, 113, 139, 190, 192, 193, 234, 295, 297
Meiners, MR, 79, 89, 96, 270, 272, 277
Mental health programs, 201–206
  clinics, 145, 152
  community mental health centers, 202–206
  mental health therapies, 202, 205–206
Mental status, 25, 41, 120, 124, 169–170, 172, 182, 188, 218, 234, 240
  day care, 146, 148, 150–151, 157, 159
  geriatric assessment, 190–197
  long-term care demonstrations, 322, 326–328, 334, 337
Mercer, SO, 235, 237, 255, 265
Merriam, S, 202, 205
Meyer, M, 166
Michigan, 117, 118
Miller, DB, 239, 240
Miller, LS, 325, 334, 343
Miller, MG, 342
Minnesota, 271, 275, 308, 312–313
Minorities, 69, 216, 222, 263; *see also* Risk factors, race as
Mitchell, J, 39, 49
Mitchell, JB, 129, 131, 295, 298
Mobility, 191, 193–194, 233, 243
  aids for, 31–32
Monk, A, 87
Monroe County Long-Term Care Program, 344
Moon, M, 78
Mor, V, 66, 173, 174
Morale, 41, 124, 133, 172, 196–197, 209, 301, 302,
Morales-Martinez, F, 150, 154
Morbidity, 20, 22, 116, 200, 212, 361
  compression of, 20
Morris, J, 38, 47, 48, 275
Moscovice, I, 308, 311, 312
Mossey, J, 23, 290, 292, 294
Mortality, 21, 23, 185, 187, 209, 212
  day care, 151, 158–159
  geriatric assessment, 195–197
  home care, 116, 128, 129, 130–132, 134, 136, 139, 141, 142, 358
  long-term care demonstrations, 322, 324–326, 328, 331–333, 337
  nursing homes, 237, 238, 239, 286, 289, 294, 300, 303, 361
  protective services, 207–208
Multiperson Senior Citizens Project, 315, 316, 317, 325, 336, 337, 340, 343

National Center for Health Statistics, 22, 24, 26, 270
National Center for Health Services Research, 10
National Council on Aging, 69
National Governors' Association, 347

National Home Caring Council, 56
National Institute on Aging, 10, 22, 71
National Long-term Care Channeling Demonstration, 91, 307, 315, 317, 318–319, 332–334, 335, 337–344, 371
National Long-Term Care Survey, 22, 78
National Nursing Home Survey, 18, 22, 24, 54, 268, 354
National Support Program, 181, 183
Need for long-term care, 12–52, 353–355
  extent of, 22–24
  forecasting, 15, 51
  needs assessment, 12
Nelson, JR, 97
Nestle, M, 165
Netting, FE, 179, 180
Newman, S, 233, 236
New York, 180, 249, 275; *see also* ACCESS, Nursing Home Without Walls
New York City, 40, 118, 127, 159; *see also* New York City Home Care Project
New York City Department for the Aging, 165, 166
New York City Home Care Project, 316, 318, 326, 334, 336, 338
Nielson, M, 129, 130, 135
NNHS, *see* National Nursing Home Survey
Nocks, BC, 329, 334
Noelker, LS, 42
Nurick, L, 178, 180
Nurses, 56, 58, 60; *see also* Geriatric nurse practitioners
Nurses' aides, 262–263
Nursing home admissions/discharges, *see* Acute care and long-term care, Utilization of service
Nursing home community councils, 258, 266
Nursing Home Without Walls, 315, 316, 318, 324, 334–336, 340
Nursing homes, 24, 25–32, 76, 77, 79, 223–278, 375–376; *see also* Intermediate care facilities, Skilled nursing facilities, Reimbursement
  access to, 90–91
  bed supply of, 54–56, 92, 93, 356
  goals of facility care, 225–228
  interventions in, 228–239
  ownership of, 55, 56
  predictors of well-being in, 228–245
  quality of care, 225, 245–261
  regulation, 250–253, 261–262
  risk of entering, 25–32
  staffing/administration, 225, 248–249, 254–258, 260–266
Nutrition, 219; *see also* Meals and meal programs, 165–168
Nutritionist, 112, 156

OARS instrument, 13–14, 16, 18, 25, 34, 185, 188
Occupational therapists, 112, 191–192, 246, 261

Occupational therapy, 148, 156–157, 191
Office of Economic Opportunity (OEO), 187
Ohio, 274
Oktay, JS, 169, 172
Older Americans Act, 5, 9, 69, 70, 75, 78, 86, 87, 91, 164, 181, 346
 Title III-B, 123
 Title III-C, 166–167
Ombudsman program, 86, 87, 88, 237, 247
Omnibus Budget Reconciliation Act of 1981, 56, 80, 91, 203–204, 266, 347
On Lok Project, 315, 316–317, 327, 334, 337, 340
Oregon, 174, 341, 345, 347–348
Oregon F16 Waiver Project, 314
Orr, LL, 142
Oster, C, 155, 156, 161
Outpatient care, *see* Ambulatory care

PaCS, *see* Patient Care and Services
Packwood, T, 175, 177
Pain control
 and home care, 133
 and hospice, 198, 200, 201
Palmer, HC, 145
Palmore, E, 26
Papsidero, JA, 315, 317
Paraprofessionals, 112, 113, 129, 264
Parkinson's disease, 181
Patient Care and Services, 86
Patten, S, 175, 179
Pelham, AO, 343
Pennsylvania, 312–313
Pennsylvania Domiciliary Care Program, 168, 171
Perceived health, 129, 134
Personal care, 20, 105, 112, 113, 117, 118, 124, 131, 148, 158, 159, 164, 168, 171, 214, 290
Personal care attendents, 129
Personal time dependency, 17, 47
Pet-assisted therapy, 229, 231, 235, 242, 245
Peters, B, 343
Peters, R, 207
Pharmacists and nursing homes, 265, 299, 301, 304
Physical therapists, 112, 131, 246, 261, 263
Physical therapy, 134, 148, 156–157, 191–192
Physicians, 24, 76, 77, 79, 202, 261, 279, 306, 311, 313, 340, 345
 geriatric assessment services, 190–197
 home care, 113, 122, 125, 131, 133, 138
 visits, 22, 295, 296–299
Piktialis, DS, 346, 347
Pinkerton, A, 331
Polich, CL, 86
Poliquin, N, 190
Poulshock, SW, 42, 49
Pre-admission screening, 90–91, 154, 307–313, 348, 363

Preferences, 98–100, 142, 277, 357, 371
Price, LC, 323
Professional standards review organizations (PSROs), 268, 281, 282, 302
Prognostic adjustment factor (PAF), 276
Project OPEN, 316, 318, 328, 334–336, 338
Project Renew, 179–180
Protective social services, 163–164, 206–208, 360
Psychogeriatric day hospitals, 153, 154
Psychosocial programs, 205; *see also* Nursing homes, interventions
Psychotherapy, 229, 231; *see also* Nursing homes, interventions

Quality assurance efforts, 105–106; *see also* Quality of care
Quality of care, 85–88, 93, 368, 377, 380; *see also* Nursing homes, Reimbursement, 266–267, 269–270, 271
 steps in assuring, 85–86
Queens Medical Center, Honolulu, 169, 173
Quinn, J, 322
Quinn, MJ, 97, 206

Rainey, LC, 201
Ralston, PA, 220, 221, 222
Rationing and long-term care, 369–370
Reality orientation therapy, 148, 205, 228–229, 230–231, 238, 361
Reichstein, KJ, 66
Reifler, BV, 191
Reimbursement; *see also* Costs of long-term care, Social health maintenance organizations
 diagnosis-related groups (DRGs), 58, 93–94, 175, 273
 home care, 121, 147
 Medicaid, 85–86, 87, 89, 93, 94, 266–267, 268–271, 272
 Medicare, 267, 268, 272, 273
 nursing homes, 225, 266–278, 298, 361
  case mix, 89, 93, 273–275, 277, 361
  flat-rate, 267–270
  outcome-based, 273, 275–277
  prospective, 266–271, 284
  retrospective systems, 266–271
 prospective payment, 93–94
Reminiscence, 60, 205, 229, 231, 236; *see also* Nursing homes, interventions
Remotivation therapy, 205; *see also* Nursing homes, interventions
Residential care homes, 66, 173; *see also* Adult foster care, Board and care
Resocialization therapy, 205; *see also* Nursing homes, interventions
Resource utilization groups (RUGs), 273
Respite care, 60–61, 112, 143, 163–164, 175–180, 327, 329–330
Retired Senior Volunteers (RSV), 185–186, 187
Retsinas, J, 243, 244
Rickards, S, 343

Rinehart, BH, 152, 155
Risk factors, 13, 25–32
  age as, 13, 17, 19, 25–32
  disability as, 25–32
  gender as, 25–32
  home care risk, 48, 121, 124
  living arrangements as, 25, 27–31
  marital status as, 25, 27–31
  mental status as, 26, 30, 31–32
  nursing home risk, 25–32, 282
  poverty as, 25, 29
  race as, 20, 25–28, 31
  social support as, 26, 32
Rochester, NY, 133
Roos, NP, 23, 290, 291, 294
Rosenfeld, AS, 121, 127
Royal Victoria Hospital, Montreal, 198
Rubenstein, LZ, 189, 196, 197
Ruchlin, HS, 167, 171, 217, 315, 317

Sager, AP, 141
St. Christopher's, London, 198
Salend, E, 207
San Diego Long-term Care Project, *see*
  Project OPEN
Sauer, WJ, 33
SCAN, 345–346
Scanlon, W, 19
Schlenker, RE, 93, 137, 142
Schneider, BW, 20, 342
Schneider, MJ, 220, 222
Schulz, R, 229, 234, 238, 239, 240
Schuman, JE, 193, 194
Section 2176, Omnibus Budget Reconcilia-
  tion Act, 356
Segal, JL, 295, 297
Seidl, FW, 320
Seltzer, MM, 344
Seltzer, MS, 344
Senile dementia, 9, 60, 104, 150, 154, 175,
  181, 182, 190–192, 193, 206, 230,
  232, 286, 289, 354–355
Senior centers, 69–70, 108, 215, 220, 221–
  222, 229, 232, 236, 237
Senior Companion Program, 185, 186–188
Seniors Plus, 345
Service mix, 8, 105–106, 111
Shanas, E, 33
Shapiro, E, 25, 29, 32, 46, 291, 292, 294
Share-a-Fare, 216, 221
Sherwood, S, 169, 171, 209, 212, 215,
  217, 314, 315, 317
S/HMO, *see* Social health maintenance
  organization
Shopping, 122, 127, 130, 140
Simpson, DF, 341
Skellie, A, 321
Skilled nursing facility (SNF), 54, 55, 88,
  93, 104, 120, 126–127, 141, 159,
  176, 178, 252, 267, 269, 272, 289,
  297
Sklar, BW, 328
Sloane, P, 191
Smits, HL, 268, 272
SNF, *see* Skilled nursing facility
Snyder, B, 43, 50

Snyder, LH, 241
Social activity, 69, 132, 209, 147, 170,
  172–173, 212, 220, 231, 232–233,
  243
Social health maintenance organizations,
  95, 307, 335, 344–346; *see also* On
  Lok
Social network, 38, 48
Social security, 5, 71, 313, 347, 368
Social support, 25, 33, 124, 125, 126, 191,
  204, 284–285, 343; *see also* Informal
  caregivers
Social workers, 58, 60, 207, 343; *see also*
  Multidisciplinary teams
  foster care, 168–169, 171, 173
  home care, 112, 124, 131, 133–134
  nursing homes, 246, 255, 261, 263, 265,
    299
Soldo, BJ, 14, 29, 31, 32, 33, 36, 46
Solon, JA, 233, 236, 295, 296
Somers, AR, 368
Sonberg, P, 181
South Carolina, *see* South Carolina Long-
  term Care Project
South Carolina Long-term Care Project,
  316, 318–319, 329, 334–335, 337,
  340
Spalding, J, 99, 249, 261, 263
Sparer, G, 136, 139
Speech therapy, 112, 156–157
SSI, *see* Supplemental Security Income
Stark, AJ, 287, 288, 289, 290
Stassen, M, 25, 315, 316
Stein, S, 239, 243
Steinberg, RM, 341
Stephens, SA, 79
Sterthous, LM, 343
Stoller, EP, 37, 48
Stone, R, 66
Strain, LA, 146
Stroke patients, 130, 157
Strokes, 104, 156, 181, 218, 230, 241, 359
Struyk, RJ, 209, 210
Stryker, R, 256, 265
Supplemental Security Income, 5, 65, 71,
  118, 166, 168, 171
Supply of long-term care services, 53–70,
  80
  adult day care, 59–60
  board and care, 65–66
  home health agencies, 56–58
  housing for the elderly, 62, 63, 65
  nursing homes, 54–56
  senior centers, 69–70
Support groups, 108, 175
Survival, *see* Mortality

Targeting, 106, 108, 221, 280, 342, 348,
  370–372
Teaching hospitals, 282–283, 284, 299
Teaching nursing homes, 259, 266
Teams, multidisciplinary, 149, 198, 302
  geriatric assessment, 193–197
  home care, 129, 133
  long-term care demonstrations, 311, 319,
    320–333

Telephone
  monitoring, 131, 210, 215, 217
  reassurance, 122, 134, 141, 142, 167
Terminal care, 112; see also Hospice care
Texas ICF Project, 314–315
Thompson, JF, 301, 304
Thorburn, P, 270, 272
Title III-B, see Older American's Act
Title III-C, see Older American's Act
Title XIX, 247
Title XX, 71, 74, 77, 91, 120, 346
Tobin, S, 165
Tomita, SK, 97
Townsend, A, 38, 48
Transfer trauma, 239, 240, 304
Transportation, 20, 119, 122, 127, 148,
  155–156, 167, 171, 215, 216, 344,
  359
Travelers Employee Caregiver Survey, 40,
  49
TRIAGE, 91, 316, 322, 334, 336
Tulloch, AJ, 195, 197
Tydeman, A, 237

United East End Settlements, 214
United States Senate Special Committee on
  Aging, 65, 67, 70, 76, 77, 79, 92
Urban Systems Research and Engineering,
  Inc., 65, 209, 210
Utilization of services, 22, 33
  according to age, 20, 24
  adult day care, 59–60
  home care, 39, 48
  hospitals, 22, 24
  nursing homes, 24
  physician visits, 22

VA, see Veterans Administration
Vandivort, R, 169, 173
Veterans Administration, 71, 78, 170, 200,
  315
  and geriatric assessment, 192, 196–197
  and home care, 117, 121, 125, 127, 129,
    131, 162
  and nursing homes, 233, 246, 248, 260,
    301–302
Vetter, NJ, 196, 197
Vincente, L, 26

Virginia, 148, 154, 308, 309, 310
Visiting nursing services, 119, 136, 139,
  142
Visiting Nurse Association, 57, 58, 137,
  141, 142
VNA, see Visiting Nurse Association
Volunteer programs, 112, 134, 163–164,
  185–189, 360

Wachtel, TJ, 29
Waivers, see Medicare, Medicaid
Wallace, J, 152, 155
Wallace, R, 42, 50
Wallach, HF, 233, 236
Wallingford Wellness Project, 218, 221
Wan, T, 34, 46
Washington, 341
Washington Community Based Care Pro-
  ject, 315
Wasylenki, DA, 202, 204
Waxman, HM, 202, 257, 265
Weatherization assistance, 63
Weiland, D, 301, 303
Weiler, P, 145, 147, 154, 156, 157, 161,
  162
Weissert, WG, 13, 18, 26, 27, 29, 31, 32,
  35, 46, 129, 132, 145, 146, 155, 158,
  161, 162, 270, 272, 314, 315, 316,
  317, 333, 336, 337
West Virginia, 271, 274
White, M, 207, 342
Widmer, G, 119, 126
Willemain, TR, 295, 297
Williams, C, 259, 266
Williams, J, 57, 58, 59, 77
Winograd, IR, 202, 203
Wisconsin, 315, 316, 318, 320, 336
Worchester Home Care Project, 315
Worthy, EH, 185

Yocom, B, 175

Zarit, SH, 45, 50, 205, 206
Zawadski, RT, 162, 315, 316
Zimmer, A, 181, 183
Zimmer, JG, 129, 133
Zimmerman, D, 87, 252, 262